Lippincott's Pathophysiology Series

HEMATOLOGIC PATHOPHYSIOLOGY

Editor
Fred J. Schiffman, M.D.
Professor of Medicine
Department of Medicine
Brown University School of Medicine
The Miriam Hospital
Providence, Rhode Island

With 16 additional contributors

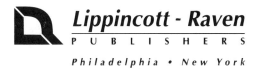

Lippincott - Raven
P U B L I S H E R S
Philadelphia • New York

Acquisitions Editor: Richard Winters
Developmental Editor: Delois Patterson
Manufacturing Manager: Dennis Teston
Production Manager: Cassie Moore
Production Editor: Emily Harkavy
Cover Illustrator: Patricia Gast
Indexer: Kathy Unger
Compositor: Maryland Composition
Printer: Courier-Kendallville

Printed in the United States of America

9 8 7 6 5 4 3 2 1

Library of Congress Cataloging-in-Publication Data
Hematologic pathophysiology / [edited by] Fred J. Schiffman : with 16 additional
    contributors.
          p.   cm. — (Lippincott's pathophysiology series)
    Includes bibliographical references and index.
    ISBN 0-397-51536-7
    1. Blood—Pathophysiology. 2. Blood—Diseases. I. Schiffman, Fred J. II. Series.
    [DNLM: 1. Hematologic Diseases—physiopathology. WH 120 H4866 1998]
  RB 145.H425 1998
  616.1´5071—dc21
  DNLM/DLC
  for Library of Congress   97-46468
                                                       CIP

To my father Harry, my mother Belle, and my brother Robert
—my first, continuing, and best teachers.

To Drs. Saul Farber, Samuel Thier, and Charles Carpenter
—inspirational role models and mentors
who made it all possible.

To Gerri, Josh, Jessica, Jake, and Judd
—my wife and children who make it all worthwhile.

CONTENTS

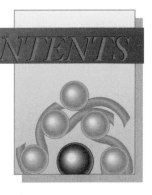

CONTRIBUTORS

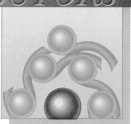

Nancy Berliner, M.D.

Associate Professor of Medicine
Department of Internal Medicine
Yale University School of Medicine
333 Cedar Street
New Haven, Connecticut 06520–8021

Angelina C. A. Carvalho, M.D.

Professor of Medicine
Department of Medicine
Brown University School of Medicine;
Chief of Hematology
Providence Veterans Administration
  Medical Center
830 Chalkstone Avenue
Providence, Rhode Island 02908–4799

Cynthia E. Dunbar, M.D.

Senior Investigator
Hematology Branch
National Heart, Lung, and Blood
  Institute
National Institutes of Health
9000 Rockville Pike
Bethesda, Maryland 20892–1652

Daniel E. Dunn, M.D., Ph.D.

Attending, Hematology and BMT
  Services
Hematology Branch
National Heart, Lung, and Blood
  Institute
National Institutes of Health
9000 Rockville Pike
Bethesda, Maryland 20892–1652

Stephen G. Emerson, M.D., Ph.D.

Francis C. Wood Professor of Medicine
Chief, Hematology-Oncology Division
Department of Medicine
University of Pennsylvania School of
  Medicine
3600 Spruce Street
Philadelphia, Pennsylvania 19104–4283

Timothy P. Flanigan, M.D.

Associate Professor of Medicine
Department of Medicine
Brown University School of Medicine
The Miriam Hospital
164 Summit Avenue
Providence, Rhode Island 02906

Mitchell E. Horwitz, M.D.

Clinical Associate
Department of Hematology
National Heart, Lung, and Blood
  Institute
National Institutes of Health
9000 Rockville Pike
Bethesda, Maryland 20892–1652

James A. Hoxie, M.D.

Professor of Medicine
Department of Medicine
University of Pennsylvania School of
  Medicine
415 Curie Boulevard
Philadelphia, Pennsylvania 19104

Eric M. Mazur, M.D.

Associate Clinical Professor of Medicine
Department of Internal Medicine
Yale University School of Medicine
Yale/Norwalk Hospital
24 Stevens Street
Norwalk, Connecticut 06856

Peter McPhedran, M.D.

Professor of Laboratory Medicine and
    Medicine
Departments of Laboratory Medicine
    and Internal Medicine
Yale University School of Medicine
Yale-New Haven Hospital
20 York Street
New Haven, Connecticut 06504

Natalie Ortoli–Drew, B.S., M.T. (A.S.C.P.)

Supervisor of Clinical Hematology and
    Lecturer in Laboratory Medicine
Departments of Laboratory Medicine
    and Clinical Hematology
Yale University School of Medicine
Yale-New Haven Hospital
20 York Street
New Haven, Connecticut 06504

Jayanthi Parameswaran, M.D.

Attending Physician
Department of Medicine
Newport Hospital/Aquidneck Medical
    Associates
Memorial Boulevard
Newport, Rhode Island 02840

Bharat Ramratnam, M.D.

Assistant Instructor of Medicine
Department of Medicine
Brown University School of Medicine
Chief Medical Resident
The Miriam Hospital
164 Summit Avenue
Providence, Rhode Island 02906

Michal G. Rose, M.D.

Post Doctoral Fellow in Hematology
Department of Medicine
Yale University School of Medicine
333 Cedar Street
New Haven, Connecticut 06520–8021

Alan G. Rosmarin, M.D.

Associate Professor of Medicine
Department of Medicine
Brown University School of Medicine
The Miriam Hospital
164 Summit Avenue
Providence, Rhode Island 02906

Fred J. Schiffman, M.D.

Professor of Medicine
Department of Medicine
Brown University School of Medicine
The Miriam Hospital
164 Summit Avenue
Providence, Rhode Island 02906

Lawrence N. Shulman, M.D.

Associate Professor of Clinical
    Medicine
Harvard Medical School;
Department of Adult Oncology
Dana-Farber Cancer Institute
44 Binney Street
Boston, Massachusetts 02115

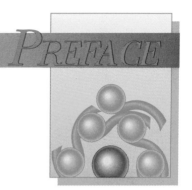

*H*ematologic Pathophysiology is designed for students or physicians who wish to obtain an overview of hematology. It is based upon pathophysiologic principles and is bolstered by case presentations and discussion of actual patient problems. The authors believe that it is useful to articulate hematologic facts that are immediately reinforced by real life patient-centered dilemmas. The purpose is to enliven what may otherwise be dry hematologic details by placing them side-by-side with relevant clinical situations.

We hope to show what the reader must know at a molecular level in order to thrive clinically. We strive to emphasize the scientific underpinning that is necessary for the successful clinical practice of hematology.

With the case presentations and discussions, we wish to convey a sense of realism, immediacy, and excitement about the practice of hematology. We want the illustrative cases to tell a memorable story, reinforce principles, and stimulate the reader to understand what is going on at a basic level in order to manage patients most efficiently.

Most chapters are organized according to a plan that first outlines normal hematologic physiology, followed by the approach to the patient in order to juxtapose the scientific techniques and clinical aspects.

The life cycle, structure and physiology of red blood cells, as well as their abnormalities, are presented to the reader. White blood cells and platelets are handled in a similar fashion. This is followed by a discussion of hemostasis, bone marrow disorders, and hematologic malignancies. In each section, illustrative cases are presented and analyzed. The chapter describing Clinical Laboratory Hematology is designed to enhance, amplify, and reinforce information presented in the previous chapter. Its tabular format allows easy access to and retrieval of information regarding hematologic laboratory testing. The appendices are a respository for normal hematologic values and miscellaneous information linking the individual chapters.

While there has been a genuine effort to make chapters uniform in approach, style, and length, an attempt was made to respect each author's individuality and creativity. We also encouraged "cross-talk" between the chapters while blending them into a coherent hematologic overview. Chapters do vary in basic scientific content, types of graphics, and overall length, mainly dictated by hematologic topic choice and the desire to explicate difficult hematologic principles more clearly and completely.

Thus, our mission is to provide an accessible, comprehensive pathophysiologic approach to the diagnosis and treatment of hematologic disease. Using vivid patient stories and illuminating visual aids, we hope to strengthen the message of how the knowledge of hematologic precepts can and should guide the care of patients with hematologic disease.

Fred J. Schiffman, M.D.

ACKNOWLEDGMENTS

I am grateful to Ms. Eleanor Aloisio for her outstanding secretarial and stylistic skills in preparing the manuscript for publication.

I thank Mr. Richard Winters, Ms. Delois Patterson, and Ms. Emily Harkavy at Lippincott–Raven Publishers for making all aspects of this endeavor productive and enjoyable.

Special gratitude is offered to the physician/scientists whose laboratories and lives I have been privileged to enter: Drs. Michael Freedman, Marco Rabinovitz, Ed Cadman, and Leon Weiss have been generous with their knowledge and spirit, and have shaped the way I view medicine and life in general.

I appreciate the careful review and insightful comments of Joshua Schiffman who read the entire manuscript with the eye of a medical student/poet.

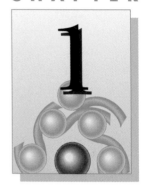

Hematopoiesis: The Development of Blood Cells

Stephen G. Emerson

INTRODUCTION

All the cells observed in the adult peripheral blood derive from the the bone marrow, through an extraordinary process termed *hematopoiesis*. This process results in the maintenance of a variety of blood cells, with each class possessing unique features and distinct lifespans. Our current understanding of this process is embodied in a theory called the stem cell model of hematopoiesis. This model forms the foundation for all our present thinking about normal hematopoiesis, pathologic hematologic disease states, and hematologic therapies.

Stem Cell Theory. Unlike other tissues of mesodermal origin, which as a rule have little turnover in their constituent cell populations, the cellular components of the blood are constantly undergoing cell death and replacement by new cells (Fig. 1-1). Whereas red blood cells circulate for approximately 4 months, platelets last only about 1 week, and granulocytes are viable for less than 10 hours. It is estimated that every day 1×10^{11} blood cells are lost to wear and tear, and are replaced with an equal number of new blood cells. To fulfill the continual need for replacement blood cells, hematopoiesis occurs actively throughout life. As a consequence, the blood-forming tissues are among the most mitotically active, along with the gastrointestinal epithelium, testes, and epidermis. The recognition of this high turnover rate for blood cells has led to the development of the stem cell theory of blood cell development and maintenance, or hematopoiesis. In the course of this chapter, we will examine this theory in detail, as well as its implications for clinical practice.

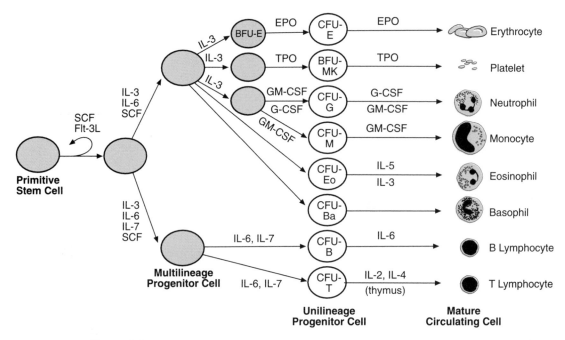

Figure 1-1. Hierarchical model of hematopoiesis and lymphopoiesis including important cytokines.

Hematopoietic Growth Factors. One of the most exciting advances in the study of hematopoiesis in the last decade has been the investigation of the role of hematopoietic-specific polypeptides in the control of the process of blood cell differentiation. These hematopoietic hormones, also known as hematopoietic growth factors, appear to control every step in the process of the development of new blood cells. At the present time, we know principally a group of such hematopoietic growth factors that are stimulatory to hematopoietic stem cells and their progeny. However, some inhibitory factors have been discovered that appear to play an equally important role in the negative control of this process. Other hormones that are felt to have primarily nonhematopoietic functions are also known to affect the production of new blood cells. In this chapter we will describe concisely the role of both stimulatory and inhibitory hematopoietic growth factors.

Hematopoietic Microenvironment. The term *hematopoietic microenvironment* refers to the "stromal" elements of the organs in which hematopoiesis occurs, that is, the cellular and noncellular elements that do not directly give rise to the blood cells but that provide a three-dimensional structural matrix in which the hematopoietic stem cells and their progeny proliferate and differentiate until their migration into the bloodstream. The role of the hematopoietic microenvironment in the control of the development of blood cells is felt to be of paramount importance in the process of hematopoiesis. Both the stromal cells and their secreted matrix proteins appear to influence the process of hematopoiesis as profoundly as the soluble, secreted hematopoietic growth factors. A summary of current understanding of the contribution of the hematopoietic microenvironment will be included in this chapter.

HEMATOPOIESIS IN THE EMBRYO AND FETUS

Role of the Yolk Sac. The fertilized egg develops the beginnings of blood tissue while still in the embryonic stage (Fig. 1-2). The first step toward development of this blood tissue is believed to occur in the yolk sac, where undifferentiated cells called mesoblasts are found and are thought to have migrated there from the primitive streak of the embryo. The mesoblasts are highly mitotically active and will subsequently differentiate into cells called *primitive erythroblasts,* which are clearly related to the mature blood cells of the adult, as well as into cells called *primitive endothelial cells* that give rise to vascular channels in the yolk sac. Within hours after migration, the yolk sac mesoblasts have generated primitive erythrocytes through a process of cell division and differentiation. Most of these cells are nucleated, but a minority are nonnucleated, and all synthesize hemoglobin and thus lend a reddish color to the

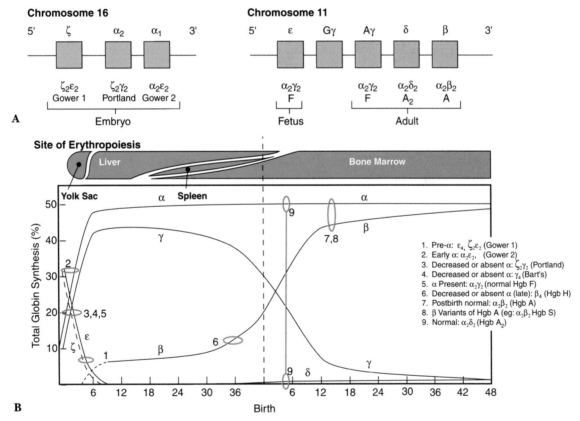

Figure 1-2. (**A**) The globin gene clusters on chromosomes 16 and 11. In embryonic, fetal, and adult life, different genes are activated or suppressed. The different globin chains are synthesized independently and then combine with each other to produce the different hemoglobins. The γ gene may have two sequences, differing by whether there is a glutamic acid or an alanine residue at position 136 (Gγ or Aγ, respectively). (From Hoffbrand AV, Pettit JE. *Essential Hematology,* 3rd ed. Cambridge, Mass.: Blackwell Scientific Publishing; 1993.) (**B**) Developmental sequence of location of hematopoiesis and hemoglobin synthesis. The lassos connect globins that associate under normal and abnormal circumstances. (After Brown MS. *Fetal and Neonatal Erythropoiesis in Developmental and Neonatal Hematology.* New York: Raven Press; 1988. From Handin RI, Stossel TP, Lux SE, eds. *Blood: Principles and Practice of Hematology.* Philadelphia: JB Lippincott, 1995.)

clumps of yolk sac cells where blood cells form. The clumps of hemoglobinized cells are visible to the naked eye, hence the name *blood islands* to describe these localized areas of embryonic hematopoiesis in the yolk sac. Megakaryocytes, the cells which produce platelets, are also found in the blood islands and are presumably derived from the mesoblasts. Other mesoblasts appear to differentiate into a type of cell called the hemocytoblast.

A second stage of hematopoiesis in the yolk sac occurs in the embryos of some mammals. In human embryos, this second stage is present but is not as vigorous as in rabbits, the mammal in which the embryogenesis of blood cells has been most extensively studied. In the second stage of yolk sac hematopoiesis, hemocytoblasts differentiate into definitive erythroblasts, which subsequently synthesize hemoglobin and are called *definitive* or *secondary normoblasts*. The latter may lose their nuclei and become definitive erythrocytes. Vascular channels form in the blood islands and eventually connect to form a network of blood vessels. This network of primitive blood vessels earlier contains the primitive erythroblasts and hemocytoblasts, and later, definitive erythroblasts and erythrocytes. By the end of the third week of embryonic development in the rabbit, all the hematopoietic activity of the blood islands has subsided and the process of hematopoiesis has shifted to the liver.

The Embryonic Body Mesenchyme. An additional role in early embryonic hematopoiesis is played by primitive mesenchymal cells in the body cavity itself, particularly in the anterior precardiac mesenchyme. Small numbers of mesenchymal cells of the body cavity develop into erythroblasts, megakaryocytes, granulocytes, and phagocytic cells analogous to their counterparts in the adult. Quantitatively, the number of cells produced is small, and large accretions of blood cells similar to the blood islands of the yolk sac do *not* form in the body cavity mesenchyme. Stem cells localized among these non–yolk sac hematopoietic cells likely play a major role in the subsequent generation of fetal and postnatal hematopoiesis, although the relative contributions of yolk sac and non–yolk sac primitive stem cells to later hematopoiesis is uncertain.

Emergence of the Liver as the Principal Site of Hematopoiesis in the Embryo. Beginning at around the 12-mm stage of the human embryo (6 weeks of age), hematopoiesis begins to shift to the embryonic liver (Fig. 1-2). The liver soon becomes the dominant site of hematopoiesis and remains active in hematopoiesis until birth. As the endodermal cords of the liver primordium grow into the septum transversum, they encounter wandering mesenchymal cells with the morphologic appearance of lymphocytes. These small, round, lymphocytoid cells called *lymphocytoid wandering cells* subsequently are trapped between the primordial liver endodermal cords and the endothelial cells of ingrowing capillaries. They give rise to hemocytoblasts similar to those of the yolk sac. These hemocytoblasts soon form foci of hematopoiesis similar to the blood islands of the yolk sac, wherein secondary erythroblasts are formed in large numbers. Secondary erythroblasts subsequently divide and differentiate into definitive erythrocytes through the progressive acquisition of hemoglobin and loss of the cell nucleus. Although definitive erythrocytes may be seen in the liver at 6 weeks of age, they do not emerge into the circulation in any great number until much later. Thus by the fourth fetal month, the majority of circulating erythrocytes in the embryo are secondary (definitive) erythrocytes. Megakaryocytes also appear to form from the hemocytoblasts in the embryonic and fetal liver. Granulocytic cells are found in the embryonic liver but appear to develop not from the hemocytoblasts but perhaps directly from the lymphocytoid wandering cells themselves.

The Embryonic Bone Marrow and Myelopoiesis. Bone formation in the embryo occurs at varying times for different bones. The earliest bones to form are the long bones of the appendicular skeleton. Initially, a cartilaginous model of each bone is formed. The central core of the diaphysis of each long bone subsequently becomes ossified, and soon an area of bone resorption develops, followed by the ingrowth of mesenchymal cells from the periosteum. These mesenchymal cells are accompanied by the ingrowth of capillaries. The mesenchymal cells continue to increase in number by continued influx of other mesenchymal cells as well as by division of those already within the newly forming marrow cavity. They also elaborate a noncellular ground substance, or matrix, that fills the developing marrow cavity. Cells morphologically similar to the hemocytoblasts of the liver and yolk sac develop from these early marrow mesenchymal cells. As in the yolk sac and liver, these give rise to megakaryocytes and erythroid cells, as well as myeloid cells, including neutrophils, basophils, and eosinophils. The embryonic marrow differs markedly from the earlier centers of hematopoiesis in that the generation of myeloid cells is especially vigorous and dominates the embryonic marrow hematopoietic activity. The process of formation of the early myeloid cells, or *myelopoiesis,* occurs first in the central portion of the marrow cavity and spreads outward eventually from there to include the entire marrow cavity. Erythropoiesis occurs slightly later in the embryonic marrow and is generally admixed with the process of myelopoiesis. Small foci of erythropoiesis can thus be seen among the many maturing cells of myeloid lineage. After birth, hematopoiesis ceases in the liver, and the bone marrow continues to be the principal site of hematopoiesis for the remainder of life.

Hematopoiesis in the Spleen of the Embryo and Fetus. The last major site of hematopoiesis to form in embryonic life is the spleen. Although the spleen itself forms much earlier, circulating hematopoietic progenitors and precursors begin to populate the spleen, beginning around the fourth fetal month in humans. Probably as the result of its large blood volume, the fetal spleen thus becomes a center of erythropoiesis until the time of birth, when splenic erythropoiesis gradually ceases. Although some myelopoiesis occurs in the embryonic and fetal spleen, it is relatively insignificant in comparison. Much later, during the fifth month of gestation, the white pulp of the spleen forms by differentiation of mesenchymal cells that have grouped around the splenic arterioles. The formation of the splenic lymphocytes appears to occur as a process completely separate from the origin of erythropoiesis in this organ.

Other Sites of Hematopoiesis in the Embryo and Fetus. The embryonic thymus develops as an outgrowth of the third branchial pouch. The thymic epithelium is invaded by wandering mesenchymal cells that begin multiplying rapidly and differentiating into lymphocytes. During this process, small numbers of erythroid and myeloid cells are formed in the thymus, but the primary process is that of lymphopoiesis. The lymphocytes formed in this organ will constitute a distinct class of lymphocytes with a special function: that of cellular-mediated immunity. (See later.)

The lymph nodes develop as outpouchings from the primitive lymphatic vessels that become surrounded by accretions of mesenchymal cells. Subsequently, these seem to round up and become similar in appearance to the lymphocytes of the adult. A few of the mesenchymal cells give rise to cells of other lineages, such as erythrocytes, granulocytes, and megakaryocytes, but this is a transitory phenomenon; as in the thymus, the principal process is lymphopoiesis.

Summary of Embryonic and Fetal Hematopoiesis. In all the hematopoietic organs of the embryo and fetus, a similar process takes place (Fig. 1-2). Circulating primitive hematopoietic stem cells lodge in a particular tissue niche, by processes still not clearly understood; at these niches they differentiate into cells recognizable as hematopoietic precursors. These embryonic hematopoietic precursors appear to be capable of multilineage differentiation, but at any one site the process of hematopoiesis may be dominated by the formation of a particular lineage, presumably under the influence of the local environment. The various sites of embryonic hematopoiesis seem to be active only at specific times during development. They follow a pattern of programmed involution, except for the bone marrow, which continues as the principal location of hematopoiesis in the adult. The lymph nodes, spleen, thymus, and other lymphatic tissues continue to be active in lymphopoiesis in the adult as well.

HEMATOPOIESIS IN THE ADULT

After birth, primitive pluripotent stem cell development and myelopoiesis occur in the bone marrow, whereas lymphopoiesis occurs in the thymus, spleen, and lymph nodes. Under certain conditions of pathologic stress, myelopoiesis reenacts its fetal expression in the spleen and liver as well. The major site of hematopoietic activity shifts gradually from the liver and spleen to the bone marrow cavities of nearly all bones of the axial and appendicular skeleton. The marrow acquires a reddish color like that of blood once hematopoietic activity begins, reflecting the vigorous production of erythrocytes that contain hemoglobin. The bone marrow cavity serves primarily as a site for the production of nonlymphoid blood cells, whereas lymphopoiesis in the adult occurs primarily in the spleen, lymph nodes, thymus, and gut-associated lymphoid tissue, including the tonsils, adenoids, and Peyer's patches. Thus when examined with the light microscope, the adult marrow will be seen to be composed primarily of erythroid and myeloid precursor cells, together with scattered megakaryocytes. There is also a population of cells known as "stromal cells" that are crucial for the maturation of the precursor cells and release of the fully differentiated cell types into the circulation.

BONE MARROW

The bone marrow provides a number of domains or hematopoietic inductive microenvironments to allow for the production of red blood cells, white blood cells, and platelets (Fig. 1-3). Stromal cells such as reticular cells and barrier cells form locules or enclosures as a physical expression of the fragile microenvironment which also includes endosteal (lining) cells, lymphoid cells, osteoblasts, osteoclasts, macrophages, and their soluble growth factors (cytokines). These create and maintain the "soil" for nurturing the "seed" hematopoietic stem cells and their progeny.

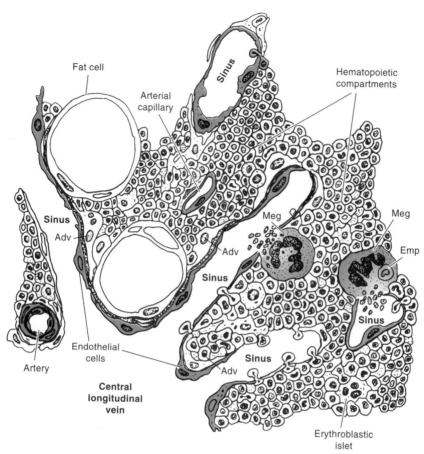

Figure 1-3. Schematic cross-sectional view of bone marrow showing hematopoietic and vascular compartments. *Adv* indicates adventitial cells. (See text for their important role in hematopoietic control.) *Meg* indicates a megakaryocyte. *Emp* shows a white cell entering the cytoplasm of a megakaryocyte—a phenomenon known as emperipolesis. (Redrawn from Weiss LP. *Cell and Tissue Biology*, 6th ed. Baltimore, Munich: Urban & Schwarzenberg; 1988.)

There are, therefore, many vulnerable loci for development of lesions in hematopoiesis.

The vascular compartment of the bone marrow contains vascular sinuses, which are large, thin-walled veins. The vascular sinuses are the dominant structure of this compartment. Blood cells from the hematopoietic compartment enter vascular sinuses (see later) and travel from the periphery of the vascular compartment to the central veins and ultimately the general circulation. Arteries flow into the capillaries, which then rejoin venous sinuses directly. Unlike the spleen, the circulation is "closed." (See later.)

The endothelium of vascular sinuses is sheathed by an incomplete basement membrane about which lie adventitial cells. These cells are large, branched, stromal reticular cells that provide a scaffolding in the hematopoietic compartment. They cover and uncover vascular endothelial cells to help regulate cell passage from the hematopoietic to the vascular compartment and can become fatty adipocytes (or accumulate gelatinous material) and thereby control hematopoietic compartment volume.

Hematopoietic compartments surround venous spaces and demonstrate developmental stages of all three cell lines. Arterial vasculature and accessory cells are also present. The myeloid-to-erythroid cellular ratio is approximately $3:1$. Red blood cell development may be organized as erythroblastic islets that consist of central macrophages surrounded by differentiating and proliferating erythroblasts. The islet lies directly against the vascular sinus, and constituent cells have a particular array whose hierarchy is determined by their maturity: Reticulocytes and orthochromatophilic pronormoblasts (the most differentiated erythroid precursors) press directly upon the vascular sinus endothelial cells, whereas the earlier precursors are most remote from the sinuses. Macrophages are situated so that they interact physically with erythroid cells prepared to phagocytize nuclei and nuclear remnants and to deliver cytokines locally to developing red blood cells. Barrier cells also assist in sequestering the erythroblastic islet. Megakaryocytes deliver cytoplasmic fragments (platelets) through vascular sinus endothelial apertures. Additionally, the lung may play an important role in megakaryocyte maturation and platelet production. Granulocytes develop into metamyelocytes before their transmural passage. Metamyelocyte microvilli clear adventitial cells from the basal surface of endothelial cells before they penetrate and pass through to the lumen of the vascular sinus. As noted previously, there are many sites and opportunities for problems to arise with hematopoiesis. These may be due to physical, metabolic, chemical, infectious, or inflammatory or immunologic causes. (See Chapter 7.)

As each individual ages, the marrow of bones of the appendicular skeleton gradually loses its red appearance and is transformed into yellow marrow, a reflection of the progressive replacement of hematopoietic tissue by adipose tissue. Thus by early adulthood, the long bones no longer bear red marrow but are replaced completely by nonhematopoietic yellow marrow, and the primary sites of red marrow are confined to the sternum, ribs, vertebrae, and pelvis. Although the stimulus for this progressive transformation of red to yellow marrow is unknown, in pathologic conditions associated with vigorous hematopoietic activity, the transformation may fail to take place and the red marrow may actually expand into bones not normally associated with hematopoietic activity, such as the diploic cavities of the cranial bones. The liver, spleen, and lymph nodes may also be locations of "extramedullary hematopoiesis" in such situations. An extreme example occurs in individuals with thalassemia major, a disease in which erythropoiesis is unusually brisk throughout life, resulting in a characteristic expansion of the marrow spaces of all the cranial bones and long bones. This is so pronounced that the diploe of the calvarium has a characteristic "hair-on-end" appearance in x-rays of the skull. Maxillary bone marrow hyperplasia results in a characteristic facies with prominent cheekbones and malocclusion of the teeth because the maxilla is disproportionately larger than the mandible (see Chapter 3).

SPLEEN

A glandular glob tucked in
behind the stomach's rumbling
fundus, beneath the diaphragm's

sturdy curve, bumped
by the transmitted thumps
of the heart's motor, lodged

in a noisy corner, this
was supposed to be the seat
of passion. The small elliptical

garbage bag of the belly
eats up old cells, used blood,
maybe that's the source

of melancholy, the regret
of a necessary cannibal,
guilt over excess spite,

the constant biting. It atones
by hatching, a little brood
hen clacking her beak

over new cells that keep
their mother's nature,
consuming foreign bacterial bits

arriving in the dark gland.
A filter between artery and vein,
microscopic channels or blood

pools, small unwalled seas
hold the mysteries, deep
in the visceral red pulp.

Alice Jones, M.D.
Oakland, CA*

The spleen is located in the left upper quadrant of the abdomen. It is associated with several other organs and has renal, colonic, pancreatic, and diaphragmatic surfaces. In the adult, it weighs approximately 150 g with pea- to plum-sized accessory spleens present in the gastrolineal ligament, greater omentum, and elsewhere. Although considered an organ of mystery since antiquity, its functions have now been better characterized. Its structure and blood flow provide a unique and elegant basis for many of its now well-defined tasks (Fig. 1-4). A capsule composed of dense connective tissue sends out a rich trabecular network into the substance of the spleen. Little muscle is present in the capsule, unlike other animals, which can expand and contract spleen size. The parenchyma is called the *splenic pulp*, which is divided into red pulp comprised largely of *splenic sinuses* and thin plates of cellular tissue, called *splenic cords*, lying between the sinuses. Although pulp is composed of clusters of lymphocytes, it assumes two formations. One is predominantly made up of T-lymphocytes (thymus derived) and accessory cells and forms a cylindrical sheath surrounding the central artery. The white cells are called the periarterial lymphatic sheath (PALS). B-lymphocytes (the term *B cell* is derived from the bursa of Fabricius, a hindgut organ required for B-cell processing and maturation in birds; human bone marrow may be the analog) form nodules within the PALS. The PALS central artery tapers as it emerges from the sheath and enters the white pulp, where it terminates as a capillary connecting directly with the venous sinus or sprays its blood into the red pulp whose cells leisurely percolate and eventually meander to the venous sinus.

The *marginal zone* of the splenic pulp is located at the junction of red and white pulp. It is the site where the process of filtering and cell sorting are initiated. The

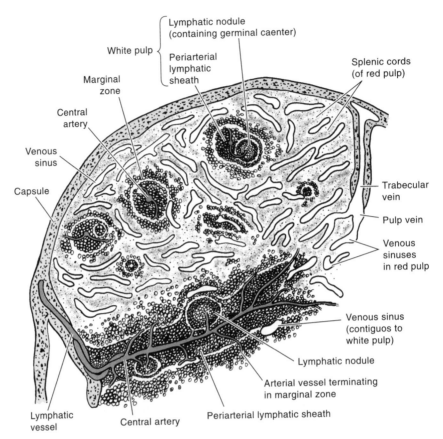

Figure 1-4. Organization of the human spleen presented schematically. (See text for description of blood flow and cell distribution.) Redrawn from Weiss L, Tavassoli M. Anatomical hazards to the passage of erythrocytes through the spleen. *Seminars in Hematology* 7:732, 1970.

path of blood flow in the spleen is important for splenic function to occur properly. Blood enters the spleen via the splenic artery passing through the hilus. Trabecular arteries are derived from the splenic artery; they then divide into central arteries that run in the center of the cylindrical PALS. As noted earlier, termination of central arteries is either direct or indirect with venous sinuses. After entering splenic sinuses, blood leaves via pulp veins that meet with trabecular veins, and the latter exit from the hilus of the spleen by the splenic vein route.

Lymph flow in the spleen runs counter to arterial flow and in the same direction as venous flow, but the lymphatics of the spleen are not as highly developed as other animals. Barrier cells described by Weiss are "intensely activated, rapidly mobilized fugitive fibroblastic cells" that are of stromal cell lineage. Although their function is still mysterious, their central location suggests that they could have multiple functions, including blood vessel sheathing, development of blood/tissue barriers, concentration of regulatory factors, sealing off of immunologically competent tissue after the immune response is initiated, concentration of regulatory factors, enclosure of hematopoietic colonies, concentration of hematopoietic factors, and protection against parasites. Such cells are also present in other hematopoietic and immunologic tissue, where they may function in a fashion similar to that in the spleen.

The spleen has many important functions, several of which are directly determined by the complex blood flow path. In contrast to the lymph nodes, which react to regional antigenic challenge by receiving lymphatic fluid, the spleen tests and immunologically interacts with blood that comes from the entire body. However, a plasma-skimming function occurs, as branches of central arteries take off at right angles, allowing plasma to be sieved before blood reaches the red pulp. Various filtration beds are made up of reticular cells and reticular fibers as well as other cell types of stromal origin, including macrophages, interdigitating cells, and follicular dendritic cells. Barrier cells also help comprise the filtration apparatus. As noted earlier, the periarterial lymphatic sheaths, marginal zone beds, and red pulp also serve as filtration beds along with the venous sinus endothelial cells. (See later.) The filter beds allow the spleen to recognize, cull, and remove cells that are defective or old and worn out. Particulate inclusions such as Howell-Jolly bodies, Heinz bodies, bacteria, parasites, and iron granules (Table 3-3) are removed via the spleen's pitting function. Iron reutilization, pooling of platelets, polishing of red cells, blood volume regulation, early and (occasionally pathologic) hematopoietic function, and immune functions are all part of the spleen's complex job.

The spleen also functions as a primary bacterial filter, or sponge, during early stages of the inflammatory response. When episodic bacteremic showers occur, the spleen traps bacteria by ingestion into macrophages. Venous sinus endothelial cells (VSEs) form a specialized tissue that blood cells encounter and must successfully traverse as they leave the spongy mesh of the red pulp on their way to the splenic vein. The VSEs have unique antigenic characteristics and motility powers that allow them to test abnormal or aged cells or those containing bacteria (e.g., polymorphonuclear leukocytes) or parasites or protozoa (e.g., RBCs) as the cells pass between the fingerlike cells' interendothelial slits. This physical barrier and the netlike basement membrane serve as a locus for cellular interactions and permit macrophages to interface with detained cells and "grope" their surfaces and interiors for imperfections and particulate matter that are subsequently ingested by them (Figs. 1-5 and 1-6).

Not only are the trapped bacteria processed by macrophages and their antigens directly presented to the lymphocytes in the spleen, stimulating specific antibody production, but macrophage engulfment itself acutely reduces the bacterial load in the circulation. This latter function is itself extremely important, as several of the polysaccharides on the surface of both gram-negative and gram-positive bacteria are powerful systemic toxins. If not sequestered in macrophages, these bacterial antigens may directly trigger the alternative complement cascade, even before an antibody response can be mounted, which could lead to vasodilation and increased capillary permeability, and ultimately shock and death.

In addition to this role as a highly complex filter, the spleen serves as a "super" lymph node, developing large numbers of B-cell clones in the presence of T cells (about 80% of spleen cells are B cells, about 15% are T cells). In addition to the generation of T-cell-dependent B-cell responses, the spleen appears to be the major site of T-independent B-cell development. This development is extremely important for the body's response to carbohydrate antigens expressed on capsules of bacteria such as *Streptococcus pneumoniae, Hemophilus influenzae,* and *Neisseriae meningitidis.*

T cells and B cells interact in the PALS and lymphocyte nodules within the PALS. Antibody-producing cell clusters consisting of B cells, plasma cells, helper and suppressor T cells, macrophages, and other accessory cells form the center of lymphatic nodules as germinal centers.

Finally, the spleen serves two related, nonimmune, mechanical functions. The

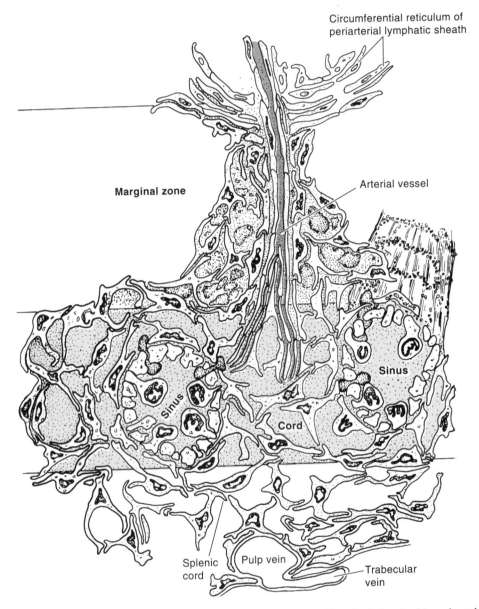

Circumferential reticulum of
periarterial lymphatic sheath

Marginal zone

Arterial vessel

Sinus

Sinus

Cord

Splenic
cord

Pulp vein

Trabecular
vein

Figure 1-5. Schematic view of splenic artery leaving the periarterial lymphatic sheath white pulp and entering red pulp. The splenic artery is shown entering a splenic cord and bifurcating between two sinuses. (Redrawn from Weiss L. *The Cells and Tissues of the Immune System.* Englewood Cliffs, N.J.: Prentice-Hall; 1972.)

spleen serves as a reservoir for platelets released by the bone marrow. Normally, this function results in only a small fraction of the body's platelet mass being retained in the spleen at any one time. However, if the spleen is increased in size, up to 90% of the body's platelet mass can be found within the spleen. Platelets in the spleen appear to be in equilibrium with the circulating pool of platelets, which slowly exchange their location.

The spleen also retains red cells, but here the process is less passive and more dynamic. Senescent, antibody-coated, or damaged red cells are trapped in the

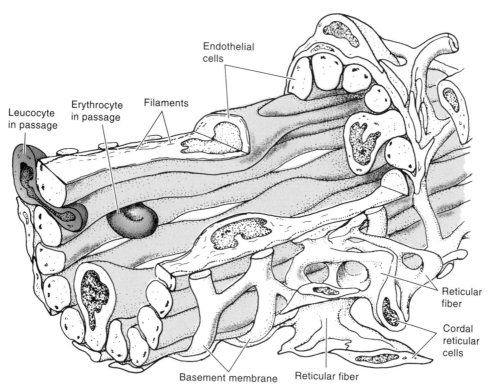

Figure 1-6. Human splenic sinus in red pulp showing the rodlike endothelial cells in three dimensions with filaments at basilar service that control interendothelial slit size. Basement membrane is fenestrated, allowing passage of red and white cells through the endothelial cells. (See text for details of red blood cell passage.) (Redrawn from Chen LT, Weiss L. *Am J Anat* 1972;134:425.)

spleen, where they are either directly removed or partially repaired, or "remodeled," by VSE cells and splenic macrophages. Remodeled red cells can then recirculate, and remaining abnormalities are sensed by the spleen and are removed quickly upon subsequent splenic recirculation. In the laboratory, red blood cells with pits, pocks, and craters are detected by special microscopic techniques when there is splenic hypofunction or asplenia. Nuclear remnants called Howell-Jolly bodies are detected (Table 3-3) in circulating red blood cells by standard light microscopy in Wright's stained blood smear when the spleen functions poorly or in the post-splenectomy state. It must be emphasized that patients whose spleens are dysfunctional or absent carry lifelong risk for overwhelming bacterial sepsis, especially from encapsulated bacterial organisms. In addition, these individuals suffer worse clinical outcomes when infected with parasitic organisms such as malaria or babesia.

The spleen may enlarge for a variety of reasons. Functional overactivity, called *hypersplenism*, often accompanies structural enlargement. Hypersplenism may be characterized by the spleen's voraciousness for the body's own cellular elements, resulting in cytopenias. There may also be pain from splenic enlargement or infarction, and early satiety may occur as the spleen encroaches upon the stomach. Splenic enlargement may come about from a variety of pathophysiologic mechanisms, which include endothelial or immune system hyperplasia from infectious diseases, or immune disorders. Enlargement from altered splenic blood flow occurs in hepatic cirrhosis, splenic, hepatic or portal vein thrombosis. Primary or metastatic tumors, extra-medullary hematopoiesis, or abnormal material infiltrating the spleen, as in amyloidosis or storage diseases such as Gaucher's disease and hemangiomas or cysts also cause splenic enlargement. The decision to surgically remove a hypersplenic, enlarged, diseased, or bleeding spleen is not an easy one since splenectomy renders the patient immunologically handicapped for life.

The full range of causes of functional and anatomic hyposplenism includes congenital absence, splenectomy, myelofibrosis and other myeloproliferative disorders, impaired vascular supply to the spleen, immune or autoimmune disorders such as lupus or rheumatoid arthritis, celiac disease and inflammatory bowel disease, invasive tumors, systemic amyloidosis, nephrotic syndrome, mastocytosis, and the neonatal state.

Peripheral blood consequences of hyposplenism include transient thrombocytosis and the presence of Howell-Jolly bodies (nuclear remnants in red cells), as well as surface pits and pocks resulting from lack of splenic conditioning of red cells. Target cells and acanthocytes are also seen in the absense of the spleen (Table 3-3). Clearance of encapsulated bacteria is reduced, as mentioned earlier. Response to antigenic challenge, including some vaccines, is altered. Susceptibility to overwhelming parasitic infections such as babesia and malaria is a consequence of asplenia.

LYMPH NODES

Lying in the course of lymphatic vessels are lymph nodes which are small, oval, or kidney-shaped structures that are 0.1–2.5 cm long. They are connected to the circulation by afferent lymphatic vessels that run into the greater curvature of the node and efferent lymphatic vessels that exit from the hilum (Fig. 1-7). Valves in lymphatic vessels ensure unidirectional lymph flow. At the hilum are entering arteries and exiting veins. A fibrous capsule encloses each node, and trabeculae extend into the parenchyma. Specialized meshwork or filtration beds composed of reticular cells and fibers receive T- and B-lymphocytes from the recirculating lymphocytic pool. T-lymphocytes comprise the peripheral area of lymph nodes and are concentrated in the interfollicular zone (between primary and secondary follicle areas) and

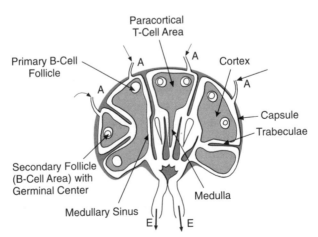

Figure 1-7.   Schematic lymph node structure. Lymph flows into lymph nodes *via* afferent lymphatics (A) and leaves lymph nodes *via* efferent lymphatics (E). B cell areas are primary and secondary follicles in lymph node cortex; while T cells are concentrated in paracortical areas. Heavy arrows show direction of lymph flow. (Redrawn from Isselbacher KJ, et al, eds. *Harrison's Principles of Internal Medicine,* 13th ed. New York: McGraw-Hill, 1994.)

in the paracortical area. T cells in lymph nodes are CD4-helper types (80%) and CD8-suppressor types (20%). B-lymphocytes in the lymph node cortex are contained within primary and secondary lymphoid follicles. Interdigitating reticular cells (veiled or dendritic cells) may be identical to the Langerhans cells of the epithelium that travel to lymphatic tissue with newly collected antigens.

Each lymph node then is composed of an aggregate of B-lymphoid follicles, each follicle representing the expansion of a small number of B-cell clones. Grouped around these follicles are seas of T-lymphocytes that function both in concert with the B cells and on their own. Specialized cell-interaction molecules are expressed on the T cells that directly surround the follicles, which serve as T-cell–B-cell adhesion molecules and help mediate T–B interaction in antibody maturation and secretion.

Barrier cells of fibroblastic origin variously aggregate to create blood pathways and sequestration sites. Macrophages work in concert with barrier cells to control infectious diseases and participate in the immune response. The afferent lymphatic vessels that contain lymph, antigens, lymphocytes, and macrophages connect with subcapsular space. Lymph and its contents then go to paracortical and medullary areas, medullary sinuses, and finally efferent lymphatic vessels. Arterial circulation delivers T cells from thymus and B cells from bone marrow to lymph nodes. B and T cells enter the interior of the lymph node while they are on their exit route in the lymph node venules, whose high endothelial cells recognize and direct lymphocytes into the lymph node. The structural and cellular makeup of lymph nodes allows for interactions of antigen and lymphocytic cells, which sets up optimal activation of the immune response.

Lymph nodes may increase in size because of a variety of normal but perhaps exaggerated immune responses as well as several clearly pathologic states. They include the following: (a) Increased blood flow and cellular makeup as part of the immune response; (b) frank infections or inflammation of the lymph node itself (lymphadenitis); (c) macrophage or storage cell engulfment of metabolic debris or end products in certain storage diseases; (d) neoplastic involvement by primary or metastatic lymphoreticular or solid tumors.

THYMUS

The thymus lies in the anterior mediastinum. Soft and bilobed in character, it is 10–15 g at birth, rapidly increasing to 20–40 g, and does not change in weight dramatically thereafter, although the amount of lymphoid tissue gradually decreases with age and the gland becomes fatty but still immunologically active. The thymus develops in the eighth week of embryonic life from branchial pouches 3 and 4 as an epithelial organ populated by thymocytes (T cells) that derive from bone marrow prothymocytes. T-cell markers characterize states of T-cell development in the thymus. The gland forms lobules because of capsular septations. There is a cortex and medulla in each lobule (Fig. 1-8). The cortex contains 95% of thymic lymphocytes, but supporting epithelial cells are also present (epithelial reticular cells). Prothymocytes enter thymic parenchyma high in the cortex and move deeper toward the corticomedullary junction, maturing as they travel. They interact with stromal cells (epithelial reticular cells, reticular cells, barrier cells, and macrophages) that instruct the developing T cells to permanently distinguish self from nonself.

The medulla contains 5% of thymic lymphocytes. These are mature T cells. Most cellular elements here are polyhedral epithelial cells. These cells may assume an irregular, circumferential, lamellated appearance with central necrosis, calci-

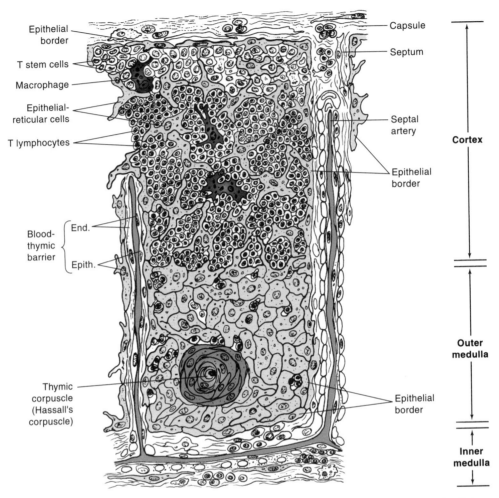

Figure 1-8. Thymic lobule schematic diagram. Cortex, outer medulla, inner medulla, and cellular components are shown. (See text for details of lymphocyte array and flow.) (Redrawn from Weiss, L, ed. *Cell and Tissue Biology: A Textbook of Histology*, 6th ed. Baltimore, Munich: Urban and Schwartzenberg; 1988.)

fication, and cyst formation. Such structures are called thymic or Hassall's corpuscles and represent the end stage of thymic–medullary–epithelial differentiation. At the corticomedullary junction or in the medulla, T-lymphocytes enter veins or lymphatics and circulate to the spleen, and then to the recirculating lymphocyte pool. Approximately 95% of lymphocytes die within the thymic cortex, so that only 5% are released as immunologically competent cells (Fig. 1-9).

In summary, thymic T-cell development occurs predominantly during childhood and adolescence. After the second decade the thymus is largely involuted, although some thymic activity still occurs in adulthood. Certain aspects of early T-cell development appear to occur outside the thymus as well, perhaps in lymph nodes, but the details of this process are uncertain. Once thymocytes develop into mature T cells, these cells circulate throughout the body. Much of their immune function occurs in lymph nodes, where they induce B cells to mature and develop into anti-

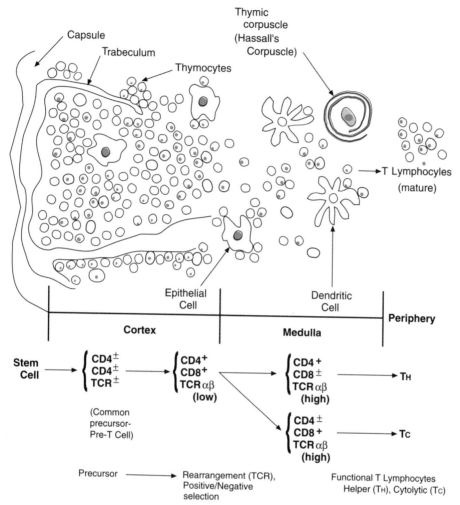

Figure 1-9. Structure of the thymus. Immature thymocytes mature from the cortex toward the medullary region. TCR $\alpha\beta$ molecules are depicted. (TCR$\gamma\delta$ cells are rare.) CD, cluster designation; TCR, T-cell receptor; $\alpha\beta,\alpha\beta$ molecules of TCR; *low, high* denote levels of $\alpha\beta$ expression. (Redrawn from Nichols WS, Kipps TJ. Structure and function of other lymphoid tissues. In: Beutler E, Lichtman MA, Coller BS, Kipps TJ, eds. *Williams Hematology*, 5th ed. New York: McGraw-Hill; 1995, 45.)

body-secreting plasma cells, whereas other aspects of T cell immune function occur in nonlymphoid tissue sites.

The thymus is thus responsible for the induction of T-cell maturation and development of the ability of T cells to distinguish self from nonself. The gland involutes with normal aging, stress, and disease. It may hypertrophy, induced by triiodothyronine (T3) prolactin and growth hormone. Rarely, following chemotherapy for systemic malignancy, the chemically and hormonally suppressed gland may rebound and assume a worrisome but benign larger size. The gland itself may be involved with thymomas—tumors that have important immunologic sequelae and may be associated with such diseases as myasthenia gravis or pure red blood cell aplasia (Chapter 7). Occasionally, thymomas may be malignant and locally invasive; they rarely give rise to distant metastatic disease.

THE STEM CELL MODEL OF HEMATOPOIESIS

The cell that gives rise to all other types of blood cells, the stem cell, is so rare that it has never been morphologically identified with certainty (Fig. 1-1). Rather, the existence of stem cells is inferred by functional assays that demonstrate the ability of single cells to generate multiple hematopoietic lineages. Thus stem cells are currently defined not by their appearance but by their function. Stem cells are known to be extremely rare, although quantifying them is somewhat imprecise because of different degrees of rigor applied to the definition of what constitutes a stem cell. The most generous estimate is that stem cells occur in human bone marrow with a frequency of 1 per 1 million nucleated bone marrow cells; more conservative estimates place this figure at 1 per 10 million.

The tremendous production rate of hematopoietic cells requires that roughly every other day the bone marrow produce as many cells as it contains. To maintain this rate throughout life, the bone marrow must possess cells that can generate vast numbers of mature cells continuously (i.e., without losing the ability to do so). This self-renewal ability is critical to the concept of the stem cell. At present there are two theories about how this might occur. According to the first, every stem cell division is asymmetric, producing one undifferentiated stem cell and one more differentiated cell that is committed to produce mature blood cells. In the second theory, each stem cell division produces either two additional stem cells or two more mature cells. The stem cell pool is thus maintained not by precise asymmetric divisions within each stem cell but by a balance between the number of stem cell divisions yielding more stem cells and divisions yielding more mature cells.

At the point the stem cell leaves the self-renewing pool to populate the differentiating pool, it still appears morphologically as a primitive blast cell and retains the capacity to produce cells of all lineages. With each subsequent division, the daughter *progenitor cells* become more and more restricted in their commitment to the production of specific blood cell lineages. That is, if one isolates progenitor cells and permits them to propagate and differentiate, they will generate collections of cells that are of only one or a few lineages. The more differentiated the progenitor cell, the fewer lineages are produced and the smaller the number of cells produced. These concepts, which have been supported by several decades of *in vivo* and *in vitro* experiments, have now defined the hierarchical stem cell model of hematopoiesis (see Fig. 1-1).

The Hematopoietic Microenvironment. If they are maintained in a simply nutritive environment, stem cells will die without differentiating or dividing. To support the process of hematopoietic self-renewal and differentiation, stem cells and their progeny must be maintained in the close proximity of nonhematopoietic mesenchymal cells, called *stromal cells*. These cells—which are composed of a heterogeneous group of fibroblasts, endothelial cells, osteoblasts, and adipocytes—line the endosteal surfaces in the bone marrow cavity. They appear to supply two closely related requirements for the hematopoietic cells—soluble hematopoietic growth factors and membrane-bound attachment molecules.

The hematopoietic growth factors (HGF), or colony stimulating factors (CSF), are a class of glycoprotein hormones that obligately regulate the division and differentiation of hematopoietic cells. These hormones are required for survival, proliferation, differentiation, and function of all the hematopoietic cells. Although initially discovered as spontaneously secreted products of T-cell tumors, it is clear that these hormones are normally the products of bone marrow stromal cells as well as T-lymphocytes and monocytes.

CSFs are produced in a two-tiered process. First, small amounts of certain CSFs (interleukin 6 [IL-6], granulocyte–macrophage colony stimulating factor [GM-CSF], stem cell factor [SCF]) and flt-3 (Flt-31) ligand are produced constitutively by bone marrow stromal cells, probably in response to stimulation by plasma proteins. The production of these CSFs is responsible for basal hematopoiesis, which maintains blood counts in the normal ranges (Fig. 1-1).

CSF secretion is greatly increased above the basal levels in response to infection. Bacterial and viral products activate monocytes, which then secrete interleukin 1 (IL-1), tumor necrosis factor alpha (TNF-α), and granulocyte colony stimulating factor (G-CSF), as well as their own macrophage colony stimulating factor (M-CSF). These products in turn stimulate additional CSF secretion. IL-1, together with antigenic stimulation of specific receptors, activate T cells to secrete GM-CSF and interleukin 3 (IL-3). IL-1 and TNF-α each stimulate fibroblasts and endothelial cells in the bone marrow stromal microenvironment to increase endothelial cell secretion of IL-6 and GM-CSF, and to secrete large quantities of G-CSF. These hematopoietic growth factors (cytokines) thereby directly increase the numbers of circulating neutrophils, monocytes, and plasma cells and activate these cells when they mature. The generation of each specific lineage of mature blood cells is regulated in this manner by a specific set of hematopoietic growth factors. Although the sets of hematopoietic growth factors that induce specific mature blood cell subsets overlap, each is characteristically distinct.

Erythropoiesis. The final stages of erythroid differentiation are regulated largely by erythropoietin (EPO), a glycoprotein produced in response to tissue hypoxia in the fetal liver and adult kidney. Of the 18 or so cell divisions that take place during the time a stem cell generates a mature red blood cell, erythropoietin strongly induces the final 8–10 divisions. The transcription of the erythropoietin gene in renal peritubular endothelial cells and hepatoblasts is regulated by oxygen-sensitive transcription factors that up-regulate gene expression with declining O_2 delivery. Overproduction of erythropoietin, observed in some cases of renal cell carcinoma and hepatoma, leads directly to erythroid polycythemia (Chapter 3).

The preceding cell divisions, which give rise to erythropoietin-sensitive erythroid progenitor cells, are largely independent of erythropoietin. These proliferation and maturation events are instead induced by granulocyte–macrophage colony stimulating factor (GM–CSF) and stem cell factor (SCF), both of which are produced locally within the marrow microenvironment by bone marrow stromal cells. In addition, these steps can be specifically amplified by the secretion of IL-3 by activated T-lymphocytes.

Granulopoiesis. Much like erythroid differentiation, the final stages in neutropoiesis and monopoiesis are induced by granulocyte colony stimulating factor (G-CSF) and macrophage colony stimulating factor (M-CSF), respectively. The early divisions, which direct multipotential progenitors to become committed to individual lineages, are regulated by the synergistic interactions of GM-CSF, SCF, and IL-3. As described earlier, although there is a constant level of basal secretion of CSF secretion by bone marrow stromal fibroblasts that line the marrow endosteal surfaces, the secretion of GM-CSF and G-CSF is dramatically up-regulated in the presence of inflammation in response to the secretion of IL-1 and TNF-α by monocytes.

For the production of eosinophils, interleukin 5 (IL-5), as well as, to a lesser extent, IL-3 and GM-CSF play major inductive roles. Basophils and mast cells are directly stimulated by SCF and IL-3. In both of these instances, the initial afferent signals that trigger the release of these cytokines is not yet well understood.

Megakaryopoiesis. The earliest stages in the development of megakaryocytic progenitor cells appear to also be induced by thrombopoietin (TPO), in conjunction with SCF. TPO itself also induces terminal maturation of megakaryocytes and platelet budding. In contrast, interleukin 11 (IL-11) may play a major role in platelet budding, with comparatively minor influences on megakaryocyte generation and development per se. (For further discussion of this topic see Chapter 5.)

B Lymphopoiesis. As with the myeloid lineages, the development of B cells begins with the differentiation of pluripotent stem cells into undifferentiated but committed B-cell progenitors. The initial stages in the proliferation and differentiation of these B-cell progenitors are induced by interleukin 7 (IL-7) and SCF. Once recognizable pre–B cells and B cells are generated, further differentiation and divisions are induced by stimulation through the immunoglobulin antigen receptor, through the Fc receptor, and through stimulation by soluble interleukin 4 (IL-4) and IL-6. Once antibodies producing plasma cells are generated, additional proliferation and antibody secretion are stimulated by IL-6 and GM-CSF.

T-lymphopoiesis. Once pre–T cells undergo the complex processes of negative and positive selection in the thymus that generate self- and non-self-discrimination, the resulting mature T cells are subject to antigen- and cytokine-induced activation and expansion. Stimulation with an antigen plus interleukin 2 (IL-2), or with an antigen plus costimulation with accessory macrophages or dendritic cells that express B7-1 or B7-2, leads to the direct activation of both CD4+ and CD8+ T cells.

THE CLINICAL USE OF HEMATOPOIETIC GROWTH FACTORS

Since the first human hematopoietic growth factors were cloned and isolated 8 years ago, preclinical and clinical trials have rapidly led to their introduction into the clinic for routine and experimental use. At the present time, erythropoietin, G-CSF, and GM-CSF have all been approved for human use by the Food and Drug Administration, and IL-3, SCF and IL-6, TPO, and Flt-3 ligand have begun the first phases of human testing.

Erythropoietin. The anemia of renal failure is the primary condition that is directly responsive to treatment with EPO. Appropriate doses given three times weekly lead to prompt reticulocytosis, as long as the patients have sufficient iron, folate, and B_{12} stores and have no other source of ongoing inflammation that would suppress erythropoiesis. The major side effect of such treatments is hypertension, especially if the hemoglobin level rises too high. The introduction of EPO therapy has made thousands of renal dialysis patients nontransfusion dependent and has greatly improved the quality of their lives.

Other anemias in the setting of such chronic diseases as cancer, AIDS, and rheumatologic diseases present a second group of conditions that also can respond to EPO. However, the doses required are greater than for patients with renal failure, and even at high doses the responses are variable. In general, the higher the baseline EPO level circulating in the patient's plasma, the less the chance of response to EPO therapy.

A third, growing area of application of EPO therapy is to *autologous donation* of red blood cells prior to elective surgery. By administering EPO under a controlled setting, hematologists can stimulate a mild erythrocytosis (high red blood cell count), which allows removal of blood without causing severe anemia. In this way it is possible to store several units of red blood cells prior to any elective surgery, thus eliminating the need for and risk of allogeneic red cell transfusion. The only limitations on this therapy are the organizational abilities of hematologists and blood banks. Given the large number of blood products required for urgent and emergent surgeries, allogeneic donation and blood transfusion will always be essential. However, for the increasing number of elective conditions requiring RBC support, autologous, EPO-stimulated donation will be relied upon more often.

Granulocyte Colony Stimulating Factor. When the peripheral neutrophil count is depressed, increased levels of circulating granulocyte colony stimulating factor (G-CSF) can be detected by sensitive assays such as ELISA. However, the amount of G-CSF produced is suboptimal to stimulate rapid granulopoiesis. With additional G-CSF, supplied as a pharmaceutical product, the neutrophil count will recover more rapidly and to a higher level. The first major setting in which G-CSF therapy has been applied has been in chemotherapy-induced neutropenia. Delivery of G-CSF subcutaneously, beginning approximately 1 week following chemotherapy, helps lessen the length of chemotherapy-induced leukopenic periods. Controlled studies have now shown that such treatment helps to prevent infections and hospitalizations. The only major side effect observed with G-CSF is bone pain, which occurs in 10–15% of patients and can be easily controlled with analgesics. A cautionary note: G–CSF therapy use, which has allowed physicians to use higher doses of chemotherapy (greater dose intensity), has not yet led to total elimination of disease and significantly greater survival.

Pharmacologic doses of G-CSF are also effective in raising the neutrophil count in several cases of chronic neutropenia, such as congenital neutropenia (Kostmann's disease), idiopathic neutropenia, and immune-mediated neutropenias, such as T-lymphoproliferative disease. In these cases, however, the doses of G-CSF required can be substantially higher, and the responses are not as uniform. In addition, recent studies suggest that as many as 15% of congenitally neutropenic patients treated with G-CSF will go on to develop secondary acute myeloid leukemia. Whether the development of leukemia is caused by the stimulation of the abnormal marrow cells with the high levels of G-CSF is unknown, but this is certainly a cause for concern.

Granulocyte-Macrophage Colony Stimulating Factor. Like G-CSF, granulocyte-macrophage colony stimulating factor (GM-CSF) increases the neutrophil count *in vivo*. However, it has a substantially broader range of activity, and it increases the monocyte count and eosinophil count. Some studies have also reported increases in reticulocytes and platelets. Given its broad spectrum of activity, GM-CSF has been approved by the FDA for acceleration of recovery of hematopoietic function following bone marrow transplantation. In this setting GM-CSF clearly shortens the time to recovery, resulting in notably decreased morbidity of the transplantation procedure.

In addition, GM-CSF almost certainly has the same salutary effect as G-CSF in preventing and treating chemotherapy-induced nadirs. Although it is possible that its spectrum of side effects (chills, fevers, third-spacing of plasma) might make its use in this setting more problematic than G-CSF, at this time there has been no side-by-side comparison of GM-CSF with G-CSF in any setting.

One recent application of GM-CSF and G-CSF that deserves particular comment is that of progenitor cell mobilization. In the first clinical trials of GM-CSF, it was found that although the density of bone marrow progenitor cells rose slightly, the density of circulating progenitor cells rose dramatically, often by a factor of 50–100 over baseline. Later, very similar data were obtained for G-CSF (and the same is probably true for IL-3, EPO, and SCF). Based upon these data, bone marrow transplant physicians have found that they have needed fewer peripheral blood collections (leukophoresis) to obtain transplant donor stem cells. (See Chapter 8.) (These harvested stem cells are used subsequently to support bone marrow reengraftment following therapy that has ablated bone marrow in an attempt to rid the body of all neoplastic cells.) Although many questions remain regarding the cause and the meaning of this growth factor effect, as well as the role of progenitor cell mobilization in transplantation, the application of hematopoietic growth factors to "hemotherapy" in transplantation medicine raise exciting possibilities for the decade ahead.

SELECTED READING

Bannister L. Haemolymphoid system. In: Peter L. Williams, ed. *Gray's Anatomy.* Edinburgh: Churchill Livingstone; 1995:1400–1442.
A vividly written and illustrated section in a world-famous anatomy book, surprising in its depth and clarity as it describes the functional anatomy and physiology of bone marrow, spleen, lymph node, and thymus.

Bonilla, MA, Gillio AP, Ruggiero M et al: Effects of recombinant human G-CSF on neutropenia in patients with congenital agranulocytosis. *N Engl J Med* 1989;320:1574.
This study, along with Eschbach et al. (1987) and Nemunaitis et al. (1991) demonstrated the clinical efficacy of EPO, G-CSF and GM-CSF in clinical hematology-oncology. They provide the first evidence that physicians can, by providing pharmacologic doses of natural hematopoietic hormones, improve patient well-being.

Bowdler AJ, ed. *The Spleen: Structure, Function and Clinical Significance.* New York: Chapman and Hall Medical, Van Nostrand Rheinhold; 1990.
Comprehensive review of many aspects of splenic anatomy and physiology.

Emerson SG, Sieff CA, Wang EA, et al. Purification of fetal hematopoietic progenitors and demonstration of recombinant multipotential colony stimulating activity. *J Clin Invest* 1985;76:1286.
The first purification of human hematopoietic stem cells and progenitors.

Eschbach JW, Egrie JC, Downing MR et al: Correction of the anemia of end stage renal disease with recombinant human erythropoietin. *N Engl J Med* 1987;316:73.
This study, along with Bonilla et al. (1989) and Nemunaitis et al. (1991), demonstrated the clinical efficacy of EPO, G-CSF, and GM-CSF in clinical hematology-oncology. These three studies provide the first evidence that physicians can improve patient well-being by providing pharmacologic doses of natural hematopoietic hormones.

Ford CE, Hamerton JL, Barnes DWH, Loutit JF. Cytological identification of radiation chimeras. *Nature* 1961;177:452.

This study and Till (1961) gave the first experimental evidence for the hierarchical stem cell model of hematopoiesis, the model that has been developed and upheld over the past 35 years.

Guba SC, Sartor CI, Gottschalk LR, et al. Bone marrow stromal fibroblasts secrete IL-6 and GM-CSF in the absence of inflammatory stimulation. *Blood* 1992;80 : 1190–1198.
This study demonstrates the production of tiny but significant quantities of IL-6 and GM-CSF by normal human bone marrow stromal fibroblasts.

Haynes BF. Enlargement of lymph nodes and spleen. In: Isselbacher KJ, et al., eds. *Harrison's Principles of Internal Medicine*, 13th ed. New York: McGraw-Hill; 1994 : 323–329.
A succinct and authoritative discussion of disorders of lymph nodes and spleen.

Henry PH, Longo DL. Enlargement of lymph nodes and spleen. In: Fauci AS, et al., eds. *Harrison's Principles of Internal Medicine*, 14th ed. New York: McGraw-Hill; 1998:345–351.
An up–to–date approach to patients with lymphadenopathy and splenomegaly.

Holzer H, Biehl J, Antin P, et al. Quantal and proliferative cell cycles: how lineages generate cell diversity and maintain fidelity. *Prog Clin Biol Res* 1983;134:213.
The classical description of the balanced stem cell replication model, with its implications for normal hematopoiesis as well as disease states such as leukemia and bone marrow failure.

Lemischka IF, Raulet CH, Mulligan RC. Developmental potential and dynamic behavior of hematopoietic stem cells. *Cell* 1986;45:917.
A fascinating article raising the possibility that stem cells might wink on and off throughout an individual's lifetime.

Nemunaitis J, Singer JW, Buckner CD, et al. Long-term follow-up of patients who received recombinant human granulocyte-macrophage colony stimulating factor after autologous bone marrow transplantation for lymphoid malignancy. *Bone Marrow Transplant* 1991;7:49.
This study, along with Eschbach et al. (1987) and Bonilla et al. (1989), demonstrated the clinical efficacy of EPO, G-CSF, and GM-CSF in clinical hematology-oncology. The three studies provide the first evidence that physicians can improve patient well-being by providing pharmacologic doses of natural hematopoietic hormones.

Nichols WS, Kipps TJ. Structure and function of other lymphoid tissues. In: Beutler E, Lichtman MA, Coller BS, Kipps TJ, eds. *Williams Hematology*, 5th ed. New York: McGraw-Hill; 1995:43–48.
A clear explanation of lymphoid tissue physiology.

Sills RH. Hyposplenism. In: Pochedly C, Sills RH, Schwartz AD, eds. *Disorders of the Spleen: Pathophysiology and Management.* New York: Marcel Dekker; 1989:99–144.
Helpful tables regarding hyposplenism are found in this text.

Stockman JA. Splenomegaly: diagnostic overview. In: Pochedly C, Sills RH, Schwartz AD, eds. *Disorders of the Spleen: Pathophysiology and Management.* New York: Marcel Dekker; 1989:217–238.
A good overview of causes of splenomegaly and how to diagnose them.

Till JE, McCulloch EA. Direct measurement of the radiation sensitivity of normal mouse bone marrow cells. *Radiat Res* 1961;14:213.
This study and Ford (1961) gave the first experimental evidence for the hierarchical stem cell model of hematopoiesis, the model that has been developed and upheld over the past 35 years.

Tsai S, Sieff CA, et al. Stromal cell associated erythropoiesis. *Blood* 1986;67:1418.
A beautiful paper showing erythroid cells developing on fibroblastoid and monocytic adherent cells. The first study demonstrating the intimate and dynamic physiologic association of erythroid cells with their stromal microenvironment, in real time.

Weiss LP. *Cell and Tissue Biology: A Textbook of Histology*, 6th ed. Baltimore: Urban and Schwarzenberg; 1988.
A gem of a text edited by an acknowledged master of cell and tissue biology. It is vividly written and lavishly illustrated with diagrams and photomicrographs that enhance luminescent prose.

Weiss LP. Functional organization of hematopoietic tissue. In: Hoffman RH, et al., eds. *Hematology: Basic Principles and Practice,* 2nd ed. New York: Churchill Livingstone; 1995:193–206.
An up-to-date survey of the anatomy and physiology of hematopoietic tissue; especially edifying and clarifying, as it treats the blood flow in hematopoietic tissues.

Weiss LP. The structure of hematopoietic tissues. In: Handin RI, Lux SE, Stossel TP, eds. *Blood: Principles and Practice of Hematology.* Philadelphia: JB Lippincott; 1995: 155–169.
A brief treatise on the structure and function, anatomy, and physiology of hematopoietic tissue by one of the world's most articulate experts in the field, especially coherent in its discussion of splenic blood flow as a basis for the spleen's myriad tasks.

Williams DA. The stem cell model of hematopoiesis. In: Hoffman R, Benz E, Shattil S, Furie B, Cohen H, Silberstein L, eds. *Hematology: Basic Principles and Practice.* Baltimore: Williams & Wilkins; 1995:180–192.
Probably the best current comprehensive view of hematopoiesis published within the last few years.

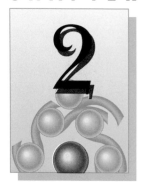

Clinical Approach to the Patient with Hematologic Problems

Fred J. Schiffman

Patients with hematologic disease may visit their physicians with concerns or manifestations that directly relate to their blood disorder. Alternatively, their complaints may represent an underlying illness that is the real cause of their hematologic problem. For example, a patient may tell the physician about shortness of breath, and the physician may discover a low hematocrit after a blood count is performed. This anemia may explain the cardiovascular symptomatology, but now the *cause* for the anemia (perhaps gastrointestinal bleeding from a peptic ulcer or colon carcinoma) must be pursued aggressively. Anemia, in fact (as well as most other hematologic problems), should always serve as a starting point for the search for the pathophysiologic state underlying the hematologic symptoms or signs. Much as a cutaneous rash may represent either a trivial alteration in skin biology or a profound perturbation in a fundamental body process, hematologic findings or disease may have benign or life-threatening causes that must be uncovered and addressed by the clinician.

The tables in this chapter outline elements of the medical history and physical examination as they apply to hematologic illness. In the first two columns, topics in the medical history or components of the physical examination are listed, and in the third column, the pathophysiologic significance is discussed. Disease associations or clues to etiology are also given. (For graphic representation of some of these entities see the complete and clearly illustrated chapter by Mitus and Rosenthal, which is cited in "Selected Reading.")

Once the history and physical examination are completed and the peripheral blood smear and bone marrow are reviewed (see later), along with other pertinent laboratory data, a working diagnostic hypothesis should be developed that must integrate many complex variables. A clear, creative, but patterned approach to diagnostic formulation should be constructed, as WB and ED Shelley have so well articulated in the initial chapters of their text. (See "Selected Reading.")

As the clinician moves serially from the history to the physical examination and then to the laboratory, more information will be discovered that may make it necessary to *return* to the bedside or examining room to recheck symptoms. Additional questions, more comprehensive or obliquely angled ones, may need to be asked. Initially omitted components of the physical examination should now be done, and other focused maneuvers may be necessary to reconcile the incremental data that are revealed as the pursuit for further information runs its course. In fact, it may be necessary to return to the patient several times to deal with the new data. Recurrently interacting with the patient has its own obvious rewards, but using these occasions to review and rework "established facts" can sometimes mine and deliver a diagnostic nugget that turns everyone's thinking around. Furthermore, after the initial history is taken, patients are often "primed" by questions asked by other health care workers; therefore later inquiries often elicit data not originally obtained.

Once diagnostic entities are more fully established, clinicians may tend to *not include* or *actively exclude* other diagnostic possibilities, even if subsequently obtained data do not fit with the working hypothesis or if therapy based on the working hypothesis does not produce the desired outcome. Thus the clinician falls prey to the common but dangerous phenomenon of "early closure." Caught in this mind set, the clinician may not consider the following:

1. The simultaneous occurrence of an additional pathophysiologic process. (For example, in a patient with hemolytic anemia whose hematocrit fails to rise with blood transfusions, a second etiology for continuing anemia such as gastrointestinal blood loss must be considered in addition to continued destruction of red blood cells.)
2. The uncommon presentation of a common illness. (For example, in a patient who presents with changes in cognition but without anemia, the possibility of B_{12} deficiency must be considered.)
3. The common presentation of an uncommon illness. (For example, in a patient with petechiae and joint aches who has thrombocytopenia a collagen vascular disease such as systemic lupus erythematosus could well be the cause; however, a more unusual etiology such as Henoch Schonlein purpura should also be added to the list of diagnostic possibilities.)

It is recommended the reader consult the informative book *Differential Diagnosis* by Barondess and Carpenter for further discussion of the approach to the patient and insights into diagnostic reasoning and strategy.

Hematologists have been somewhat quaintly, if not operationally, defined as physicians who themselves look at peripheral blood smears under the microscope. It would seem that club membership is easy to obtain, but unfortunately most physicians do not meet admission standards. It must be emphasized that there is no substitute for the patient's own physician reviewing the peripheral blood smear. Fragments of data may be made whole; poorly formed ideas may be focused, amplified, and enhanced; and subliminal cues may be elevated to a plane of perceptibility as the clinician who knows the patient best looks at the peripheral blood smear.

Just as the approach to the patient requires a structured set of guidelines for optimal extraction and processing of information from the bedside or examining room encounter, the approach to review of the peripheral blood smear requires observational rigor and forced interplay of morphologic data with those derived from history taking and the physical examination. Once again, the return to the bedside or examining room to obtain, clarify, reconcile, or develop new information is spurred by the discovery of clues in the form of size, shape, or inclusion abnormalities (in red blood cells, white blood cells, or platelets) that were optically grasped while scanning peripheral blood smear slides. For example, the finding of microspherocytes may suggest that the patient's history of gallbladder disease might have its root in hereditary spherocytosis. A more detailed family medical history could reveal a similar pattern in relatives, whereas a more careful look at the ankles of the patient may reveal traces of ulcerations, also part of the hereditary spherocytosis complex. Conversely, a history of gastrectomy and subtle neurologic findings should drive the clinician-cum-hematologist to the microscope in a quest for the macro-ovalocytes and hypersegmented polymorphonuclear leukocytes that would suggest B_{12} deficiency as an etiology for the patient's problems even in the absence of anemia.

Guidelines for review of the peripheral blood smear for all clinicians include the following:

1. Develop an approach.
2. Know how a blood smear is made (see Chapter 11).
3. Know what the stains stain (methylene blue stains acidic structures blue; eosin stains alkaline structures red).
4. Find the sweet spot (the area where there is little or no artifact).
5. Begin at low power (looking for overall pattern, frequency, and distribution of blood cells abnormalities; for example, clumping of red blood cells [as seen in cold agglutinin disease]; frequency of smudge cells [a chronic lymphocyte leukemia marker]).
6. Look at all three cell lines (red blood cells, white blood cells, platelets) one at a time. Be disciplined; don't get distracted. (See Chapters 3–5 and the appendix for normal and abnormal morphological features of all three cell lines.)
7. Be a detective.
8. Don't try to identify every cell.
9. Look at many fields.
10. Pay attention to overall configuration, color, consistency/internal structure, shape, size.

Guidelines for review of bone marrow aspirate specimens for the advanced clinician and include the following:

1. Develop an approach.
2. Know how a bone marrow smear is made.
3. Know what the stains stain (methylene blue stains acidic structures blue; eosin stains alkaline structures red).
4. Find the sweet spot (the area where there is little or no artifact).
5. Begin at low power (looking for overall architecture, tumor, cellularity, fat, heterogeneity, granuloma, fibrosis, lymphoma, infiltrates, megakaryocyte, myeloid-to-erythroid ratio).
6. Examine many fields.
7. Look at all three cell lines (erythroid, myeloid, megakaryocyte) one at a time. Be disciplined; don't get distracted.

8. Be a detective.
9. Don't try to identify every cell.
10. Examine many fields on many different slides.
11. Pay attention to dysmyelopoiesis, megaloblastic changes, lymphocytes and plasma cells, abnormal cells (e.g., Gaucher cells).

It is beyond the scope of this chapter to discuss the indications for and analysis of other, more specialized hematologic tests. It is hoped that the paradigms presented earlier will serve as a model for such test ordering and interpretation. Chapter 11 should be of some assistance here.

The tables of selected symptoms and signs as they apply to the hematologic illness have been designed to follow a history-taking and physical examination format. This compilation should assist the clinician in the overall care of the patient as symptoms and signs are recorded, analyzed, integrated, and reintegrated as more specialized hematologic data are revealed and treatment is begun.

SELECTED READING

Barondess JA, Carpenter CCJ. *Differential Diagnosis*. Philadelphia: Lea & Febiger; 1994.
A wonderfully insightful text about all aspects of differential diagnosis and more. A classic.

Braverman IM. Skin signs of systemic disease, 2nd ed. Philadelphia: WB Saunders; 1981.
A classic text which clearly illustrates and discusses many of the dermatologic findings presented in this chapter.

Berger TG, Silverman S. Oral and cutaneous manifestations of gastrointestinal disease. In: Sleisenger MH, Fordtran JS, eds. Gastrointestinal Disease. Pathophysiology/Diagnosis/Management, 5/e. Philadelphia: WB Saunders; 1993:268–285.
This chapter contains a very useful table on oral and cutaneous manifestations of GI disease, many of which are related to hematologic problems.

Degowin EL, Degowin RL. Bedside diagnostic examination, 5th ed. New York: McGraw-Hill; 1994.
A small gem in its fifth edition. Very useful introductory chapters.

Grover SA, Barkun AN, Sackett DL. Does this patient have splenomegaly? *JAMA* 1993;270:2218–2221.
An authoritative synthesis of this group's previous work on bedside assessment of splenic enlargement.

Henry PH, Longo DL. Enlargement of lymph nodes and spleen. In: Fauci AS, et al, eds. *Harrison's Principles of Internal Medicine*, 14th ed. McGraw–Hill; 1998: 345–351.
An up–to–date approach to patients with lymphadenopathy and splenomegaly.

Mitus AJ, Rosenthal DS. History and physical examination of relevance to the hematologist. In: Handin RI, Lux SE, Stossel TP, eds. *Blood: Principles and Practice of Hematology*. Philadelphia: JB Lippincott; 1995:3–21.
A clear and comprehensive treatise, well written and beautifully illustrated, on the approach to the history and physical examination.

Shelley WB, Shelley ED. Advanced dermatologic diagnosis. Philadelphia: WB Saunders; 1992.
Far more than a dermatology text, this book is a masterful approach to dermatologic diagnosis and diagnostic reasoning and strategies in general.

Williams WJ. Approach to the patient. In: Beutler E, Lichtman MA, Coller BS, Kipps TJ, eds. *Williams Hematology*, 5th ed. New York: McGraw-Hill; 1995:43–48.
A detailed review of how the patient with hematologic illness ought to be approached from a history and physical examination standpoint.

TABLE 2-1. *SELECTED SYMPTOMS, SIGNS, AND OTHER DATA AS THEY APPLY TO HEMATOLOGIC ILLNESS*

COMPONENTS OF HISTORY	DATA/SYMPTOMS/SIGNS	PATHOPHYSIOLOGIC SIGNIFICANCE
CHIEF COMPLAINT	Reason patient sought medical attention	Serves as an important clue with which to begin making a differential diagnosis.
HISTORY OF PRESENT ILLNESS	A temporally and physiologically correct story of the patient's illness with little editorializing by the physician. Includes dates and quantitation of key symptoms whenever possible. Includes sense of severity and urgency. Provocative palliative factors, quality, region, severity, and temporal characteristics of symptoms should always be sought.	Allows the physician to organize thoughts about the patient's illness.
	May be important to include medications in every HPI.	Any drug at any time can cause illness, especially of the hematologic variety.
	Include systemic and constitutional symptoms such as fevers, sweats, chills, itch, and weight change.	Important to assess if patient's illness has significant impact on the body as a whole. Often serious hematologic and oncologic illnesses are accompanied by constitutional systems.
PAST MEDICAL HISTORY	Medications/drugs (prescription, over-the-counter, and illicit)	This is of critical importance for consideration of any hematologic illness. Any drug any time can cause hematologic disease. Nonprescription drugs bought in supermarkets or drugstores must be included in data gathering. Illicit medications and their routes of administration are of importance.
	Allergies	May be important especially with respect to a diagnosis of eosinophilia.
	Hospitalizations	Past serious illness may give clues to current hematologic disease. Obtaining data from previous hospitalizations or physicians' office records is always of importance, since laboratory values can be followed serially.
	Accidents/injuries/trauma	Data from these events are of critical importance, especially if there was splenectomy, since there are myriad hematologic and immunologic consequences. Foreign bodies, especially lead bullet fragments (may cause lead poisoning and sideroblastic anemia), must be asked about. How a patient fared with trauma may provide useful hemostatic stress data.

(continued)

TABLE 2-1. (continued)		
COMPONENTS OF HISTORY	**DATA/SYMPTOMS/SIGNS**	**PATHOPHYSIOLOGIC SIGNIFICANCE**
PAST MEDICAL HISTORY (continued)	Surgical operations	Gastrectomy and ileectomy may interfere with nutrient absorption (e.g., iron, vitamin B_{12}). Short bowel syndrome causes malabsorption of nutrients of many varieties. How a patient tolerated surgery, especially wisdom teeth extraction, may provide hemostatic stress data (a profound hemostatic challenge).
	Serious illnesses and their treatments	HIV, TB, other infectious diseases; kidney, liver GI, pulmonary, cardiac, rheumatologic, neurologic disease, and their treatments may all impact upon hematologic status.
	GYN: Menarche, menstrual periods with characteristics, miscarriages, abortions, births, perinatal, hemorrhagic or thrombotic problems, menopause	Indicates hemostatic problems. The lupus anticoagulant and other antiphospholipid syndromes may be associated with miscarriages and abortions. Reasons for hysterectomy causing surgical menopause may be clues to underlying malignancies. Menstrual irregularities may indicate endocrinologic abnormalities that have hematologic implications.
	Childhood illnesses	Joint hemorrhage or epistaxis may give clues to hemostatic disorders. Intussusception after age 2 is a clue to Henoch-Shonlein purpura.
	Immunizations	The lack of immunizations may be associated with development of adult illnesses that have hematologic implications. Vaccines given to immunosuppressed patients can cause problems (e.g., live vaccines in CLL patients).
	Transfusions	May be associated with the development of alloantibodies and hemolytic transfusion reactions. May transmit viral, bacterial, and parasitic disease.
	HIV risk factors	These should always be sought specifically: Illicit parenteral drug use, life style/sexuality/blood transfusions.

FAMILY MEDICAL HISTORY	Ages and causes of death or serious illness in family members, causes of hospitalizations, complications of hospitalizations (e.g., hemorrhage/thrombosis). The pedigree should always be sketched out and may graphically reveal the pattern of inheritance.	Many hematologic illnesses are transmitted in characteristic genetic fashion: disorders that cause anemia, thrombocytopenia, and leukopenia. Many coagulation disorders are transmitted quite typically, and disorders of thrombosis may be considered when there has been arterial or pulmonary embolism in family members, recurrently or at an early age.
	Ethnicity and country of origin	Important for many hematologic illnesses (e.g., sickle cell anemia, thalassemia, GGPD deficiency), and it should be recalled that men or women may change names because of whim or marriage and the true ethnic origin of the patient may be masked.
	Illnesses in family	Disease in family members of genetic or infectious nature or caused by home exposure may be of extraordinary importance. For example, the presence of a faulty furnace, causing carbon monoxide poisoning, resulting in the patient's erythrocytosis, may have been clued earlier by the presence of somnolence or erythrocytosis in family members. Conversely, the presence of hematologic disease in the patient should trigger the physician to search for similar diseases in family members (e.g., erythrocytosis from carbon monoxide exposure, hereditary coagulation disorders, hemochromatosis, hereditary spherocytosis).
SOCIAL AND PERSONAL HISTORY	Lifestyle: homosexual, heterosexual, monogamous, marital status	These bear upon consideration of sexually transmitted diseases, especially HIV.
	Occupational and environmental exposures	Toxins, dusts, fumes, gases, chemicals associated with the workplace or home may offer important clues for many varieties of hematologic illness. The associations of the defoliant Agent Orange with lymphomas; lead poisoning with anemia; benzene with aplastic anemia and leukemia; heavy metals and pesticides with various hematologic illnesses have been established.

(continued)

TABLE 2-1. *(continued)*

COMPONENTS OF HISTORY	DATA/SYMPTOMS/SIGNS	PATHOPHYSIOLOGIC SIGNIFICANCE
SOCIAL AND PERSONAL HISTORY *(continued)*	Travel	Exotic diseases, especially parasitic illnesses, may be acquired through travel. Local endemic areas such as Cape Cod, Nantucket, and Martha's Vineyard may suggest to the physician babesiosis-associated hemolytic anemia. Also, contact with those who have recently come from foreign countries, or ingestion of imported foods may be a clue to the acquisition of hematologic illness. Additionally, the treatment of exotic disease with certain medications may trigger hematologic illnesses (quinine-associated hemolytic or thrombocytopenic states).
	Pets	Psittacosis (from birds) and salmonellosis (from reptiles) have hematologic complications. Asplenic patients have more serious illness from the bacteria DF2 (*Capnocytophagia canimorsus*) and *Eikenella corrodens* (associated with dogs). Cat scratch fever, a lymphoma mimicker, is associated with feline pets, as is toxoplasmosis.
	Diet	Often overlooked in the general medical history but critical for many hematologic illnesses. Iron, folate, B_{12} and other B vitamins, as well as vitamin K may be eliminated in certain diets. Conversely, too much vitamin intake may be a cause of hematologic problems, which may have cellular as well as hemostatic implications. Certain dietary aberrations such as clay eating (geophagia) and ice eating (pagophagia) may be manifestations of iron deficiency.
	Habits, hobbies, avocations	Long-distance runners, karate kickers, conga drum beaters may have exertion-induced hemolytic anemia. Exposure to glues or solvents or paints from artistic endeavors may cause hematologic disease.
	Drugs (especially illicit)	Any drug, any time can cause hematologic problems, although there are common associations with certain medications. Both cellular and coagulation disorders are described. Use of nonprescription (supermarket and drugstore) medications must always be asked about.

Alcohol

Careful history must be obtained sensitively. Coagulation disorders, anemia, thrombocytopenia are associated with alcohol's acute toxic effect on the bone marrow, or there may be long-term effects on the liver from parenchymal disease and portal hypertension. Pain in affected lymph node regions occurs after alcohol ingestion in patients with Hodgkin's disease.

Cigarette smoking

The association of cigarette smoking with several malignancies is well known. Tumor-associated anemia, erythrocytosis, leukocytosis, thrombocytopenia, thrombocytosis, and hyper- or hypocoagulability may be seen. Cigarette smoking itself may cause leukocytosis.

REVIEW OF SYSTEMS

Integument: SKIN: color, pigmentation, temperature, moisture, eruptions, pruritus, scaling, bruising, bleeding. HAIR: color, texture, abnormal loss or growth, distribution. NAILS: color changes, brittleness, ridging, pitting, curvature.

Patients may report dry skin and dry, fine hair with brittle nails in iron deficiency anemia. Patients may report coarse skin in myxedema. Itching occurs in some patients with Hodgkin's disease, mycosis fungoides, and polycythemia vera after bathing. (See Physical Examination for other specific skin and nail changes and their pathophysiologic significance.)

Lymph nodes: enlargement, pain, suppuration, draining sinuses, location.

(See "Physical Examination" for enlargement of lymph nodes and their pathophysiologic significance.)

Bones, joints, muscles: fractures, arthritis, pain, swelling, stiffness, migratory distribution, degree of disability, muscular weakness, wasting or atrophy. Night cramps.

Bone pain may signal involvement with neoplasm such as multiple myeloma, lymphoma, or metastatic disease, especially affecting the vertebral column. Bone pain may occur in hemoglobinopathies, especially hemoglobin SS, SC disease. Sternal pain may be a symptom of leukemia, especially CML. Joint pain caused by pseudogout (chondrocalcinosis) may be a clue to hemochromatosis. Acute gout from hyperuricemia may be a clue to underlying myeloproliferative disorders, high-grade lymphomas, acute leukemias. Joint problems may be a signal of rheumatoid arthritis, and Felty's syndrome, Henoch-Schonlein purpura, and the arthropathy of hemophilia. Left shoulder pain may be a symptom of splenomegaly or splenic infarction (referred pain). A history of leg cramps may trigger a question about quinine ingestion, a cause of thrombocytopenia or anemia.

(continued)

TABLE 2-1. *(continued)*

COMPONENTS OF HISTORY	DATA/SYMPTOMS/SIGNS	PATHOPHYSIOLOGIC SIGNIFICANCE
REVIEW OF SYSTEMS *(continued)*	*Hematopoietic system:* anemia (type, therapy, and response), lymphadenopathy, bleeding (spontaneous, traumatic, familial). *Endocrine system:* history of growth, body configuration, and weight. Size of hands, feet, and head, especially changes during adulthood. Hair distribution. Skin pigmentation. Weakness. Goiter, exophthalmos, dryness of skin and hair, intolerance to heat or cold, tremor. Polyphagia, polydipsia, polyuria, glycosuria. Secondary sex characteristics, impotence, sterility, treatment. Diagnosis of and treatment for endocrine disorders in the past.	A history of any type or any hematologic disease in the past should raise suspicion about present complaints. Many endocrinologic disorders have hematologic associations. **RBC:** Anemia may accompany peptic ulcer, Zollinger-Ellison syndrome. A normochromic, normocytic anemia often accompanies panhypopituitarism. Hypothyroidism may be associated with a macrocytic anemia ($\pm$ B_{12} or folate deficiency) or more commonly a normochromic, normocytic anemia. Hypothyroidism is also associated with a hypochromic microcytic anemia from iron malabsorption or menorrhagia. Severely thyrotoxic patients may display a normochromic, normocytic, or hypochromic anemia. Pernicious anemia with antiparietal cell antibodies occurs in approximately 3% of patients with Graves' disease. Patients with adrenal insufficiency have a mild normochromic, normocytic anemia. Patients with Cushing's disease may display a mild erythrocytosis with hemoglobin levels of 1–2 g% higher than normal. Primary hyperparathyroidism is associated with a normochromic, normocytic anemia in about 20% of patients. Iron deficiency anemia may occur in hyperparathyroidism complicated by peptic ulcer disease. **WBC:** Leukopenia may be noted in hypopituitarism. Thyrotoxicosis patients may show leukopenia or granulocytopenia, and treatment with methimazole or propylthiouracil may cause agranulocytosis. Cushing's syndrome patients may show eosinopenia. Lymphocytosis and eosinophilia may be seen in Addison's disease, and leukocytosis may be seen in diabetic ketoacidosis. Glucocorticoids cause a leukocytosis and thrombocytosis.

Allergic and immunologic history: dermatitis, urticaria, angioneurotic edema, eczema, hay fever, vasomotor rhinitis, asthma, migraine, vernal conjunctivitis. Sensitivity to pollens, foods, danders, or drugs. Previous skin tests and their results. Results of tuberculin tests and others. Desensitization, serum injections, vaccinations, and immunizations.

Allergic disorders may be associated with eosinophilia.

Head: headaches, migraine, trauma, vertigo, syncope, convulsive seizures.

May be from anemia or polycythemia, invasion of the CNS with leukemia or lymphoma, infection such as cryptococcosis or tuberculosis. Brain hemorrhage (parenchymal, subarachnoid, epidural, or subdural) with underlying coagulopathies may cause CNS symptoms, too.

Eyes: visual loss or color blindness, diplopia, hemianopsia, trauma, inflammation, glasses (date of last eye examination).

Profound anemia can cause retinal ischemia or infarction, resulting in blurred vision or blindness. Coagulopathies can cause retinal infarction (hypercoaguable states) or hemorrhage (hypocoaguable state). Double vision or visual field defects can be seen with CNS lymphomas or other malignancies, as they affect brain parenchyma or cranial nerves.

Ears: deafness, tinnitus, vertigo, discharge from the ears, pain, mastoiditis, operations.

Severe anemia may cause a roaring, rushing, pounding, or ringing in the ears in the anemic patient. Difficulty hearing may occur in children with sickle cell anemia.

Nose: coryza, rhinitis, sinusitis, discharge, obstruction, epistaxis.

Epistaxis may signal coagulopathy due to coagulation cascade defects or platelet problems. AV malformations such as those seen in the Osler-Weber-Rendu syndrome may present with nosebleeding. Anosmia or olfactory hallucinations may occur in pernicious anemia. Tumors involving the olfactory bulb can cause anosmia.

Mouth: soreness of mouth or tongue, symptoms referable to teeth.

Sore tongue may be seen in pernicious anemia or iron deficiency anemia. A large tongue may be seen in myxedema or amyloidosis. Painful gums may be seen with the infiltration of acute monocytic leukemia; mucosal ulcerations are seen in neutropenic patient. Dry mouth may be a complaint associated with hypercalcemia from hematologic malignancies such as multiple myeloma.

(continued)

TABLE 2-1. *(continued)*

COMPONENTS OF HISTORY	DATA/SYMPTOMS/SIGNS	PATHOPHYSIOLOGIC SIGNIFICANCE
REVIEW OF SYSTEMS *(continued)*	*Throat:* hoarseness, sore throats, tonsillitis, voice changes.	Hoarseness may be caused by recurrent laryngeal nerve involvement associated with neck or upper chest lymphoreticular lesions. Sore throat may be associated with infectious mononucleosis. Voice change can be seen with retropharyngeal hematomas caused by a coagulopathy.
	Neck: swelling, suppurative lesions, enlargement of lymph nodes, goiter, stiffness, and limitation of motion.	Report of neck swelling may be a sign of thyromegaly, lymphadenopathy, or superior vena cava syndrome.
	Breasts: development, lactation, trauma, lumps, pains, discharge from nipples, gynecomastia, changes in nipples.	Report of breast mass may signify a primary malignancy or lymphomatous deposits, extramedullary hematopoiesis, or plasmacytoma involvement.
	Respiratory system: pain, shortness of breath, wheezing, dyspnea, nocturnal dyspnea, orthopnea, cough, sputum, hemoptysis, night sweats, pleurisy, bronchitis, tuberculosis (history of contacts), pneumonia, asthma, other respiratory infections.	Shortness of breath may signify anemia. Hemoptysis may be a sign of coagulopathy, infection in the compromised host, or AV malformations of Osler–Weber–Rendu disease. Cough may be a symptom of mediastinal involvement with lymph nodes or tumor or infection in the neutropenic host. Pleural, airway parenchymal involvement must be considered.
	Cardiovascular system: palpitations, tachycardia, irregularities of rhythm, chest pain, exertional dyspnea, paroxysmal nocturnal dyspnea, orthopnea, cough, cyanosis, ascites, edema. Intermittent claudication, cold extremities, phlebitis, postural or permanent skin color. Hypertension, rheumatic fever, chorea, syphilis, diphtheria. Drugs such as digitalis, quinidine, nitroglycerin, diuretics, and other medications.	Anemia or polycythemia causing problems with oxygen delivery may present with a variety of cardiovascular system complaints. The hypercoagulable state can cause arterial or venous thrombosis and also embolic disease. Many cardiovascular diseases and drugs have associated hematologic implications.
	Gastrointestinal system: appetite, changes in weight, dysphagia, nausea, eructations, flatulence, abdominal pain or colic, vomiting, hematemesis, jaundice (pain, fever, intensity, duration, color of urine and stools), stools (color, frequency, consistency, odor, gas, cathartics), hemorrhoids. Change in bowel habits.	Anorexia is a nonspecific complaint seen with many systemic illnesses. It may be a presenting complaint of lymphomas and leukemias, or it can be due to secondary effects of hematologic diseases, including hypercalcemia or azotemia. Early satiety may indicate gastric outlet problems or splenomegaly. Abdominal pain may have a variety of causes that range from hepatosplenic enlargement (associated with a myriad of hematologic diseases), obstruction of GI tract, retroperitoneal hemor-

REVIEW OF SYSTEMS
(continued)

rhage, effects of chemotherapy, rare hematologic illnesses such as Henoch-Schonlein purpura, acute intermittent porphyria, and more common and problematic illnesses such as sickle cell disease where vaso-occlusive crises may be manifested by abdominal pain. A history of GI bleeding should signal a search for coagulopathy or neoplasm of the GI tract. Constipation may indicate GI neoplasm or metabolic disorders such as hypercalcemia. Symptoms of malabsorption may indicate lymphomatous involvement of the GI tract. Dysphagia may be seen with iron deficiency anemia and the sideropenic esophageal web syndromes that carry the eponyms of Patterson–Kelly and Plummer–Vinson. Esophagogastric neoplasms may bleed and cause anemia.

Genitourinary system: color of urine, polyuria, oliguria, nocturia, dysuria, hematuria, pyuria, urinary retention, urinary frequency, incontinence, pain or colic, passage of stones or gravel. *Menstrual history:* age of onset, frequency of periods, regularity, duration, amount of flow, leukorrhea, dysmenorrhea, date of last normal and preceding periods date and character of menopause, postmenopausal bleeding. *Pregnancies:* number, abortions, miscarriages, stillbirths, chronologic sequence, complications of pregnancy. Birth control measures. *Venereal history:* sexual activity. Chancre, bubo, penile discharge. Diagnosis and treatment of venereal diseases.

Red urine may be a sign of bleeding in the GI tract from an underlying coagulopathy. However, dark reddish coloration in the urine can signify hemoglobinuria, myoglobinuria, porphyrinuria, food or drug ingestion. A history of red urine must always be followed up with a microscopic examination of the urine and more specialized tests. As noted earlier, a menstrual and pregnancy history is critical in the evaluation of coagulopathies. Erectile dysfunction or bladder problems may be an indicator of hematologic malignancies involving the nervous system. Pernicious anemia causes a variety of neuropsychiatric problems, including genitourinary ones. Kidney stones may be a sign of hypercalcemia or hyperuricemia, which may be associated with hematologic malignancies. History of persistent erection (priapism) may occur in leukemia or sickle cell disease.

(continued)

TABLE 2-1. *(continued)*

COMPONENTS OF HISTORY	DATA/SYMPTOMS/SIGNS	PATHOPHYSIOLOGIC SIGNIFICANCE
REVIEW OF SYSTEMS *(continued)*	*Nervous system: cranial nerves*	Complaints of tingling (paresthesias) may be an indicator of pernicious anemia, hematologic malignancies, amyloidosis, multiple myeloma, or drugs used to treat hematologic disorders. (See physical exam for some specific examples of physical neurologic sign linkage with specific pathophysiology.)
	Psychiatric history	Psychiatric complaints may be the presenting feature of many hematologic illnesses: In anemia and polycythemia, oxygen delivery to the brain is impaired. Coagulation disorders may predispose to epidural, subdural, subarachnoid, or parenchymal hemorrhages that have neuropsychiatric associations. The brain and its coverings may be involved with leukemia or lymphoma cells. Pernicious anemia may cause "megaloblastic madness" as one of its lesser understood effects. Some types of porphyria have neuropsychiatric involvement (acute intermittent porphyria). Hematologic malignancies may cause hypercalcemia leading to neuropsychiatric problems.

TABLE 2-1. *(continued)*

COMPONENTS OF PHYSICAL EXAMINATION	DATA/SYMPTOMS/SIGNS	PATHOPHYSIOLOGIC SIGNIFICANCE
VITAL SIGNS	Pulse rate and regularity	*Tachycardia* may signify problems with oxygen delivery from anemia or be associated with pulmonary embolism caused by hypercoagulability. It may also be a sign of pericardial disease where there has been pericardial hemorrhage or involvement with tumor, causing tamponade or constriction.
	Respiration rate	*Tachypnea* may signify anemia, airway, pleural, or lung parenchymal involvement with hematologic malignancies or pleuropulmonary infection in the immunocompromised host.
	Temperature (oral/rectal)	*Temperature elevation* may be a sign of many primary hematologic disorders, especially the hematologic malignancies and myelofibrosis. It may also be a sign of a secondary effect due to infection or inflammation caused by an obstructing neoplasm. Infection associated with the immunocompromised host may cause fever, but temperature elevation will be less marked in those on corticosteroids or in immunosuppressed patients, the elderly, or diabetic patients.
	Blood pressure	*A low blood pressure* may be a sign of hemorrhage caused by coagulopathy. In addition, pericardial disease (see earlier) or septic shock associated with the immunocompromised host may cause low blood pressure.
SKIN	Turgor, texture, pigmentation, cyanosis, telangiectasia, petechiae, purpura, ecchymoses, infection, lesions, hair, nails, mucous membranes	*SKIN COLOR* is very important in hematologic illness. Pallor commonly accompanies anemia. With the hand open, the palm creases should be pink if the hemoglobin is greater than 7 g%. *TURGOR, TEXTURE:* In iron deficiency anemia, the texture of the *skin is dry*, hair is dry and fine, and *nails are brittle* and spoonshaped (koilonychia). Myxedema may present with *dry, coarse, and scaly skin*.

(continued)

TABLE 2-1. (continued)

COMPONENTS OF PHYSICAL EXAMINATION	DATA/SYMPTOMS/SIGNS	PATHOPHYSIOLOGIC SIGNIFICANCE
SKIN (continued)		**COLOR, PIGMENTATION: jaundice** may be seen with a variety of hematologic illnesses involving the liver or can be caused by hemolysis (indirect, unconjugated bilirubin). The **lemon-yellow color** of pernicious anemia is due to a combination of jaundice and pallor. **Blue eyes, blonde, or early-graying hair** is associated with pernicious anemia. **A bronze, grayish pigmentation** is seen in hemochromatosis. **Peripheral or acral cyanosis** is seen in tips of nose, ears, fingers, and toes with cryoglobulins or cold agglutinins. **Peripheral and central cyanosis** (blue lips, tongue) are seen in cardiopulmonary disorders where there are 5 g of reduced hemoglobin. In states such as polycythemia, the total red cell mass is increased, and often more than 5 g of hemoglobin are reduced. Where there are 1.5–2 g of methemoglobin, cyanosis is apparent, and a brownish cyanosis is seen with only 0.5 g of sulfhemoglobin. **Red skin** and a variety of skin rashes may occur with cutaneous T-cell lymphomas, CLL, some lymphocytic lymphomas, and graft versus host disease. The skin may be **cyanotic or, rarely, cherry red** with carbon monoxide exposure. **Patches of hypopigmented skin (vitiligo)** may be a sign of antibodies against melanocytes — part of the autoimmune disorder with which pernicious anemia is associated. **LESIONS, RASHES: Telangiectasia** may indicate liver disease or disorders such as Osler-Weber-Rendu disease or Bloom's syndrome. **Giant hemangiomas** will occur in Kasabach-Merritt syndrome, which is associated with disseminated intravascular coagulation. The **reddish purple raised lesions** of Kaposi's sarcoma are associated with HIV infection.

Petechiae are a sign of qualitative or quantitative platelet disorders, blood vessel or skin abnormalities, or vasculitis. (They are seen in perineal distribution with corkscrew hairs in scurvy.) They may be associated with dysproteinemia. ***Purpura*** has similar causes (with the addition of sepsis, as is seen in the Waterhouse-Friderichsen syndrome of meningiococcemia). When purpura occurs in the mouth as blood blisters (or wet purpura), it may signal dangerously low levels of platelets. Periorbital and perirectal purpura may be a sign of amyloidosis. ***Ecchymosis*** is a sign of a variety of coagulation disorders and may occur in specific distributions (Grey Turner's [flanks] or Cullen's [periumbilical] signs indicate retroperitoneal and intra-abdominal hemorrhage, respectively). ***Necrotic skin lesions*** may be a sign of DIC with purpura fulminans, cryoproteins, cold agglutinins, warfarin- or heparin-induced skin necrosis. ***Chloromas***, which appear as indurated skin tumors, are collections of leukemic myeloblasts. Sweet's syndrome is a febrile neutrophilic dermatosis in the setting of acute leukemia. Hairy cell leukemia, angio-immunoblastic lymphadenopathy, urticaria pigmentosa all have skin manifestations. Many gastrointestinal disorders, some related to hematologic disease, have oral and cutaneous manifestation's. (See Berger and Silverman's chapter in "Selected Reading.") ***Skin infections*** are associated with leukopenia or qualitative leukocyte abnormalities such as Chediak–Higashi syndrome, chronic granulomatous disease, and Job's syndrome. ***Mucocutaneous candidiasis*** may occur with myeloperoxidase deficiency. Skin lesions of several varieties have been described in the hypereosinophilic syndrome. Leg ulcers may be seen commonly in sickle cell anemia and hereditary spherocytosis. The ***hand-foot syndrome*** is seen in 15% of children with sickle cell anemia. It is characterized by red, painful, nonpitting swelling over the distal extremities.

NAILS: Changes in the nails, especially ***kolionychia*** (spoon nails) may be a sign of iron deficiency.

(continued)

TABLE 2-1.	*(continued)*	
COMPONENTS OF PHYSICAL EXAMINATION	**DATA/SYMPTOMS/SIGNS**	**PATHOPHYSIOLOGIC SIGNIFICANCE**
SKULL	General description	Prominence of frontal and parietal bones (frontal bossing) and other facial abnormalities are seen in sickle cell anemia and thalassemia, where the marrow cavities are expanded to keep up with hemolysis. Fanconi's anemia, Bloom's syndrome, and hereditary spherocytosis, plasmacytomas, and eosinophilic granulomas all may have skull manifestations.
EYES	Extraocular motion	Extraocular motion may be affected by metabolic disorders such as pernicious anemia or porphyria. Additionally, hemorrhage, masses from hematologic malignancies causing direct pressure, paraneoplastic states, or infections associated with the immunocompromised hosts may affect eye motion.
	Pupillary examination	Pupillary size and response are influenced by the same pathophysiologic mechanisms as extraocular motion.
	Sclera and conjunctiva	*Conjunctival pallor* may indicate anemia, *Suffusion* may be from polycythemia or superior vena cava syndrome. Jaundice may be detected by scleral and conjunctival examination. *Proptosis* may signal hyperthyroidism orbital lymphoma, chloroma, neuroblastoma, extramedullary hematopoiesis. *Pingueculae* may be a sign of Gaucher's disease. Other scleral abnormalities may indicate collagen vascular disease or lymphoma. *Irregular, comma-shaped, or corkscrew conjunctival blood vessels* may be seen in sickle cell anemia.
	Cornea	*Kayser-Fleisher ring* of Wilson's disease is a corneal abnormality seen with the slit lamp. (Wilson's disease has an associated hemolytic anemia.) The *band keratopathy* of hypercalcemia seen at 3 and 9 o'clock positions on the cornea is associated with hypercalcemia, which may be seen as an accompaniment of hematologic malignancies. It occurs in these positions because

calcium and carbon dioxide from the air interact to form calcium phosphate in those corneal positions exposed with open eyelids. **Gray or brown crystals** may be associated with paraprotein deposition seen in plasma cell dyscrasias.

Uveitis may be a sign of sarcoidosis or vasculitis.

Vitreous hemorrhage may be seen with hereditary or acquired coagulation disorders. **Retinal hemorrhage, infarction (Roth's spot)**, and **exudate** may occur in patients with anemia and thrombocytopenia as well as other coagulopathies.

Changes in retinal veins occur in hyperviscosity syndromes **(crossing changes, tortuosity,** and **"box carring"** or **"sausage linking"),** sickle cell anemia, and thalassemia. Sickle cell anemia has characteristic retinal changes that may progress and cause blindness. So-called **black sunburst** and **salmon patch hemorrhages** as well as **angioid streaks** may be seen. In hemoglobin SC disease, neovascularization takes the form of **"sea fans."** Sickle cell–thalassemia syndrome also has retinal abnormalities. Hyereosinophilic syndrome has a choroidal disorder associated with it. Leukemia may affect any ocular tissue by direct infiltration of leukemic cells or secondary effects of the malignancy or its treatment. Pernicious anemia mainly affects the afferent visual system, causing **optic neuropathy, vision change,** including **color discrimination abnormalities (dyschromatopsia).**

Tophaceous gout signifying a variety of hyperproliferative hematologic disorders may be present on the pinna. Tinnitus or other noises in the ear may be associated with anemia or polycythemia vera. **Hearing loss** may occur with sickle cell anemia.

A **smooth, beefy red, painful tongue** may indicate B_{12} or iron deficiency. Mucosal ulcerations may be a sign of neutropenia; tonsillar enlargement may be caused by mononucleosis or lymphoma. **Blood blisters or wet purpura** is a sign of thrombocytopenia.

(continued)

Uvea
Fundiscopic exam

EARS
Inspection; acuity

MOUTH, NOSE AND THROAT
See "Review of Systems" (earlier)

TABLE 2-1. *(continued)*		
COMPONENTS OF PHYSICAL EXAMINATION	**DATA/SYMPTOMS/SIGNS**	**PATHOPHYSIOLOGIC SIGNIFICANCE**
NECK		*Thyroid enlargement* may signify primary thyroid disease or lymphomatous involvement. See below for lymphadenopathy.
LYMPH NODES	Lymphadenopathy (node greater than 1 cm in diameter) is of great importance to the hematologist. Critical questions that need to be asked include, "Is the palpable mass indeed a lymph node?" "How long has the lymphadenopathy been present?" "What is the character of the enlarged node itself?" "Is the lymphadenopathy localized or generalized?" "Are there associated systemic or localizing symptoms or signs?" "Are there unusual epidemiologic clues?" Important associations include pain, evidence of inflammation, pace of lymphadenopathy.	Many disorders may underlie the etiology of lymphadenopathy, including infectious, dermatopathic, inflammatory, metabolic, storage diseases, drug-associated illnesses, and malignant conditions, both primary and metastatic. After 1–2 months if no diagnosis is forthcoming, biopsy of the lymph node should be undertaken. (See Chapter 1.)
BREASTS		Mass may signify primary malignancy or lymphomatous involvement, plasmacytosis, or extramedullary hematopoiesis. Gynecomastia in the male may be linked with testicular atrophy associated with liver disease of many types, including hemochromatosis. It may also be a sign of primary tumor in the male or secondary to a remote functional tumor or medication.
CHEST	Inspection	Suffusion of the upper chest with dilated blood vessels may be a sign of the superior vena cava syndrome from neoplastic involvement of the superior vena cava. Sternal tenderness may be a sign of leukemic or lymphomatous infiltration of the bone marrow in this region.
	Palpation	Rib, scapula, vertebral, or sternal tenderness may be a sign of leukemic: lymphomatous or carcinomatous infiltration of the bone or bone marrow in this region.
	Percussion	*Percussion:* Dullness to percussion as well as changes in tactile fremitus may indicate pleural disease seen with many hematologic disorders, including lymphoreticular malignancies, which can cause pleural effusions. Addi-

Auscultation	tionally, mediastinal involvement with lymphadenopathy may cause pleural effusions, or infections in the immunocompromised host may cause them. Dullness to percussion may also signify consolidation.

Auscultation: Ascultatory changes in the form of decreased or increased breath sounds may be a sign of pleural effusions or consolidation in the pulmonary parenchyma with hematologic associations as described for pleural effusions (see earlier). Rales and rhonchi are helpful physical examination signs that may indicate pulmonary consolidation even before x-ray changes occur. The acute chest syndrome seen in sickle cell anemia has as its basis infection or pulmonary infarction. Pulmonary infarction may come from emboli of necrotic bone marrow in hemoglobinopathies. Pulmonary embolism may be a sign of an underlying hypercoagulable state, as seen in protein C, S, or antithrombin III deficiency or with the antiphospholipid syndrome. Additionally, pulmonary embolism and venous thrombosis can be seen in the hypercoagulable state associated with certain disseminated malignancies. Lymphomatous or leukemic involvement of pulmonary parenchyma may cause consolidation with classical signs or may be associated with a variety of pulmonary infections, especially in the immunocompromised host, leading to pleural or lung parenchymal disorders. |
CARDIOVASCULAR SYSTEM	Pulse rate and blood pressure (see "VITAL SIGNS" earlier)
	Chest wall inspection and palpation
	Pericardial rub
	Jugular venous examination: External jugular venous abnormalities may be seen with superior vena cava syndrome with cardiac tamponade or constrictive pericarditis caused by hematologic neoplasms.

An active precordium may be a sign of anemia.

Pericardial disease has an important differential diagnosis for hematologic disorders. (See under Jugular venous examination.) |

(continued)

TABLE 2-1. *(continued)*

COMPONENTS OF PHYSICAL EXAMINATION	DATA/SYMPTOMS/SIGNS	PATHOPHYSIOLOGIC SIGNIFICANCE
CARDIOVASCULAR SYSTEM *(continued)*	Murmurs	Flow murmurs may be heard with anemia. Tumor plop is characteristic of left atrial myxoma. S_3 and other signs of congestive heart failure may be a sign of anemia. Right-sided heart failure caused by pulmonary hypertension may be associated with erythrocytosis, especially of the secondary variety. Neoplastic involvement of pericardium, myocardium, and endocardium gives signs of pericarditis, cardiomyopathy, or valvular disease.
ABDOMEN	Inspection	***Distention:*** The presence of abdominal distention may indicate ascites associated with peritoneal or hepatic involvement with hematologic malignancy. Ascites may occur with Budd–Chiari syndrome (hepatic vein thrombosis), which is associated with hypercoagulabulim. ***Venous pattern:*** The venous pattern of the abdomen and direction of venous flow may indicate portal or hepatic vein obstruction. Hepatic or inferior vena cava obstruction is seen in hypercoagulable states, especially polycythemia vera, where the Budd–Chiari syndrome is caused. ***Ecchymosis:*** Flank ecchymosis (Grey Turner's sign) and periumbilical ecchymosis (Cullen's sign) are seen with retroperitoneal and abdominal hemorrhage, respectively. Coagulation disorders may underlie these hemorrhagic problems.
	Auscultation	***Reduced bowel sounds*** occur with anatomic obstruction or in the functionally obstructive states associated with vaso-occlusive crisis of sickle cell disease, pernicious anemia, acute intermittent porphyria, hypercalcemia (associated with hematologic malignancies).

	Percussion and Palpation	***Hepatomegally*** has many associations with hematologic disease, and careful percussion and palpation exam should always be done. The detection of splenomegaly is a key part of the focused hematologic abdominal examination. The most reliable method is described by Grover *et al.* (see "Selected Reading.") and involves percussion of Traube's space and palpation in the region of the lower abdominal and costal margin with the patient in the supine position. For the hematologist, the causes and effects of splenomegaly are myriad and have as their basis infectious, inflammatory, congestive, hematologic, malignant, storage, and many miscellaneous disorders. (See Chapter 1.)
EXTREMITY EXAMINATION	Signs of deep venous thrombosis (e.g., cords and Homan's signs). Signs of arterial thrombosis	The presence of ***arterial or deep venous thrombosis*** may indicate a hypercoagulable state and should be sought for carefully in patients with systemic hematologic disease.
	Joint examination	***Arthritic disorders*** of many kinds as well as collagen vascular diseases with joint manifestations have many important hematologic associations. The presence of arthritis may be clue to these. Additionally, ***chondrocalcinosis*** may be a sign of hemochromatosis, and ***gout*** may be a manifestation of many hematologic disorders where there is rapid cellular turnover.
MALE GENITAL EXAMINATION	Penis	***Priapism*** may be seen with leukemia or sickle cell anemia secondary to infiltration of the corpus cavernosum with abnormal white or red cells.
	Testes	***Testicular atrophy*** may be a sign of liver disease associated with hematologic disorders, including hemochromatosis. ***Masses*** may indicate primary testicular malignancies or leukemic or lymphomatous involvement.

(continued)

TABLE 2-1. *(continued)*

COMPONENTS OF PHYSICAL EXAMINATION	DATA/SYMPTOMS/SIGNS	PATHOPHYSIOLOGIC SIGNIFICANCE
FEMALE GENITAL EXAMINATION	Ovaries	Lymphomatous involvement of ovaries may cause *enlargement*. *Bleeding from the vagina* may be an indication of coagulopathy.
RECTAL EXAMINATION		*Hemorrhoids* may be a sign of portal hypertension associated with liver disease, which has many hematologic associations (see earlier). *Mucosal abnormalities* may include epithelial neoplasia seen in HIV disease, including extranodal sites of Hodgkin's disease. *Bleeding from the GI tract* may be a sign of lymphomatous involvement of the GI tract, other primary malignancies, or underlying coagulopathy.
NEUROLOGIC EXAMINATION	Mental status, cranial nerve, sensory, motor, coordination testing	Neurologic abnormalities of many types may have hematologic disease as an underlying basis. Coagulation disorders (hemorrhagic or thrombotic), hematologic malignancies (by direct invasion or pressure or by paraneoplastic mechanism), metabolic disorders (pernicious anemia or porphyria), or infectious complications, especially in the immunocompromised host, all may underlie mental status, cranial nerve, sensory, motor, or coordination problems. Peripheral neuropathies may be caused by metabolic or hematologic disease, such as pernicious anemia, porphyria, or paraprotein abnormalities as well as associated diseases such as amyloidosis. Medications used to treat leukemias and lymphomas may cause specific neurologic problems. For example, vincristine and cisplatin cause peripheral neuropathies. High doses of cytosine arabinoside may cause Purkinje cell damage in the cerebellum and coordination disorders.

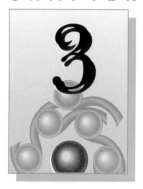

Red Blood Cells

Michal G. Rose, Nancy Berliner

RED BLOOD CELL (RBC) STRUCTURE AND FUNCTION

THE ERYTHROCYTE

The erythrocyte is a highly specialized cell whose main role is to carry oxygen from the lungs to the tissues and carbon dioxide (CO_2) back to the lungs. This role is facilitated by the cell's biconcave disc shape, which creates a large surface area for gas exchange. The RBC has a diameter of 8 μm, but its cytoskeletal and membrane structure enable it to undergo marked deformation and pass through capillaries 2–3 μm in diameter. This deformability is made possible by interactions between proteins in the membrane (band 3 and glycophorin) and proteins in the cytoplasm (spectrin, ankyrin, and protein 4.1) (Fig. 3-1). Defects in these proteins result in abnormal red cell shapes and functions (Table 3-1). The mature RBC lacks cytoplasmic organelles and a nucleus and is therefore incapable of protein and lipid synthesis, oxidative phosphorylation, and tricarboxylic acid cycling. The cell obtains most of its energy through the anaerobic Embden-Meyerhof pathway and stores it as ATP. Depending on the degree of oxidant challenge, varying amounts of glucose are diverted through the hexose monophosphate shunt to produce reducing compounds (glutathione and nicotinamide adenine dinucleotide phosphate (NADPH) (Fig. 3-2).

Approximately 98% of the cytoplasmic protein in the RBC is hemoglobin (Hb), the molecule which binds and transports oxygen. Hemoglobin (Hb) is a heterodimeric tetramer comprised of two α-like globin chains and two non-α globin chains (β, γ, or δ), conjugated to four heme moieties. Heme is a single molecule of protoporphyrin IX bound to an iron atom. Each Hb tetramer is capable of reversibly binding and transporting a maximum of four oxygen molecules.

The most common Hbs are Hb A ($\alpha_2\beta_2$, the major adult Hb), Hb F ($\alpha_2\gamma_2$, the major fetal Hb), and Hb A_2 ($\alpha_2\beta_2$, a minor adult Hb) (Table 3-2). The switch from

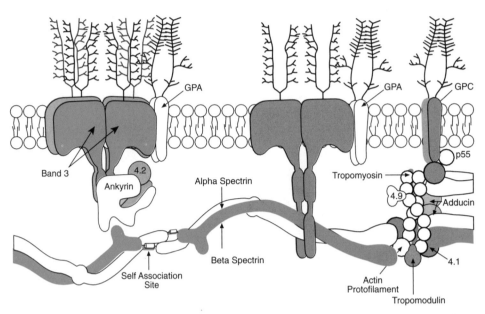

Figure 3-1. Structure of the RBC membrane. GPA, glycophorin A; GPC, glycophorin C. (Redrawn from Handin RI, Stossel TP, Lux SG, eds. *Blood: Principles and Practice of Hematology,* Philadelphia: JB Lippincott, 1995:1726.)

TABLE 3-1.	*HEREDITARY RBC MEMBRANE ABNORMALITIES*	
CONDITION	**ABNORMAL PROTEIN(S)**	**MODE OF INHERITANCE**
Spherocytosis	Spectrin, ankyrin Band 3, Protein 4.2	Autosomal dominant Recessive (rare)
Elliptocytosis	Spectrin Protein 4.1	Autosomal dominant Recessive (rare)
Pyropoikilocytosis	Spectrin	Recessive
Stomatocytosis	Na$^+$ permeability defect	Autosomal dominant

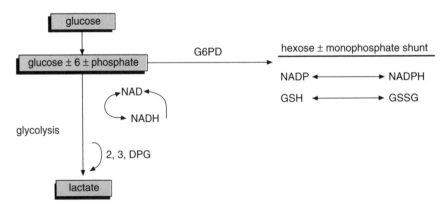

Figure 3-2. Metabolic pathways of the RBC. NAD, nicotinamide adenine dinucleotide (NADH, reduced form); 2,3, DPG, 2,3-diphosphoglyceric acid; G6PD, glucose-6-phosphate dehydrogenase; NADP, nicotinamide adenine dinucleotide phosphate (NADPH, reduced form). GSH, GSSG, reduced and oxidized glutathione.

TABLE 3-2.	*THE HUMAN HEMOGLOBINS*	
HEMOGLOBIN	**COMPOSITION**	**REPRESENTATION**
A	$\alpha_2\beta_2$	95–98% of adult Hb
A$_2$	$\alpha_2\delta_2$	1.5–3.5% of adult Hb
F	$\alpha_2\gamma_2$	Fetal Hb, 0.5–1% adult Hb
Gower 1	$\zeta_2\epsilon_2$	Embryonic hemoglobin
Gower 2	$\alpha_2\epsilon_2$	Embryonic hemoglobin
Portland	$\zeta_2\gamma_2$	Embryonic hemoglobin

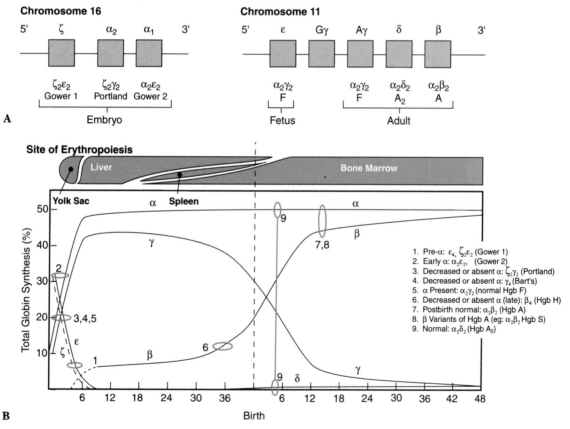

Figure 3-3. (**A**) The globin gene clusters on chromosomes 16 and 11. In embryonic, fetal, and adult life, different genes are activated or suppressed. The different globin chains are synthesized independently and then combine with each other to produce the different hemoglobins. The γ gene may have two sequences, differing by whether there is a glutamic acid or an alanine residue at position 136 (Gγ or Aγ, respectively). (From Hoffbrand AV, Pettit JE. *Essential Hematology*, 3rd ed. Cambridge, Mass.: Blackwell Scientific Publishing; 1993.) (**B**) Developmental sequence of location of hematopoiesis and hemoglobin synthesis. The lassos connect globins that associate under normal and abnormal circumstances. (After Brown MS. *Fetal and Neonatal Erythropoiesis in Developmental and Neonatal Hematology*. New York: Raven Press; 1988. From Handin RI, Stossel TP, Lux SE, eds. *Blood: Principles and Practice of Hematology*. Philadelphia: JB Lippincott, 1995.)

Hb F to A occurs around birth; by age 4–6 months, the level of fetal Hb in the blood is less than 1% (Fig. 3-3).

The O_2 dissociation curve of Hb describes the percentage of saturation of Hb with oxygen at different oxygen tensions (Fig. 3-4). The sigmoidal shape of this curve reflects the interaction among the subunits of the Hb tetramer. The major regulator of the O_2 affinity of Hb is 2,3-diphosphoglyceric acid (2,3-DPG), an intermediate product of glycolysis. 2,3-DPG decreases the O_2 affinity of Hb, resulting in a right shift of the Hb oxygen dissociation curve and augmenting O_2 delivery to tissues. A right shift is also caused by increased temperature and pCO_2 and a decrease in pH (see Fig. 3-4). Fetal Hb binds 2,3-DPG weakly and therefore has a high O_2 affinity compared with HbA.

HEMOGLOBIN GENES

Each chromosome 16 contains two nearly identical genes for α-globin, and chromosome 11 contains an almost identical pair of γ genes and one copy each of the δ gene and the β-gene. Globin is synthesized only in erythroid cells and only during the period in which these cells mature from proerythroblasts into reticulocytes. At every stage of development, α-globin genes and non-α-globin genes exhibit coordinate expression. This is critical because tetramers comprised of single Hb chains (e.g., α_4 or β_4) are relatively insoluble, and therefore balanced chain synthesis is necessary to maintain Hb as a soluble tetramer. When one Hb chain is produced in excess, as in thalassemia, it may precipitate in the RBC and damage the cell, leading to premature destruction by the reticuloendothelial system.

ERYTHROPOIESIS

Tissue culture studies have identified two kinds of early erythroid progenitors: The first is the burst-forming unit-erythroid (BFU-E), which differentiates into the colony-forming unit-erythroid (CFU-E). The latter gives rise to the proerythroblast,

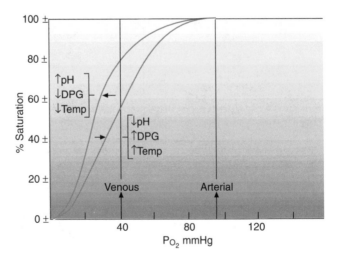

Figure 3-4. Oxygen dissociation curve of hemoglobin. Alkalosis, lower temperature, and a decrease in 2,3-DPG cause a shift to the left of the curve and an increase in oxygen affinity. Acidosis and an increase in temperature and/or 2,3-DPG cause a shift to the right and a decrease in oxygen affinity. (Redrawn from Isselbacher KJ, et al., eds. *Harrison's Principles of Internal Medicine,* 13th ed. New York: McGraw-Hill, 1994:1719, Fig. 302-4.)

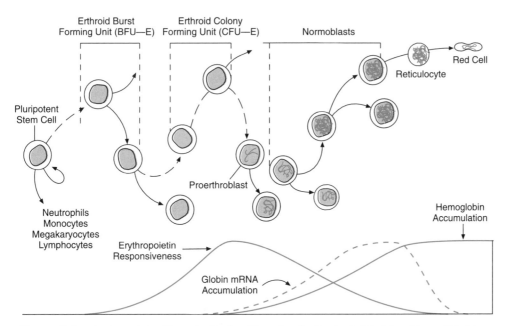

Figure 3-5. Erythropoiesis. (From Isselbacher KJ, et al., eds. *Harrison's Principles of Internal Medicine,* 13th ed. New York: McGraw-Hill; 1994:1718, Fig. 302-1. Differentiation and morphologic maturation of erythroid cells.)

the earliest erythroid precursor that can be distinguished morphologically in the marrow. After four or five mitotic divisions and morphologic changes, the proerythroblast becomes a mature enucleated erythroid cell (Fig. 3-5),which circulates in the peripheral blood for 90–120 days before being removed by the spleen and other parts of the reticuloendothelial system.

Erythropoietin, a hormone produced in the peritubular cells of the kidneys, is an obligatory growth factor for erythroid development, starting at the CFU-E stage. Its role is to maintain a red cell mass appropriate to the body's oxygen needs. A sensing device responsive to tissue oxygen content within the kidney regulates the release of erythropoietin.

APPROACH TO THE PATIENT WITH ANEMIA

Anemia is a reduction in the red blood cell mass. Since blood volume is usually maintained at a constant level, the degree of anemia can be measured either by the volume of red cells expressed as a percentage of the blood volume [the hematocrit (HCT)] or by the plasma concentration of hemoglobin. Normal values for these measurements differ between males and females because androgens increase both erythropoietin secretion and the number of hormone-responsive bone marrow precursors. At higher altitudes, where oxygen tension is lower, these values increase and the definition of anemia changes.

CLINICAL PRESENTATION

Anemia is one of the most important indicators of disease, and its cause should always be sought. The symptoms and signs of anemia reflect the level of the hematocrit, the rate at which the anemia developed, and the underlying cause. Patients with mild to moderate anemia are often asymptomatic. Anemia that develops rapidly, before compensatory mechanisms can take effect, usually causes symptoms that are more severe than those caused by anemia that has reached the same level more gradually. Patients with anemia may suffer from fatigue, dyspnea, palpitations, and poor exercise tolerance. They may feel dizzy and complain of headache or tinnitus. Severe anemia may cause anorexia, indigestion, irritability, and difficulty sleeping and concentrating. Females may have abnormal menstruation, and males may suffer from impotence and/or loss of libido. Anemia may also trigger symptoms of underlying coronary vascular insufficiency, and patients may present with chest pain and/or myocardial infarction.

Pallor is the major sign of anemia and is most easily detected in the oral mucous membranes, nail beds, conjunctivae, and creases of the palm. Other physical findings include tachycardia, a hyperdynamic precordium, and flow murmurs. Anemia caused by hemolysis and hemoglobinopathies may produce jaundice and splenomegaly (Chapter 2).

LABORATORY INVESTIGATION

The Peripheral Blood Smear

The evaluation of red blood cell morphology is a key step in the work-up of any anemia (Table 3-3). Microangiopathic hemolytic anemias and traumatic hemolysis by artificial cardiac valves cause RBC fragmentation; spherocytes are seen in autoimmune hemolysis and hereditary spherocytosis; liver disease, thalassemia, and hemoglobin C disease cause target cells; nucleated RBCs and teardrops are the hallmarks of myelofibrosis and myelophthisic processes (in which the bone marrow is damaged by invasion by carcinoma, lymphoma, fibrosis, and/or granulomata); and intracorpuscular parasites can be seen in malaria and babesiosis (Table 3-3).

The examination of white blood cells (WBCs) and platelets in the peripheral smear may also provide clues to the etiology of an anemia. Hypersegmented polymorphonuclear cells are seen in megaloblastic anemias (Table 4-1). Anemia may be the first manifestation of both the acute and chronic leukemias, which can usually be diagnosed by the presence of abnormal white blood cells in the peripheral blood. The presence of thrombocytopenia and leukopenia indicates bone marrow pathology involving all three cell lines.

Reticulocyte Count

Anemia may result from a primary failure of RBC production, acute blood loss, or accelerated RBC destruction. One of the most important means of distinguishing among these etiologies is to assess the bone marrow response to anemia. Under normal circumstances, every day about 1% of the body's RBCs are replaced by young red blood cells called reticulocytes. Because these cells still contain polyribosomal RNA, they can be detected by special stains of peripheral blood. With Wright's stain, which contains eosin and methylene blue, reticulocytes are colored a gray-purplish hue because the methylene blue stains acid substances such as RNA. More specific stains such as new methylene blue and brilliant cresyl blue precipitate RNA and demonstrate the polyribosomes of the young red blood cells as a reticular network, giving reticulocytes their name (Table 3-3).

The reticulocyte count is usually expressed as a percentage of the number of RBCs counted. This percentage can be high either because of more circulating reticulocytes or because of fewer circulating RBCs (anemia), and thus the corrected reticulocyte count is used to correct for anemia:

$$\text{Corrected Reticulocyte Count} = \% \text{ Reticulocytes} \times \frac{\text{Patient's HCT}}{\text{Normal HCT}}$$

An elevated corrected reticulocyte count indicates that the marrow is under erythropoietin stimulation, and this stimulation not only increases reticulocyte production but also causes early release of reticulocytes into the blood. Reticulocytes entering the blood under these conditions will be premature and will be detectable for more than 1 day, depending on how long it takes them to complete their maturation and lose their RNA. This period of time correlates with the level of the hematocrit: When the HCT is 45%, a reticulocyte spends only 1 day in the peripheral blood. However, when the HCT is 35%, 25%, or 15%, a reticulocyte will spend 1.5 days, 2 days, and 2.5 days, in the peripheral blood, respectively. The reticulocyte production index corrects for the longer time spent by the reticulocyte in the peripheral blood with the following formula:

$$\text{Reticulocyte Production Index} = \frac{\text{Corrected Reticulocyte Count}}{\text{Reticulocyte Maturation Time (Days)}}$$

Another way of estimating RBC production is to calculate the absolute reticulocyte count, which is the percent of reticulocytes multiplied by the RBC count. Normally, this count is between 50,000 and 60,000/μL. This determination of the absolute reticulocyte count is now available in many laboratories and will probably supersede the standard reticulocyte count.

When the cause of anemia is blood loss or destruction of blood outside the marrow, erythropoietin secretion rises, pushing the reticulocyte count above the normal level of 1% and raising the absolute reticulocyte count to greater than 100,000/μL. Absence of an appropriate reticulocytosis in the setting of anemia indicates interference with RBC production in the bone marrow, and etiologies such as nutritional deficiencies, maturation arrest, and/or bone marrow invasion should be considered.

Mean Corpuscular Volume

The mean corpuscular volume (MCV) can be estimated by review of the peripheral blood smear (Table 3-3). It is directly measured by automated cell counters (e.g., the Coulter counter) or can be calculated by dividing the hematocrit by the red cell count (Appendix 1). Measurement of the MCV is especially useful in the evaluation of the hypoproliferative anemias (anemias with a low reticulocyte count) and is used to divide these anemias into three categories: microcytic (MCV < 80 fL), normocytic (80 fL $\leq$ MCV < 100 fl) and macrocytic (MCV $\geq$ 100 fl) anemias (Table 3-4).

The mean corpuscular hemoglobin (MCH = hemoglobin/RBC number) and the mean corpuscular hemoglobin concentration (MCHC = hemoglobin/hematocrit) are two values that are calculated by the automated cell counters and add little to the information obtained from the MCV. The MCH usually parallels the MCV measurement. The MCHC is reduced in most microcytic anemias, especially when caused by iron deficiency, and is increased in hereditary or autoimmune hemolytic anemia.

TABLE 3.3	ABNORMAL RBC MORPHOLOGY AND ITS CLINICAL CORRELATES		
NAME	**MICROSCOPIC APPEARANCE**	**DESCRIPTION**	**CLINICAL SIGNIFICANCE**
1. Normal RBC		Round, 8 μ-diameter, central pallor.	Seen in normal, healthy state and normochromic normocytic anemias.
Polychromatophilic cell		Large cell, gray-purplish blue, ground-glass appearance (polychromasia/polychromatophilia). Loss of central pallor. MCV increased.	Seen in health (1% of RBC) or increased numbers where BM is responding to anemia. Polychromasia is from cytoplasmic polyribosomes that are producing hemoglobin. If supravital stain done, reticular network is visible. Cells then called reticulocytes (see later).
2. Abnormalities in Size and Shape			
Macrocyte (round)		Large cell. Central pallor less apparent. MCV increased.	Seen in liver disease (especially alcohol-induced) and postsplenectomy. Thin if viewed from side. Cell membrane lecithin/cholesterol ratio is changed.
Macrocyte (Oval) (Macro-ovalocyte)		Large oval cell with loss of central pallor. MCV increased.	Seen in peripheral blood of patients with •megaloblastic anemias. Also seen in a variety of other conditions.
Microcyte		Small cell (MCV decreased). Hypochromic if associated with iron deficiency. Central pallor increased.	Seen with •iron deficiency, and •thalassemia.

Cell	Image	Description	Associations
Spherocyte		Can be microcytic, normocytic, or macrocytic. No central pallor. Normally microcytic with MCV decreased and MCHC increased.	Seen with hereditary spherocytosis or any hemolytic anemia where membrane is removed by spleen or RES, and amount of hemoglobin remains constant.
Echinocyte (sea urchin cell) Burr cell Berry cell Crenated cell	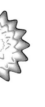	Similarly sized, equally spaced projections in RBC surface.	•Artifact •Uremia •Pyruvate kinase deficiency •Transfusion with aged RBC •Gastric cancer •Peptic ulcer with hemorrhage •Hypophosphatemia •Hypomagnesemia
Acanthocyte (leaflike cell) Spur cell		Irregularly sized and spaced projections on RBC surface.	•Abetalipoproteinemia •Alcoholic liver disease •Postsplenectomy state •Malabsorption
Bite cell (degmacyte)		Cells appear as if a bite has been taken out of them.	•G6PD deficiency •Unstable hemoglobins. Bite cells are formed when Heinz bodies are removed by RES with a portion of cell membrane and hemoglobin.
Blister cell		Cells appear as if a vesicle or blister is on surface.	•Immune hemolytic anemia. Mechanism of formation unclear.

(continued)

TABLE 3.3 *(continued)*

NAME	MICROSCOPIC APPEARANCE	DESCRIPTION	CLINICAL SIGNIFICANCE
Poikilocyte		Cells appear in bizarre shapes. Fragments are seen.	•Burns •Hereditary pyropoikilocytosis. •Myelofibrosis •Thalassemia •Iron deficiency •Megaloblastic anemia •Myelofibrosis •Myelodysplasia.
Ovalocyte or elliptocyte		Oval or elongated cell. Central pallor not appreciated. Membrane or hemoglobin abnormalities cause shape change.	•Hereditary elliptocytosis. •Thalassemia. •Iron deficiency. •Megaloblastic anemias.
Stomatocyte (mouth cell)		Bowl-shaped RBC	•Hereditary spherocytosis. •Hereditary stomatocytosis. •Neoplasm •Alcoholism •Cirrhosis •Obstructive liver disease •Na$^+$-K$^+$ membrane pump defects. Drugs.
Target cell Codocyte or bell cell		Target appearance is artifact of Wright's stain preparation. If viewed from side, cells would look like two Mexican hats brim to brim. Really, cells are bell shaped.	•Liver disease •Hemoglobinopathies C, D, and E •Thalassemia •Iron deficiency anemia •Postsplenectomy state •LCAT deficiency Because of redundant membrane, cells are resistant to osmotic fragility stress.

Schistocyte Helmet cell Fragmented cell	Cells look like helmets, tri-cornered hats, fragments.	•Microangiopathic hemolytic anemias of all causes.
Sickle cell (drepanocyte)	Cells look like sickles or holly leaves.	•Hemoglobin SS or S in combination with HbD, C, Memphis, and thalassemia
Teardrop cell (dacryocyte)	Cells resemble teardrops or tadpoles	•Myelofibrosis •Myeloid metaplasia •Myelophthisic anemias (weak or damaged marrow caused by invasion by tumor, granuloma, lymphoma, fibrosis). •Thalassemias.

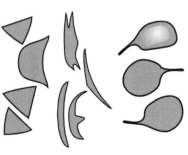

3. Red Blood Cell Inclusions with Wright's Stain

Nucleus	This is an orthochromatophilic normoblast. Last stage before nucleus is removed by RES and cell becomes reticulocyte.	Seen where there is profound anemic stress. Usually intense hemolysis or GI bleeding, especially where there is hypoxemia. Also myelophthisic conditions where there are leukoerythroblastic changes.
Howell-Jolly body	Nuclear remnant from incomplete removal of nucleus by RES. Can be distinguished from platelet overlying RBC since there is a "halo" around the platelet (see above).	Seen in asplenic states or where there is intense hemolysis and RES is "engorged." Also megaloblastic anemia.

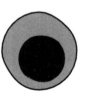

(continued)

TABLE 3.3 *(continued)*

NAME	MICROSCOPIC APPEARANCE	DESCRIPTION	CLINICAL SIGNIFICANCE
Basophilic stippling		Dispersed blue granulation from ribosomal precipitation, may be coarse in appearance.	•Lead or heavy metal intoxication •Thalassemia •Alcohol •Cytotoxic drugs
Siderotic granule (Pappenheimer body)		Dark blue granules of ferric iron. When they occur in nucleated RBC, they are called sideroblasts, and if they surround the nucleus they are called ringed sideroblasts.	•Hemolytic anemia •Sideroblastic anemia •Hyposplenism.
Cabot ring		Complete or incomplete rings or figure eights. May be granular and reddish blue. They are from mitotic spindle or nuclear membrane.	•Megaloblastic anemia.
Hemoglobin C crystal		Hexagonal or rhomboid intracellular crystals. May be curved and blunt in hemoglobin SC with lighter area between crystals.	•Hemoglobin C disease.

Malaria	Early ring forms are usually seen. They are bluish and may be incomplete with red dot(s). *P. falciparum* may be recognized by "earphone"-like configuration and also macrogametocyte banana form. Shüffner's granules seen in *P. vivax* and *P. ovale*.	•*Plasmodium falciparum, vivax, malariae,* and *ovale*.
Babesia	Parasites appear similar to malarial forms. "Maltese crosses" may be seen.	•*Babesia microti*.

4. Red Blood Cell Inclusions with Supravital Stain

Reticulocyte	New methylene blue staining results in granular filamentous structures that are stippled and diffusely basophilic.	Seen in health (1% of RBC) or increased numbers where BM is responding to anemia.
Heinz body	After incubation with acetyl phenyl hydrazine, followed by staining with crystal violet, hemoglobin is denatured and appears as blue, round precipitates. 1–4 Heinz bodies are seen in normal cells, 5 or more in pathologic states.	•G6PD deficiency •Unstable hemoglobins and other hereditary hemolytic anemias following the use of oxidizing drugs. May see bite cells formed when Heinz bodies are removed by RES.

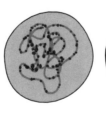

TABLE 3-4. *CAUSES OF HYPOPROLIFERATIVE ANEMIA*
Microcytic
Iron deficiency anemia
Thalassemia
Sideroblastic anemia
Lead poisoning
(Anemia of chronic disease)
Normocytic
Bone marrow failure (aplastic anemia)
Myelophthisis
Anemia of chronic disease
Endocrinopathies
Early iron deficiency
"Mixed" anemias
Macrocytic
Megaloblastic
B_{12} deficiency
Folate deficiency
Myelodysplasia
Drug-induced megaloblastic anemia
Nonmegaloblastic macrocytic anemia
High reticulocyte count
Liver disease
(Hypothyroidism)

Bone Marrow Examination

If the initial evaluation of a patient with anemia shows a low reticulocyte count, then a failure of RBC production or a hypoproliferative anemia should be strongly considered (Table 3-4). The marrow examination may demonstrate a myelodysplastic process, a leukemia, or marrow infiltration by a solid tumor (most commonly, breast, prostate, or lung). Megaloblastic changes are also evident on a marrow examination. Infections such as those caused by *Mycobacterium tuberculosis, Mycobacterium avium intracellulare,* cytomegalovirus, and histoplasma may be diagnosed by culturing a marrow sample or by typical morphology in the aspirate or biopsy specimens. An iron stain can confirm the diagnosis of iron deficiency and may demonstrate ringed sideroblasts as part of a myelodysplastic or congenital disorder. Bone marrow examination is usually of little value in the evaluation of anemias associated with reticulocytosis, since an adequate marrow response to anemia usually rules out an intramedullary defect in RBC production.

DIFFERENTIAL DIAGNOSIS OF HYPOPROLIFERATIVE ANEMIA

MICROCYTIC ANEMIAS

The differential diagnosis of microcytosis (Table 3-4) includes iron deficiency anemia, thalassemia, lead poisoning, sideroblastic anemias, and the anemia associated with chronic disease. Although anemia of chronic disease can be microcytic, it is more commonly normocytic. The most common cause of microcytosis is iron deficiency.

Iron Deficiency Anemia

Iron Metabolism. Iron exists in food either as heme or as nonheme iron. Although heme iron is usually a smaller portion of dietary iron, it is more available for absorption, with 20–30% absorbed under normal conditions. Usually less than 5% of nonheme iron is absorbed, and absorption may be even lower in the presence of dietary phytates, tannates, and phosphates. Ascorbic acid enhances nonheme iron absorption.

Iron absorption is mainly regulated by the mucosal cells of the proximal small intestine, but the mechanism is poorly understood. The rate of iron absorption is increased in iron deficiency and in patients with ineffective erythropoiesis. In patients with severe ineffective erythropoiesis, as seen in some thalassemias, increased iron absorption occurs despite plentiful total body iron, and coupled with blood transfusions, often results in clinically significant iron overload.

Iron is transported, bound to a plasma-binding protein called transferrin which binds to a specific membrane receptor. The receptor/transferrin/iron complex is internalized by developing RBCs, the iron is then released, and the transferrin/transferrin receptor compound is recycled to the cell membrane.

Ferritin is an intracellular protein that stores iron in a nontoxic form to be mobilized in time of need. Each ferritin molecule can bind up to 4,500 iron atoms, but under normal conditions only about half that amount is present on the molecule. Some ferritin is converted into hemosiderin, a water-insoluble compound that stores iron in higher amounts but in a less available form. Men and women have 50 mg/kg and 40 mg/kg iron, respectively, in their bodies. Between 28 and 31 mg/kg of iron is in hemoglobin, 4–5 mg/kg is in myoglobin, 12 mg/kg is in ferritin and hemosiderin, and the rest is in heme and nonheme enzymes (Table 3-5). The main sites of iron storage are in the liver (hepatocytes and macrophages), bone marrow, spleen, and muscle.

The iron-responsive element-binding protein (IRE-BP) binds to a regulatory site on mRNA and coordinates the expression of ferritin, transferrin, and the transferrin receptor. If the IRE-BP senses a low intracellular iron level, it triggers increased transferrin receptor synthesis and inhibits ferritin synthesis.

Etiology of Iron Deficiency Anemia. Iron deficiency anemia (IDA) is the most common cause of anemia worldwide. The most frequent cause of iron deficiency is blood loss (Table 3-6), which in most men and postmenopausal women is

TABLE 3-5. *IRON DISTRIBUTION*

LOCATION	IRON (mg/kg)
Hemoglobin	30 (men); 27 (women)
Heme and nonheme enzymes	2
Myoglobin	5
Ferritin and hemosiderin	13 (men); 6 (women)
Total	50 (men); 40 (women)

TABLE 3-6. *CAUSES OF IRON DEFICIENCY*

Blood loss
    Gastrointestinal
    Menstruation and childbirth
    Pulmonary (hemoptysis, pulmonary hemosiderosis)
    Urinary (renal disease, urologic disease, hemoglobinuria)
Malabsorption
    Gastric resection
    Pancreatic insufficiency
    Tropical and nontropical sprue
    Crohn's disease of the small bowel
    Short bowel syndrome
Increased demand
    Rapid growth (premature infants, children, teenagers)
    Pregnancy and lactation
Poor dietary intake

caused by gastrointestinal (GI) bleeding. Any man or postmenopausal woman with iron deficiency should have a full GI workup for structural GI tract abnormalities, especially malignancy. In about 15% of patients with GI bleeding, the cause cannot be found. In women of childbearing age the most common causes of iron deficiency anemia are vaginal bleeding, pregnancies, and lactation. Menstruation results in loss of about 15 mg of elemental iron per month. About 900 mg of iron are lost during a normal pregnancy and delivery, with iron transferred to the fetus and placenta, and lost during parturitional hemorrhage. Rarer causes of blood loss include recurrent hemoptysis, pulmonary siderosis, Goodpasture syndrome, and hematuria.

Iron deficiency can develop in the absence of blood loss when children are undergoing rapid growth and their increased needs are not met by adequate intake. This situation is common in newborns, especially premature infants, and in adolescents (especially menstruating young women). Malabsorption is another cause of iron deficiency, seen in patients who have undergone gastric surgery and in patients with more generalized intestinal malabsorption syndromes.

Clinical Presentation. Iron deficiency produces the signs and symptoms common to all anemias, including pallor, palpitations, tinnitus, headache, and fatigue. Rare but more specific signs and symptoms include pica, an abnormal craving for and ingestion of substances such as starch, ice, and clay (amylophagia, pagophagia, and geophagia), koilonychia, and blue sclerae. The depletion of iron in nonerythroid tissues may cause such symptoms as glossitis, angular stomatitis, and esophageal webs (Chapter 2).

Laboratory Evaluation. Although classic IDA may present as a hypochromic, microcytic anemia, most patients have a normochromic anemia early in their disease. Anemia usually precedes microcytosis, and hypochromia is the latest manifestation of worsening IDA. The reason for this preservation of the MCHC at the expense of the RBC mass until the late stages of IDA is unknown. The anemia is often accompanied by a reactive thrombocytosis. The peripheral blood smear in severe IDA demonstrates microcytosis with pale, hypochromic RBCs, and occasional elongated "pencil cells" and target cells.

Iron stores can be assessed indirectly by measuring ferritin, iron, and transferrin saturation (iron-binding capacity). The liver produces ferritin in proportion to the amount of iron available, and small amounts of ferritin are secreted into the plasma in proportion to the amount produced by the liver. Therefore the plasma level of ferritin is an important measure of the body's iron stores. A level below 12 ng/mL strongly indicates iron deficiency, but hypothyroidism and ascorbic acid deficiency can occasionally also cause low plasma ferritin. Normal levels of ferritin do not rule out iron deficiency, because ferritin is an acute phase reactant, and its level may rise during fever, infection, inflammation, liver damage, malignancy, hemolysis, and ineffective erythropoiesis. However, these conditions alone should not elevate the ferritin level to more than 50–100 ng/mL, so a ferritin above this level usually rules out iron deficiency.

Iron stores also can be assessed by measuring transferrin saturation, which is the ratio of plasma iron to transferrin concentration (iron/total iron-binding capacity). Normally, this ratio is at least 20%, but iron deficiency lowers it by decreasing plasma iron levels and increasing plasma transferrin levels. In chronic conditions such as infection, inflammation, malignancy, and liver disease, both iron and iron-binding capacity drop, but the ratio between them usually remains above 20% in the absence of iron deficiency (Figure 3-6).

Ferritin and transferrin saturation provide indirect measures of iron stores, but a definitive diagnosis of iron deficiency can be made only by an iron stain of a bone marrow aspirate or biopsy. The presence of any iron in the marrow excludes deficiency, and the complete absence of iron is diagnostic of IDA.

Therapy. The total body iron deficit can be estimated by the following formula:

$$\text{iron (mg)} = (\text{normal Hb} - \text{patient Hb}) \times \text{weight (kg)} \times 2.21 + 1,000.$$

This amount corrects the anemia and restores 1,000 mg of iron stores. Oral iron supplementation is the treatment of choice, and blood transfusions can usually

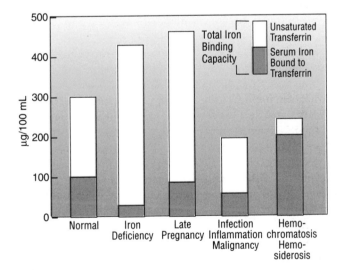

Figure 3-6. Serum iron and iron-binding capacity in various clinical conditions. (Redrawn from Isselbacher KJ, et al., eds. *Harrison's Principles of Internal Medicine*, 13th ed. New York: McGraw-Hill, 1994:1722, Fig. 303-2. Serum iron and total iron binding capacity in various disorders.)

be avoided unless the patient has evidence of cardiac ischemia or failure. When blood transfusions are necessary, they should be administered with caution in older patients with long-standing anemia because such patients usually have expanded plasma volumes, and a further increase in their intravascular volume may trigger congestive heart failure.

Oral iron is given in the form of iron salts, usually ferrous sulfate. Patients should receive 150–200 mg elemental iron per day, divided into three or four doses. About 20% of patients develop either diarrhea or constipation, and these complications can be treated symptomatically. Symptoms of gastric irritation such as nausea and epigastric discomfort are usually relieved by administering the iron with meals or reducing the dose. Often a gradual buildup of the dose will prevent these symptoms.

Parenteral iron therapy is indicated only in patients with malabsorption, the rare patients who cannot tolerate oral supplements, and patients who have chronic bleeding and whose needs cannot be met by oral supplementation alone. The main risk of parenteral treatment is anaphylaxis, which has been reported in up to 1% of patients. This reaction appears to be unrelated to dose and has been reported more frequently in women with collagen vascular disease. The anaphylactic reaction may be fatal despite treatment.

An increase in the reticulocyte count should be seen 3 to 4 days after initiating iron therapy in a patient with IDA, and reticulocytosis peaks in 10 days. The hemoglobin concentration is expected to increase by about 2 g/dL after 3 weeks of therapy. Iron supplementation is usually continued for about 4–6 months after the anemia is corrected, or until the ferritin concentration is above 50 ng/mL.

The Thalassemia Syndromes

The thalassemias are a heterogeneous group of inherited anemias characterized by defects in the synthesis of one or more of the globin chain subunits of hemoglobin. In α- or β-thalassemia, α- or β-globin synthesis is reduced or absent, respectively. The diagnosis of thalassemia is based on the quantitation of hemoglobin and globin chain fractions by electrophoresis (Chapter 11.) Severe thalassemic syndromes are associated with profound hemolytic anemia and are diagnosed early in life. However, minor thalassemic variants cause only a mild microcytic anemia and little or no hemolysis. These mild thalassemias are often misdiagnosed as IDA because of the associated low MCV.

Thalassemias are most common in the areas of the world historically afflicted with endemic malaria, including the Mediterranean shores, the Arabian peninsula, Turkey, Iran, India, and Southeast Asia. This is thought to be because the RBCs of heterozygotes for thalassemia are relatively resistant to infection with the malaria parasite.

β-Thalassemia. β-thalassemia is caused by a spectrum of mutations within the β-globin locus on chromosome 11 that affect the level of β-globin chain synthesis. More than 100 mutations have been described, resulting in disruption of all stages of gene expression, including transcription, mRNA processing, and translation. Promoter mutations leading to reduced mRNA transcription, and mutations leading to errors in mRNA splicing usually result in reduced β-chain synthesis (β^+-thalassemia), whereas nonsense mutations in the coding region causing premature termination of β-globin chains cause complete absence of β-chains (β^0-thalassemia).

The pathogenesis of β-thalassemia is related to both the inability to synthesize adequate amounts of normal hemoglobin and the presence of the relatively insoluble α-chain tetramers that form because of insufficient amount of β-chains. Inadequate hemoglobin synthesis leads to anemia with hypochromia and microcytosis, and unbalanced accumulation of the α-globin chains leads to formation of α_4-tetramers, which precipitate within developing and mature erythrocytes. The intracellular precipitates of hemoglobin signal the reticuloendothelial system to remove them from the RBC, a process that damages the cells, shortens their lifespan, and results in intramedullary RBC destruction and hemolysis. In severe thalassemic syndromes, hemolysis leads to intense erythroid hyperplasia and a massive expansion of the intramedullary spaces, causing skeletal abnormalities. In addition, ineffective erythropoiesis (the destruction of RBC precursors within the marrow) induces increased iron absorption, so that even untransfused patients with thalassemia can develop life-threatening iron overload.

The clinical syndromes associated with β-thalassemia are related to the severity of the genetic lesion, and the associated degree of β-globin chain deficiency (Table 3-7). **β-thalassemia major,** or Cooley's anemia, usually results from homozygosity for a β^0-thalassemia allele. Patients with **β-thalassemia intermedia** have significant anemia but chronic transfusion therapy is not absolutely required. They usually have inherited two β-thalassemia mutations, one mild and one severe. **β-thalassemia minor** is due to the presence of a single β-thalassemia mutation on one chromosome, with a normal β-globin gene on the other chromosome 11. These patients usually have asymptomatic microcytosis and hypochromia, and are often inappropriately treated with iron for presumed iron deficiency. The diagnosis of β-thalassemia is suggested by anemia, microcytosis, a relatively high RBC number, and normal iron studies. Peripheral smear may show bizarre and nucleated RBCs, target cells, teardrops, and inclusion bodies (Table 3-3), although in β-thalassemia minor these changes may be very mild. Hemoglobin electrophoresis reveals a compensatory elevation in hemoglobins A_2 and F.

TABLE 3-7. *THE THALASSEMIA SYNDROMES*

SYNDROME	GENETIC DEFECT	CLINICAL SYNDROME
α-Thalassemia		
Silent carrier	$\alpha-/\alpha\alpha$	None
Trait	$\alpha-/\alpha-$ or $--/\alpha\alpha$	Mild microcytic anemia
Hemoglobin H	$--/\alpha-$	Mild anemia and hemolysis; not transfusion dependent
Hydrops fetalis	$--/--$	Severe anemia, anasarca; death *in utero* or at birth
β-Thalassemia		
Minor	β^{thal} trait	Mild microcytic anemia
Intermedia	Combination of β^0 and β^+ mutations	Not transfusion dependent, iron overload
Major	Homozygous β^0	"Cooley's anemia" severe hemolysis, ineffective erythropoiesis, transfusion dependence, skeletal abnormalities, hepatosplenomegaly, iron overload

α-Thalassemia. Two nearly identical copies of the α-globin gene reside on chromosome 16. In 80–85% of cases of α-thalassemia there are one or more deletions of these four genes, and in the remainder of the cases the genes are present but dysfunctional. The clinical manifestations of α-thalassemia relate to the degree of loss of α-globin chain synthesis (Table 3-7), but they are generally milder than those of β-thalassemia. This is for two reasons: First, the presence of four α-globin genes allows for production of adequate levels of α-chains until three or four genes are lost. Significant hemoglobin chain imbalance occurs only if three of the four genes are affected. Second, aggregates of β-chains (β_4 tetramers created when there are insufficient α-chains) are much more soluble than α_4 tetramers and therefore even patients with significantly reduced α-globin synthesis have much less hemolysis and ineffective erythropoiesis in α-thalassemia than in β-thalassemia.

People with deletion or dysfunction of only **one** of the four α-genes are silent carriers and are usually recognized only as parents of children with hemoglobin H disease. (See later.) Their red cells are not microcytic, and their Hb A_2 and F levels are normal. Patients with deletions of **two** α-globin genes, either on the same chromosome (in cis, α-thal 1) or on different chromosomes (in trans, α-thal 2), are also asymptomatic but have microcytosis and hypochromia. Both α-thal 1 and α-thal 2 are common among Asians and people from the Mediterranean area; whereas in Africans, only the α-thal 2 deletion is present (Fig. 3-7).

Patients with deletions or dysfunction of **three** α-globin genes have Hb H disease. The excess β-chains form β_4 tetramers called Hb H, which can be detected as a fast-moving component on gel electrophoresis. Hb H precipitates mainly in mature RBCs, causing mild hemolytic anemia but relatively little ineffective erythropoiesis.

Patients with homozygous α-thalassemia 1 have no normal α-globin genes (all **four** genes are affected, two on each chromosome), and thus can produce no functional hemoglobin beyond the embryonic stage (in which ζ-chains serve as α-like chains). Free β-globin forms tetramers called Hb Bart's, with a very high affinity for oxygen. This hemoglobin does not release oxygen to the fetal tissues, resulting in asphyxia at the tissue level, edema, congestive heart failure, and the clinical picture of hydrops fetalis. Fetuses are either stillborn or die within hours of birth. Hemoglobin Bart's occurs almost exclusively in people from Southeast Asia, in whom the cis deletion of α-globin genes is prevalent.

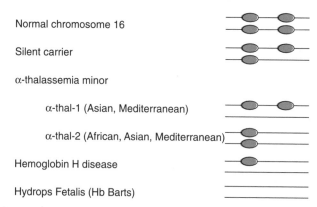

Figure 3-7. Genotypes of α-thalassemia syndromes. The gray ovals represent copies of the α-thalassemia gene.

Management of the Thalassemia Syndromes. Patients with homozygous β-thalassemia (Cooley's anemia) should be transfused to maintain hemoglobin levels of 9–10 g/dL, a regimen that results in improved growth and development and prevents severe skeletal deformities. Iron overload should be treated with deferoxamine, a water soluble compound that binds iron and enables it to be excreted in the urine. Splenectomy should be performed when patients become refractory to transfusions, but not before age 5. Bone marrow transplantation from HLA-matched siblings offers a possibility of cure. Most patients with α-thalassemia survive into adult life without transfusions or splenectomy, but splenectomy may benefit patients with significant anemia. All patients with thalassemia should be offered genetic counseling and antenatal diagnosis, as DNA diagnosis can now be performed for the vast majority of thalassemia mutations.

MACROCYTIC ANEMIAS

The macrocytic anemias are subdivided into two groups, megaloblastic anemias and nonmegaloblastic macrocytic anemias (Table 3-8) . In megaloblastic anemia, a defect in DNA synthesis causes abnormalities in cell growth and maturation that affects all dividing cells in the body. Nonmegaloblastic macrocytosis usually reflects pathology in RBC membrane lipids, and other cell lines are normal. The two main conditions in which nonmegaloblastic macrocytosis occurs are liver disease and hypothyroidism. Alcohol use may also cause macrocytosis which lasts for the lifespan of the RBC once exposure has occurred. In patients with reticulocytosis, the average MCV, as measured by automated counters, is increased because reticulocytes are larger than mature RBCs, but these patients do not have true macrocytosis.

Megaloblastic Anemias

Megaloblastic anemias are a group of disorders characterized by cells with distinct morphologic features: large, immature-looking nuclei surrounded by relatively more mature-appearing cytoplasm. The primary biochemical abnormality in these disorders is a defect in DNA synthesis: cells are arrested in the S phase of the cell cycle, with part of their DNA replicated but are unable to complete cell division. As a result, megaloblastic cells are large and have more DNA than their normal counterparts. The megaloblastic process usually affects actively dividing cells leading to pancytopenia and gastrointestinal symptoms and signs. The most common conditions causing megaloblastosis are folic acid deficiency, cobalamin (Cbl, vitamin B_{12}) deficiency, myelodysplasia (see Chapter 9) and medications that inhibit DNA synthesis (Table 3-8).

Cobalamin (vitamin B_{12}) Deficiency. Cobalamin is a complex molecule consisting of a central cobalt atom linked to four pyrrole rings and to a nucleotide. It is produced by microorganisms that contaminate roots and legumes and is present in muscle and parenchymal tissues of animals that eat these plants. Humans receive Cbl from animal protein within the diet. The total body content of Cbl is 2–5 mg, and because the obligatory daily loss is very low, the body stores are sufficient for 3–4 years if the supply of Cbl stops abruptly. (See below for discussion of the metabolism of B_{12} and folic acid.)

The process of Cbl absorption is complex. In the stomach pepsin releases the protein-bound vitamin, which is transferred to a high-affinity binder present in the

TABLE 3-8. ETIOLOGY OF MEGALOBLASTIC ANEMIA

Cobalamin (B$_{12}$) Deficiency
  Nutritional
    Vegans
    Breast-fed infants of vegans
  Malabsorption of B$_{12}$
    Pernicious anemia
    Partial or total gastrectomy
    Pancreatic insufficiency
    Zollinger-Ellison syndrome
    Bacterial overgrowth
    Disease of terminal ileum (resection, bypass, Crohn's disease, TB, lymphoma)
    Tapeworm infection (*Diphyllobothrium latum*)
  Congenital absence of B$_{12}$ binders (Immerslund-Grasbeck syndrome)
  Drugs (nitrous oxide)
Folic Acid Deficiency
  Poor intake
  Increased demand
    Pregnancy and lactation
    Prematurity
    Hemolysis
    Exfoliative dermatitis
    Rapidly growing malignancy
  Malabsorption
    Sprue
    Nontropical sprue
    Crohn's disease
    Short bowel syndrome
    Amyloidosis
Myelodysplasia and erythroleukemia
Medications
  Anticonvulsants (phenytoin, carbamazepine)
  Dihydrofolate reductase inhibitors (sulfa drugs, methotrexate)
  Chemotherapy (DNA synthesis inhibitors)
  Others

gastric secretions called transcobalamin I (TCI). The transcobalamins TCI and TCIII (also known as R-binders) are found in all secretions and in plasma. Their function in these fluids is unknown, but they are thought to be involved with storage of Cbl. Intrinsic factor (IF), another protein with lesser affinity for Cbl, is secreted from the parietal cells of the stomach and is delivered to the second part of the duodenum together with the Cbl–TCI protein complex. Pancreatic proteases then degrade the R-protein and Cbl is transferred to IF. The IF–Cbl complex travels to the distal ileum, where it is absorbed through membrane-associated receptors. In the blood Cbl is bound to transcobalamin II (TCII), a transport protein that mediates Cbl uptake into target tissues by receptor-mediated endocytosis.

    Etiology of Cobalamin Deficiency. Nutritional Cbl deficiency is rare and seen only in patients on long-standing vegan diets, which exclude all animal products (Table 3-8). Breast-fed infants of vegans may also develop Cbl deficiency.

The most common cause of Cbl deficiency is pernicious anemia (PA), an autoimmune disease characterized by atrophy of the gastric parietal cells and the absence of IF and hydrochloric acid secretion. The name PA was introduced by Biermer in 1872, but the pathophysiology was not explained until the 1920s. The term PA is now reserved for that once fatal condition resulting from defectice secretion of intrinsic factor by the gastric mucosa. PA is usually a disease of the older population but is seen in all ages and affects all races with an incidence of 25/100,000 persons above age 40 per year. There appears to be a genetic component to PA, and it is also associated with other autoimmune diseases, such as Graves' disease, Hashimoto thyroiditis, vitiligo, Addison's disease, hypoparathyroidism, and adult-onset hypogammaglobulinemia. More than 90% of patients with PA have detectable antiparietal cell IgG antibodies in their serum, but these antibodies are also found in about 50% of patients who have atrophic gastritis without PA. Anti-IF antibodies, however, are found in the serum of only about 60% of patients with PA, but they are highly specific for the disease.

Because of the complex process of Cbl absorption and uptake, many lesions of the gastrointestinal tract can lead to Cbl malabsorption and deficiency (see Table 3-8). Such deficiencies usually arise only after 4–10 years of malabsorption, as the body stores of Cbl are significant and obligatory losses are minute. Bacterial overgrowth may lead to Cbl deficiency, because the bacteria sequester the vitamin. Rarer causes of Cbl deficiency include congenital defects in IF molecules, IF receptors, and postreceptor processes, and congenital absence of transcobalamin II. Rare inborn defects of Cbl metabolism have also been described.

Folate Deficiency. Folates are B vitamins present in leafy vegetables (beans, lettuce, spinach, broccoli), fruits, mushrooms, and animal protein. However, they are destroyed by prolonged cooking, and thus fresh fruit and vegetables are their best dietary source. After ingestion, folates interact with small intestine brush-border-associated binding proteins and undergo uptake and methylation. Folate is loosely bound to plasma proteins in the blood, and is rapidly taken up by cells. Serum levels of folate are maintained by the diet and by an intact enterohepatic circulation. Abrupt interruption of folate intake leads to deficiency within 3 weeks. External biliary drainage may result in a folate deficiency within hours.

Etiology of Folate Deficiency. Inadequate intake is the most common cause of folate deficiency, and it tends to occur in patients who are generally malnourished, such as alcoholics, narcotic addicts, and elderly patients who consume very little fresh fruits or vegetables (Table 3-8). Folate deficiency may develop in the setting of rapid cell turnover, when increased demands are not met by dietary intake. This is seen in pregnancy, in patients with acute or chronic hemolysis, and in patients with exfoliative dermatitis. Patients on hemodialysis also have increased folate needs, because folate is lost during dialysis. Malabsorption of folate is found in small intestine diseases such as tropical and nontropical sprue and Crohn's disease.

Other Causes of Megaloblastosis.

Drugs and Toxins. Drugs cause megaloblastic anemia through several mechanisms. Some, such as methotrexate, a powerful inhibitor of dihydrofolate reductase; pentamidine, trimethoprim, triamterene, and pyrimethamine are folate antagonists. Chemotherapeutic agents such as purine analogs (azathioprine, 6-mercaptopurine, 6-thioguanine), pyrimidine analogs (5-fluorouracil, cytosine arabinoside), and others (procarbazine, hydroxyurea) inhibit DNA synthesis directly. Anticonvulsants (phenytoin, barbiturates) cause folate deficiency by unclear mechanisms, and alcohol interferes with folate metabolism. The antivirals zidovidine and acyclovir both cause significant megaloblastic anemia by unclear mechanisms. Nitrous oxide oxidizes Cbl and may cause an acute megaloblastic state characterized by rapidly developing thrombocytopenia and/or leukopenia in the absence of anemia.

Myelodysplasia and Erythroleukemia. Megaloblastic erythropoiesis is seen in refractory anemia, acquired sideroblastic anemia, and other forms of myelodysplasia. Megaloblastosis and bizarre erythroid maturation are one of the hallmarks of erythroleukemia (di Guglielmo syndrome).

Metabolism of B_{12} and Folic Acid. Cbl serves as a cofactor for two intracellular enzymes. In the mitochondria it is a coenzyme for methylmalony CoA mutase, which catalyzes the conversion of methylmalonyl-CoA to succinyl-CoA (Fig. 3-8A). In the cytoplasm, it is a cofactor for homocysteine–methionine methyltransferase (methionine synthase), which catalyzes transfer of methyl groups from N-methyl tetrahydrofolate to homocysteine to form methionine (Fig. 3-8B).

Once in the cell, folate undergoes reduction to 5-methyl-tetrahydrofolate, which donates the methyl group to Cbl in the process of forming methionine from homocysteine (Fig. 3-8). Folate compounds are also essential in DNA synthesis by serving as single-carbon donors in the conversion of deoxyuridine to deoxythymidine. Tetrahydrofolate undergoes polyglutamation, and it is thought that this enables the folate to be retained in the cell. Cobalamin deficiency causes a "trapping" of folate in the methyltetrahydrofolate form, resulting in folate necessary for deoxyuridine synthesis and in less efficient polyglutamation, causing a leak of folate out of the cell (see Fig. 3-8B).

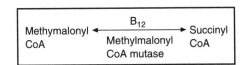

Figure 3-8(A). Mitochondrial metabolic pathway of cobalamin.

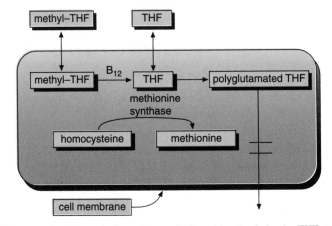

Figure 3-8(B). Cytoplasmic metabolic pathways of folic acid and cobalamin. THF, tetrahydrofolate.

Because Cbl deficiency causes megaloblastosis through a functional folate deficiency, the deficiencies of these two vitamins cannot be distinguished on the basis of blood and marrow morphology. However, only Cbl deficiency causes neurologic disease, characterized by patchy demyelination of the gray matter of the cerebrum, the spinal cord, and peripheral nerves. The explanation for this is not established. It is hypothesized that inhibition of methylmalonyl-CoA mutase (which occurs in B_{12} deficiency but not in folate deficiency) disrupts odd-chain fatty acid metabolism, resulting in abnormal fatty acid incorporation into myelin. Such abnormal fatty acids have been found in nerve biopsies of cobalamin-deficient patients. Methionine deficiency may also contribute to the neurologic syndrome by impairing production of choline-containing phospholipids.

Symptoms and Signs of Megaloblastic Anemia. When interviewing a patient with megaloblastosis, attention should be paid to the patient's diet, nutritional status, and bowel habits. Folate deficiency is suggested by a history of malnutrition, malabsorption, and alcoholism. A history of gastric surgery suggests Cbl deficiency, as does a history of neurologic or psychiatric disease. Recent drug ingestion should be noted, especially anticonvulsants, chemotherapeutic agents, folate antagonists, and nitrous oxide. A history of autoimmune disorders—such as hypothyroidism, Addison's disease, and vitiligo—suggests pernicious anemia.

On physical exam several findings may point to the diagnosis and provide clues to the etiology. Fair-skinned patients will sometimes have lemon-colored skin, caused by the combination of jaundice and pallor. Glossitis and cheilosis are common in megaloblastic anemia. Malnourished patients may have signs of other vitamin deficiencies, such as osteomalacia, dermatitis, bleeding, and infections. Patients with folate or Cbl deficiency often have increased pigmentation of nail beds and skin creases. A mild splenomegaly may develop, secondary to extramedullary hematopoiesis.

The neurologic signs and symptoms of Cbl deficiency vary in their severity. Early signs include posterior column dysfunction with loss of proprioception and vibration sense. Patients have a wide-based gait and difficulty walking. They then develop pyramidal, spinocerebellar, and spinothalamic tract disease, with muscular weakness, progressive spasticity, hyperreflexia, and scissor gait. Patients can also develop peripheral nerve damage, with loss of deep tendon reflexes, cranial nerve palsies, or loss of sphincter control. In prolonged Cbl deficiency, patients develop dementia and neuropsychiatric disease. The neurologic disease of Cbl deficiency may be present without anemia, and in fact, some studies suggest that the higher the hematocrit, the more severe the neurologic disease. Thus B_{12} levels should be part of a routine workup of dementia and neuropsychiatric symptoms. The clinical features of folate deficiency are similar to those of Cbl deficiency, but neurologic signs are absent; however, poorly defined neuropsychiatric abnormalities have been described.

Diagnosis of Folate and Cobalamin Deficiency. Macrocytosis should alert the clinician to the possibility of folate and/or Cbl deficiency, especially when the MCV is above 110. However, patients with concurrent iron deficiency, thalassemia, and anemia of chronic disease may have megaloblastosis without macrocytosis. A low reticulocyte count and mild leukopenia and thrombocytopenia also point to folate or Cbl deficiency.

The peripheral blood smear demonstrates macro-ovalocytes, anisocytosis, poikilocytosis, some basophilic stippling, and occasional nucleated RBCs (Table 3-3). Hypersegmentation of the nucleus of polymorphonuclear cells, which is caused by the defect in DNA synthesis, is unique to megaloblastic anemia, and the finding of even one cell with a nucleus of six lobes is highly suggestive of Cbl or folate deficiency (Chapter 4, Table 1). Platelets tend to be large and abnormally shaped. The bone marrow is hypercellular, with decreased numbers of megakaryocytes and abnormally large granulocyte precursors (giant bands and metamyelocytes). RBC precursors are large and demonstrate nuclear-cytoplasmic asynchrony (a nucleus that appears less mature than the cytoplasm). Patients have evidence of ineffective erythropoiesis, with indirect hyperbilirubinemia and elevated LDH from intramedullary (bone marrow) lysis of RBC.

The diagnosis of megaloblastic anemia is established by measuring blood levels of folic acid and Cbl. Folate levels can be measured either in the serum or in the RBC fraction. The serum level reflects the patient's recent intake of folic acid, and this level will be low 24–48 hours after a sudden drop in dietary folate. Conversely, normal levels may be seen in a folate-deficient patient within hours of a folate-containing meal. Hemolyzed RBCs release folic acid into the serum, falsely raising the serum folate levels even with intracellular folate deficiency. RBC folate levels are 30 times higher than serum levels and usually correlate well with tissue folate levels. However, Cbl deficiency, by impairing folate polyglutamation, may cause a cellular leak of folate, resulting in low RBC folate levels but normal serum levels.

Serum Cbl levels usually accurately reflect body stores. About 5% of patients with Cbl deficiency and neurologic and/or hematologic disease will have serum Cbl levels in the low normal range. In these patients the diagnosis can be made by measuring the urinary levels of the metabolites methylmalonic acid and homocysteine. Both are elevated in Cbl deficiency, reflecting the metabolic block of methylmalonyl CoA mutase and methionine synthase, respectively (Figs. 3-8A and 3-8B).

Once the diagnosis of Cbl deficiency has been made, a Schilling test may establish the origin of the deficiency. Radioactive Cbl is given by mouth, and this is followed by a large parenteral dose of unlabeled vitamin. This nonradioactive flushing dose is given to saturate the circulating cobalamin binding proteins TCI and TCII, so that there is maximal urine excretion of the radioactive Cbl that is absorbed from the gut. The radioactivity in a 24-hour urine should be more than 8% of the administered dose. Simultaneous oral administration of a differently radiolabeled Cbl bound to IF allows comparison of the absorption of IF-Cbl to that of free vitamin. Selective malabsorption of free Cbl that corrects with IF-Cbl is diagnostic of pernicious anemia and lack of IF. If the malabsorption is not corrected, the test may be repeated after the patient is treated with a course of broad-spectrum antibiotics to treat bacterial overgrowth, and following administration of pancreatic enzymes to rule out pancreatic insufficiency. The Schilling test requires adequate urine collection and is now less widely used, since documentation of anti-IF or antiparietal cell antibodies can establish the diagnosis of pernicious anemia without it.

Treatment of Folate and Cobalamin Deficiency. Treatment should be started after folate and Cbl levels have been drawn. Patients with Cbl deficiency secondary to pernicious anemia should receive parenteral therapy. This is usually started at a daily dose of 1 mg subcutaneously or 100 μg IV for 7 days, and then 1 mg subcutaneously once a month. Patients with normal Cbl absorption can receive oral replacement therapy at a daily dose of 1–5 mg/day. Some patients with PA may respond to oral replacement therapy at high enough doses, and this may be an alternative in patients unwilling to receive parenteral therapy. All patients receiving Cbl therapy should receive folate supplementation and should be followed for the development of iron deficiency because folate and iron will be consumed by proliferating tissues. In patients with severe anemia and megaloblastosis, the correction of cobalamin deficiency may lead to acute hypokalemia, hyperuricemia, and hypophosphatemia, because of the sudden increased proliferation of cells and turnover of DNA and proteins.

Patients with folate deficiency can be treated with a daily oral folate dose of 1–5 mg folate. Since Cbl deficiency may cause concomitant folate deficiency, it is important to make certain that the patient is not Cbl deficient before treating with folate alone. In patients with Cbl deficiency, the anemia may respond to high doses of folate; however, the neurologic disease will not improve, and delaying the appropriate therapy may cause irreversible damage.

Patients may have a dramatic improvement in their well-being shortly after receiving replacement therapy, even before an increase in hematocrit. The reticulocyte count increases in 2–3 days and peaks at day 8. A rise in the hemoglobin and hematocrit should be seen within a week, and the anemia should resolve within 2 months. Neurologic disease is not always reversible, and the potential for improvement decreases with increased duration of neurologic signs. Most patients will have maximal improvement in 6–12 months.

NORMOCYTIC ANEMIAS

The differential diagnosis of normocytic anemia is wide (Table 3-4). Macrocytic and microcytic anemias are usually normocytic at early stages of the disease, and a mixed anemia, such as combined folate and iron deficiency, may be reported as normocytic by an automated cell counter. Thus the peripheral smear should always be examined to confirm automated blood counter indices. Anemia with a normal MCV is seen in a variety of chronic diseases, as well as in disorders of primary bone marrow failure such as aplastic anemia and pure red cell aplasia. The anemia accompanying uremia, hypothyroidism, hyperthyroidism, and other endocrinopathies is usually normocytic.

Anemia of Chronic Disease

Anemia of chronic disease is seen in patients with chronic infectious or inflammatory conditions, malignancy, and autoimmune disorders. It is characterized by relatively low erythropoietin levels, a decreased marrow response to erythropoietin, and mildly shortened red cell survival. Patients have low iron and iron-binding capacity, with a transferrin saturation usually above 10%. Ferritin is an acute-phase reactant, and its levels are often increased. Bone marrow examination demonstrates adequate to increased iron stores in the reticuloendothelial system but a decreased amount of iron in RBC precursors.

Anemia of chronic disease resolves when the primary disorder is treated. In some patients, especially those with low erythropoietin levels; treatment with large doses of erythropoietin can be effective in improving the anemia. This has been shown in some malignancies (especially multiple myeloma), in HIV infection, and in some inflammatory conditions, such as rheumatoid arthritis. Erythropoietin is the mainstay of treatment of uremic anemia.

EVALUATION OF ANEMIA WITH RETICULOCYTOSIS

Hemolysis is the premature destruction of RBCs in blood vessels and/or in the vascular spaces of the reticuloendothelial system. The hallmark of hemolysis is a high reticulocyte count, as the normal bone marrow attempts to compensate for the reduced RBC mass and oxygen-carrying capacity. The only other condition causing reticulocytosis is blood loss. In evaluating a patient with suspected hemolysis, pertinent facts in the history include recent infections, all medications and drugs used; exposure to toxins, fumes, chemicals, and extreme temperatures; and a careful occupational, family, and travel history. The patient's ethnic and racial background may point to specific hereditary hemoglobinopathies and enzymopathies. Transfusions of blood and blood products should be noted. Physical findings in patients with hemolysis include pallor, jaundice, and splenomegaly. Patients with acute intravascular hemolysis such as that seen in transfusion reactions or paroxysmal nocturnal hemoglobinuria develop back pain and dark urine. Individuals with significant chronic hemolysis will develop the typical facies and skeletal changes that are caused by marrow expansion and seen also in thalassemia. Chronic hemolysis results in pigment gallstones at a young age.

Laboratory abnormalities include an anemia that is usually reported as macrocytic by electronic blood coulters, because reticulocytes are larger than mature RBCs. The peripheral blood smear is a valuable tool in the diagnosis, because the morphology of the RBC will often reflect the etiology of the destructive process (Table 3-3). Patients with hemolytic anemia and with megaloblastic anemia have indirect hyperbilirubinemia and an elevated lactic dehydrogenase. The plasma level of haptoglobin, the binder of free hemoglobin, is decreased, because once haptoglobin is bound to hemoglobin, it is rapidly cleared from the circulation by the liver. The direct antiglobulin (Coombs) test, which measures immunoglobulin and complement on the RBC surface, is positive in immune-mediated hemolysis. Patients with intravascular hemolysis will have hemoglobinuria, hemosiderinuria, and an elevation of free-plasma hemoglobin.

Hemolytic anemias may be caused by either intracorpuscular or extracorpuscular RBC abnormalities and may result from congenital or acquired conditions (Tables 3-9 and 3-10).

HEMOLYTIC ANEMIA CAUSED BY INTRACORPUSCULAR RBC ABNORMALITIES

Membrane Disorders

Hereditary spherocytosis (HS) is a heterogeneous disorder caused by mutations in genes encoding for RBC cytoskeletal membrane proteins. The disorder is almost always inherited in an autosomal dominant fashion, although autosomal recessive inheritance has been described in rare variants. The most common defects in HS are spectrin and ankyrin abnormalities; less frequently, patients may have an abnormal band 3 or protein 4.2 (Fig. 3-1). Patients with HS have a hemolytic anemia, splenomegaly, and spherocytes on peripheral blood smear. These spherocytes

TABLE 3-9. *CLASSIFICATION OF HEMOLYTIC ANEMIA*

Intracorpuscular abnormalities
    Enzymopathies
        G6PD deficiency
        Pyruvate kinase deficiency
        Others
    Hemoglobinopathies
    Membrane abnormalities
        Hereditary spherocytosis
        Hereditary elliptocytosis
        Hereditary pyropoikilocytosis
        Hereditary stomatocytosis
    Spur cell anemia
    Paroxysmal nocturnal hemoglobinuria

Extracorpuscular abnormalities
    Splenomegaly
    Autoimmune hemolytic anemia
    Microangiopathic hemolytic anemia
    Infections, toxins

TABLE 3-10. *COMMON DRUGS CAUSING HEMOLYSIS IN G6PD DEFICIENCY*

Antimicrobials
    Sulfonamides
    Nitrofurantoin
    Nalidixic acid
    Antimalarials
    Dapsone
    Chloramphenicol
    Doxorubicin

Others
    Aminosalicylic acid
    Phenacetin
    Probenecid
    Procainamide
    Vitamins C and K
    High-dose aspirin

are produced when RBCs with abnormal membrane structural proteins pass through the spleen and part of the cell membrane is removed. As a result, these RBCs lose their biconcave shape and become ball-shaped. They have a decreased cell membrane surface and are less able to undergo distention in a hypotonic solution. They therefore undergo lysis at a higher ambient osmolarity than normal RBCs, and the diagnosis of HS is made by an assay of osmotic fragility (Fig. 3-9).

Most HS patients have a compensated mild anemia, which worsens if reticulocytosis is suppressed, as may occur during infections and/or use of bone-marrow-

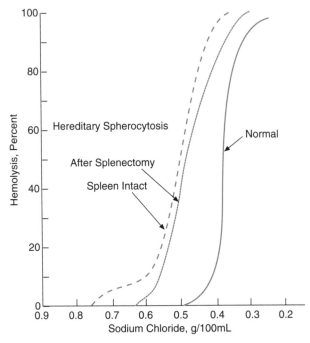

Figure 3-9. Osmotic fragility of RBC in a patient with hereditary spherocytosis before and after splenectomy. (Redrawn from Isselbacher KJ, et al., eds. *Harrison's Principles of Internal Medicine,* 13th ed. New York: McGraw-Hill, 1994:1539, Fig. 307-1. Osmotic fragility of red blood cells in hereditary spherocytosis.)

suppressive medications. Folic acid supplementation is necessary in many patients. Most HS patients also develop biliary pigment stones, which may require surgical intervention. In more severe cases, when patients have symptomatic anemia, splenectomy should be performed. This procedure decreases the degree of hemolysis and increases the RBC lifespan sufficiently to improve the anemia.

In **hereditary elliptocytosis** (**HE**), the cytoskeletal abnormalities involve sites of interactions between the cytoplasmic proteins, especially α- and β-spectrin and spectrin–protein 4.1. This results in oval or elliptical RBCs (Table 3-3) with a decreased lifespan. The inheritance is usually autosomal dominant, with most individuals remaining asymptomatic or exhibiting mild anemia and splenomegaly. A severe form of HE, called hereditary pyropoikilocytosis is characterized by autosomal recessive inheritance, severe anemia and fragmented RBC, microspherocytes, and eliptocytes on smear. The management of HE is similar to that of HS, with splenectomy reserved for patients with significant anemia.

A third RBC abnormality is **stomatocytosis,** characterized by the typical transverse slit (stoma) in RBCs on peripheral smear (Table 3-3). This condition is seen in rare hereditary disorders of membrane cation permeability; in acquired conditions such as alcoholism, neoplastic, vascular, and biliary disease; and as a rare side effect of drugs.

Acanthocytes, or **spur cells,** (Table 3-3) have membrane protrusions of varying size that are easily recognized on peripheral smear. They are found in patients with end-stage liver disease and are caused by the abnormal lipoproteins present in the plasma and RBC membrane in this condition. Acanthocytes may also be seen in the asplenic state, in severely malnourished patients, and in patients with malabsorption. Patients with abetalipoproteinemia, a congenital absence of β-lipoprotein, have similar morphologic changes on peripheral blood smear, and mild hemolysis. Uremic patients have RBCs with smaller symmetrical protrusions called **burr cells** or **echinocytes.**

Paroxysmal Nocturnal Hemoglobinuria

Paroxysmal nocturnal hemoglobinuria (PNH) is an acquired clonal disease in which hematopoietic cells lack the ability to synthesize a glycan-phosphatidylinositol (GPI) anchor that is required to bind complement regulators to the RBC membrane. The RBCs in PNH are abnormally sensitive to lysis by complement. The diagnosis can be made by demonstrating abnormal lysis of RBCs by acidic serum (HAM test) or hypotonic medium (sucrose lysis test), conditions that activate complement. Direct diagnosis can now be made by using flow cytometry to document absence of decay accelerating factor (DAF) and membrane inhibitor of reactive lysis (MIRL) on the RBC membrane. These two proteins are important regulators of complement function and are normally attached to the cell membrane by GPI.

PNH usually affects young adults and is manifested by acute episodes of back pain caused by intravascular hemolytic anemia. As the hemolysis occurs primarily in the intravascular spaces, the reticuloendothelial system does not capture all the liberated hemoglobin and iron, and this results in hemoglobinuria and/or hemosiderinuria (iron-laden urinary epithelial cells shed into the urine). Thrombotic complications (deep vein thrombosis, portal vein thrombosis, Budd–Chiari syndrome, mesenteric vein thrombosis, and thrombosis of cerebral veins) also occur in PNH and are thought to be caused by aggregation of platelets induced by the uninhibited complement activation. The disease is also associated with aplastic anemia, acute leukemia, and myelofibrosis. Patients have a normocytic anemia, mild thrombocytopenia and leukopenia, and a low leukocyte alkaline phosphatase level. Treatment is supportive. Patients should receive blood transfusions to suppress hematopoiesis of the abnormal clone, and corticosteroids are sometimes of benefit. Bone marrow transplantation should be considered in young patients, especially those with aplastic anemia or severe thrombotic complications.

RBC Enzymopathies

Glucose-6-Phosphate Dehydrogenase Deficiency. The most common abnormality of red cell metabolism is deficiency of glucose-6-phosphate dehydrogenase (G6PD), an enzyme that reduces pyridine nucleotide in the hexose-monophosphate shunt (Fig. 3-2). This pathway utilizes the metabolism of glucose to generate reduced glutathione, which protects sulfhydryl groups of hemoglobin and the RBC membrane from oxidation. In patients lacking G6PD, oxidant stresses such as infections, acidosis, and certain drugs and toxins (Table 3-10) cause precipitation of hemoglobin and intravascular hemolysis. The precipitation of hemoglobin can be visualized on peripheral smear as inclusion bodies (Heinz bodies) with a crystal violet stain. The peripheral smear may also demonstrate "bite cells," which are RBCs that have had the inclusion bodies and some adjacent membrane removed by the spleen (Table 3-3).

G6PD deficiency is an X-linked disorder, and heterozygote females only rarely have significant hemolysis. Two main clinical syndromes exist: a mild variant (seen in people of African origin) and a more severe condition (seen in people from Asia and the Mediterranean). The African variant is characterized by some reduced enzymatic activity, mostly in older RBCs. Hemolysis is usually self-limited, as reticulocytes and young RBCs have adequate enzyme levels. Patients with the Mediterranean variant may have chronic low-grade hemolysis and may develop life-threatening hemolysis when exposed to oxidant stress. For unclear reasons, these patients also develop severe hemolysis when they eat fava beans.

The diagnosis is established by measuring G6PD levels in blood, but patients who have just had an acute hemolytic episode may exhibit normal levels, reflecting the normal enzyme activity in the surviving reticulocytes and young RBCs. Treatment involves avoiding offending agents in susceptible patients and supportive care during an acute episode. Patients with chronic hemolysis may benefit from splenectomy.

Other Enzymopathies. Deficiencies of most of the enzymes of the glycolytic pathway have been reported, but of these by far the most common is pyruvate kinase deficiency. Most of these disorders are inherited in an autosomal recessive pattern, and patients have congenital, nonspherocytic hemolysis of varying degree. Treatment is supportive, with some patients requiring splenectomy.

Hemoglobinopathies

Hemoglobinopathies are disorders caused by the synthesis of abnormal hemoglobin. Like thalassemia and G6PD deficiency, common hemoglobinopathies are most prevalent among populations of the "malaria belt," because heterozygotes are relatively resistant to infection with falciparum malaria. The diagnosis of hemoglobinopathies is made by hemoglobin electrophoresis (Chapter 11).

Sickle Cell Disease. Sickle cell disease (SCD) is a common hemoglobinopathy among African-Americans, Africans, and natives of central India, the Mediterranean, and the Middle East. Hemoglobin S arises from a point mutation in the β-chain gene, that results in the substitution of valine for glutamic acid at the sixth amino acid position. Deoxygenated sickle hemoglobin has decreased solubility and may undergo polymerization, causing deformity of the erythrocyte (sickling) and hemolysis (Table 3-3).

Acute Manifestations of SCD. Sickle cell disease may cause acute abnormalities involving nearly every organ system (Table 3-11). The majority of these complications arise from episodic sickling leading to microvascular occlusion. Painful (vaso-occlusive) crises occur when deformed, sickled RBCs interact with platelets, endothelium, coagulation proteins, and other circulating factors to occlude the microcirculation. This causes tissue hypoxia, infarctions, and the characteristic recurrent pain episodes, which most commonly involve the chest, abdomen, back, and long bones. The vaso-occlusive events are often precipitated by infections, cold, exercise, pregnancy, and emotional stress. Children may suffer from a precipitous fall in hematocrit secondary to sequestration of blood in the spleen. However, recurrent splenic infarctions cause necrosis and fibrosis, and most adults with SCD are functionally asplenic. They therefore have an increased susceptibility to infections, especially with encapsulated bacterial organisms (Chapter 1).

The average RBC lifespan in a patient homozygous for sickle hemoglobin is

TABLE 3-11.	*CLINICAL MANIFESTATIONS OF SICKLE CELL DISEASE*	
ORGAN	**ACUTE MANIFESTATIONS**	**CHRONIC MANIFESTATIONS**
Pulmonary	Acute chest syndrome	Chronic hypoxemia
Genitourinary	Hematuria Papillary necrosis Priapism	Hyposthenuria Tubular defects Chronic renal failure
Neurologic	Thrombotic strokes Hemorrhagic strokes Seizures Transient ischemic attacks	Spinal disease Neovascularization, with aneurysm formation
Hepatobiliary	Right upper quadrant syndrome Viral hepatitis	Cholelithiasis Sickle hepatopathy
Skeletal	Osteomyelitis (esp. Salmonella) Bony infarcts	Avascular necrosis X-ray abnormalities (fishmouth deformity)
Ocular	Retinal ischemia/hemorrhage Retinal detachment	Proliferative retinopathy
Skin		Skin ulcers

only 17 days, compared with the normal 120 days. Patients with SCD have a chronic hemolytic anemia, with hematocrit values ranging from 18% to 32% and reticulocyte percentages around 10%. Because of the shortened RBC lifespan, patients are particularly sensitive to transient bone marrow suppression caused by infections such as parvovirus B19 (which specifically infects erythroid progenitors), pneumococcus, salmonella, Epstein-Barr virus, and others. In these settings they may develop an "aplastic crisis" characterized by a sudden drop in hematocrit, hemoglobin, and reticulocyte count. Patients may go on to develop bone marrow necrosis, with bone pain, fever, rapidly dropping counts, and a leukoerythroblastic picture in the peripheral blood. This may be further complicated by bone marrow emboli to the lungs.

Vaso-occlusive crises may cause significant morbidity and mortality when they affect vital organs. The **acute chest syndrome** is caused by sickling in the microvasculature of the lungs and is characterized by chest pain, shortness of breath, hypoxemia, fever, and infiltrates on chest x-ray. It is clinically indistinguishable from pneumonia, and all patients with the acute chest syndrome should receive antibiotic therapy (usually erythromycin, see later). The acute chest syndrome is life-threatening and is an indication for exchange transfusions and intensive monitoring.

Up to 25% of patients develop acute neurologic events, including seizures, thrombotic and hemorrhagic strokes, and transient ischemic attacks. Cerebral strokes resulting from large-vessel occlusion occur primarily in children, and 70% recur within 3 years without treatment. Stroke is an indication for long-term exchange transfusions, which have been shown to markedly decrease recurrent events. Adult sickle cell patients may develop acute hemorrhagic strokes as a result of neovascularization and aneurysm formation in the brain.

Acute genitourinary events are common in SCD. Recurrent priapism affects more than 50% of males with sickle cell disease. Priapism that persists for more than a few hours should be treated with exchange transfusions, in an effort to promote detumescence and prevent long-term complications of scarring and impotence. Surgery to decompress the corpora cavernosa may be indicated if conservative measures fail. Sickling in the renal medulla causes hematuria and papillary necrosis. However, sickle cell patients with hematuria should always be evaluated for other causes such as urinary tract infections, glomerulonephritis, tumor, and stones.

Sickle cell patients are prone to osteomyelitis, which must be differentiated from bone infarcts. The most common causative organisms include salmonella species, staphylococci, and enteric organisms. A bacterial diagnosis should be established before treatment.

Chronic Manifestations of SCD. Recurrent vaso-occlusive episodes and chronic hemolysis result in progressive dysfunction of virtually all organs (Table 3-11). Recurrent pulmonary insults usually result in a mild to moderate hypoxemia by the fourth or fifth decade of life and often leads to respiratory insufficiency and death. The acid and hypertonic renal medulla promotes sickling, and all patients with SCD develop chronic renal disease early in life. The first defect in renal function is hyposthenuria, inability of the kidney to concentrate the urine, which can be detected in the first decade of life. The inability to concentrate their urine makes sickle cell patients particularly susceptible to dehydration. Tubular defects may manifest as renal tubular acidosis and hyperkalemia. Other typical long-term complications of SCD include cholelithiasis, liver dysfunction, retinopathy, and chronic skin ulcers.

Treatment of Sickle Cell Disease. The mainstays of treatment of an acute vaso-occlusive episode are fluids, oxygen, folic acid supplementation, and narcotic analgesics. The precipitating event, which is usually an infection, should be sought and treated. Patients with symptomatic anemia and hematocrits below their baseline levels should be transfused, but their hematocrit should not be increased above 30% because the higher blood viscosity may worsen vaso-occlusive disease. Indications for exchange transfusions include acute chest syndrome with hypoxemia, stroke, bone marrow necrosis, acute ocular events, priapism, and intractable pain. The goal of exchange transfusions is usually to reduce the percent of sickle hemoglobin to less than 35%.

Infections should be treated promptly in an effort to prevent vaso-occlusive episodes and overwhelming sepsis in these functionally asplenic patients. Children are at an especially high risk for sepsis and benefit from prophylactic penicillin therapy to prevent *Streptococcus pneumoniae* infections. In adults the most common cause of pneumonia is *Mycoplasma pneumoniae* and these patients should be treated with erythromycin.

Patients undergoing surgery should be hydrated well and transfused to a hemoglobin of 10 g/dL in order to prevent perioperative morbidity. A recent multicenter randomized study concluded that this conservative transfusion regimen was as effective as an aggressive regimen of exchange transfusions to a percent hemoglobin S of less than 30% and was associated with fewer transfusion reactions.

Patients should receive polyvalent pneumococcal vaccine and yearly influenza vaccine. Other general preventive measures include routine folic acid supplementation and yearly eye checkups for retinal disease. Sexually active women should be advised about contraception and about the high risk to mother and fetus during pregnancy: Complications during pregnancy include pyelonephritis, pulmonary infarctions, pneumonia, the acute chest syndrome, post-partum hemorrhage, prematurity, and fetal death. Prophylactic exchange transfusions are controversial in pregnancy but should be considered for evidence of intrauterine growth retardation. Abortions and miscarriages may trigger an acute sickling event, and women should be monitored appropriately.

A recent randomized study has demonstrated that hydroxyurea increases the level of fetal hemoglobin in patients with SCD and reduces the number and severity of painful episodes. The higher concentration of γ-hemoglobin in the RBCs prevents vaso-occlusive episodes by forming $\alpha_2\beta^s\gamma$ tetramers, which do not polymerize and do not cause sickling. Butyric acid has similar effects on fetal hemoglobin and is being evaluated in ongoing clinical trials.

A significant number of patients with SCD develop iron overload, primarily as a result of chronic transfusions. Patients with ferritin above 2,500–3,000 ng/mL should be started on chronic chelation therapy with deferoxamine.

Health care providers should always bear in mind that sickle cell anemia is a chronic condition, and patients must cope with recurrent painful and life-threatening episodes. Management of these cases demands a willingness to provide long-term emotional support.

Sickle Cell Trait. Sickle cell trait is found in 8–10% of African-Americans, and rarely has clinical manifestations. Individuals are not anemic and do not suffer from vaso-occlusive episodes. However, they may develop hematuria, isosthenuria, and rarely, retinal complications. These individuals should receive genetic counseling about the risk of a hemoglobinopathy in their offspring if their partner carries one or more genes for SCD, hemoglobin C (see later), or β-thalassemia. Prenatal diagnosis is available for all the common hemoglobinopathies.

Other Hemoglobinopathies. In hemoglobin C, glutamic acid is replaced by lysine at the sixth amino acid of the β-globin chain. The mutation is prevalent in West Africa, and the trait is found in about 2% of African-Americans. Patients homozygous for hemoglobin C usually have a mild hemolytic anemia and require minimal therapy. Their peripheral blood smear demonstrates multiple target cells and folded RBCs, some with intracellular crystals (Table 3-3). Patients with hemoglobin SC have a milder sickling syndrome than patients with hemoglobin SS. The SC patients tend to have splenomegaly and a higher incidence of retinopathy. Patients with sickle hemoglobin and β^+-thalassemia also usually have milder disease than those homozygous for sickle hemoglobin. However, patients with sickle-β^{0-} thalassemia make no normal β-hemoglobin and have the same phenotype as patients with SS disease. Hemoglobin E is prevalent in Southeast Asia, especially in Burma and Thailand, and results from a mutation at amino acid 26 of the β-chain gene. Homozygotes are asymptomatic and have mild anemia with microcytosis and target cells. Heterozygotes have only microcytosis.

HEMOLYTIC ANEMIA CAUSED BY EXTRACORPUSCULAR ABNORMALITIES

Immune Hemolysis

In immune hemolysis, accelerated destruction of RBCs is caused by coating the cell membrane with antibodies and/or complement. Diagnosis is made by the direct antiglobulin (Coombs) test, in which antibodies against immunoglobulins and complement are mixed with the patient's RBCs. The cells are then tested for ag-

TABLE 3-12. AUTOIMMUNE HEMOLYTIC ANEMIA

TYPE	ASSOCIATED CONDITIONS	ANTIBODY CLASS	COMPLEMENT FIXING	DIRECT ANTIGLOBULIN TEST (DAT) (DIRECT COOMBS TEST)		INDIRECT ANTIGLOBULIN TEST (INDIRECT COOMBS TEST)	LOCATION OF HEMOLYSIS		COMMENTS
				IgG	Complement		RES	Intravascular	
Warm Autoimmune Hemolytic Anemia									
AIHA	Collagen vascular disease Thyroid diseases Infections CLL NHL Myeloma Hodgkin's disease Other neoplasms	Usually IgG	Occasionally	+	+/−	+	+	−	Typical findings include microspherocytes and splenomegaly. Therapy: immunosupression, splenectomy
Drug-Induced Hemolytic Anemia									
Type I Hapten drug adsorption	High dose penicillin		Rarely	+	−	+ if test RBC are incubated with drug	+	slight	Drug binds to RBC membrane. Antibody is directed against drug.

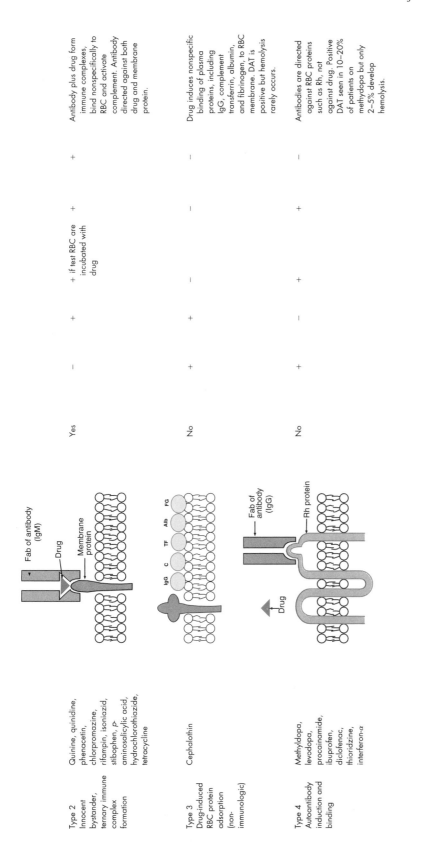

	Drugs						Comments
Type 2 Innocent bystander, ternary immune complex formation	Quinine, quinidine, phenacetin, chlorpromazine, rifampin, isoniazid, stibophen, p-aminosalicylic acid, hydrochlorothiazide, tetracycline	Yes	−	+	+ if test RBC are incubated with drug	+	Antibody plus drug form immune complexes, bind nonspecifically to RBC and activate complement. Antibody directed against both drug and membrane protein.
Type 3 Drug-induced RBC protein adsorption (non-immunologic)	Cephalothin	No	+	+	−	−	Drug induces nonspecific binding of plasma proteins, including IgG, complement transferrin, albumin, and fibrinogen, to RBC membrane. DAT is positive but hemolysis rarely occurs.
Type 4 Autoantibody induction and binding	Methyldopa, levodopa, procainamide, ibuprofen, diclofenac, thioridzine, interferon-α	No	+	−	+	−	Antibodies are directed against RBC proteins such as Rh, not against drug. Positive DAT seen in 10–20% of patients on methyldopa but only 2–5% develop hemolysis.

(continued)

TABLE 3-12. *(continued)*

TYPE	ASSOCIATED CONDITIONS	ANTIBODY CLASS	COMPLEMENT FIXING	DIRECT ANTIGLOBULIN TEST (DAT) (DIRECT COOMBS TEST)		INDIRECT ANTIGLOBULIN TEST (INDIRECT COOMBS TEST)	LOCATION OF HEMOLYSIS		COMMENTS
				IgG	Complement		RES	Intravascular	
Cold Autoimmune Hemolytic Anemia									
Cold agglutinin	Polyclonal: Mycoplasma (anti-I), IMN (anti-i), CMV, listeriosis, mumps, SBE, syphilis, collagen vascular disease. Monoclonal: Waldenstroms macroglobulinemia, lymphoma, CLL, Kaposi's sarcoma, myeloma	IgM	Yes	−	+	+/−	+ (liver and bone marrow not spleen)	+	IgM and complement bind to RBC in cold periphery (hands, feet). IgM drops off as RBC moves to warm body core, complement is left. Therapy: treat cause, plasmapheresis, avoid cold.
Paroxysmal cold hemoglobinuria	Syphilis, postviral (measles, mumps, others)	IgG (Donath-Landsteiner antibody)	Yes	+ (in cold)	+ (during attack)	+ (in cold)	+	++	Same sequence as above.

AIHA = Autoimmune hemolytic anemia; RES = reticuloendothelial system; CLL = chronic lymphocytic lymphoma; NHL = non-Hodgkin's lymphoma; RBC = red blood cells; DAT = direct antiglobulin test; IMN = infectious mononucleosis; CMV = cytomegalovirus; SBE = subacute bacterial endocarditis. (Figures redrawn from Packman CH, Leddy JP. Drug-related IHA. In: Beutler E, Lichtman MA, Coller BS, Kipps TJ, eds. Williams Hematology, 5th ed. New York: McGraw-Hill, 1995:693.)

glutination, which occurs if there is immunoglobulin or complement on the RBC membrane. The indirect antiglobulin (Coombs) test looks for the presence of antibodies in the patient's serum and is positive in about 80% of patients with immune hemolytic anemia.

Antibodies causing immune hemolysis are usually categorized into two groups, those with maximal activity at body temperature (warm antibodies, usually IgG, rarely IgA) and those with maximal activity in the cold (cold antibodies, usually IgM, occasionally IgG). Each group of antibodies is associated with several distinct clinical syndromes (Table 3-12) .

"Warm-Type" Immune Hemolytic Anemia. In "warm-type" immune hemolytic anemia, antibody production can be either primary (idiopathic) or secondary to conditions such as autoimmune diseases (systemic lupus erythematosus, anticardiolipin syndrome), lymphoproliferative disorders (chronic lymphocytic leukemia, lymphomas), drugs, and neoplasms. Idiopathic immune hemolytic anemia is most commonly seen in middle-aged women. Patients usually present with jaundice and symptoms of anemia, and about a third have an enlarged spleen. Laboratory findings include anemia and an increased reticulocyte count. The peripheral blood smear will show spherocytes, which result from the action of the spleen macrophages on the membrane of antibody-coated RBCs. Nucleated RBCs are seen when the hemolysis is brisk (Table 3-3). The absence of reticulocytosis does not rule out hemolysis because on rare occasions antibodies are directed against reticulocytes too, and/or patients may be folate or iron deficient. Patients will, however, usually have a low haptoglobin, and if the hemolysis is intravascular, an elevated plasma hemoglobin.

The diagnosis is made by the direct antiglobulin (Coombs) test, which demonstrates IgG, usually IgG_1 and IgG_3, on the RBC membrane. Both subclasses of IgG can activate complement, and in some cases complement (C3d) is also found on the RBC membrane.

Treatment of immune hemolytic anemia involves controlling the underlying condition causing the hemolysis if possible, suppressing antibody production, and/or inhibiting the clearance of antibody-coated RBCs in the spleen and liver. Corticosteroids inhibit macrophage activity and suppress antibody production, and are the first-line therapy in most patients. Immunosuppressive therapy such as cyclophosphamide, chlorambucil, and azathioprine may be used as steroid-sparing agents to suppress the antibody-producing clone. Danazol, a synthetic androgen that inhibits macrophage function and may have other nonspecific effects on the immune system, is beneficial in some patients. Intravenous immunoglobulin blocks macrophage activity and may work in selected patients. Splenectomy may be considered in patients who are steroid dependent and refractory to other therapy, and is effective in about 50% of patients.

Drug-Induced Hemolysis. Alpha methyldopa is an antihypertensive that induces antibodies against the RBC membrane in about 20% of patients. However, clinically significant hemolytic anemia in these patients is rare. Other drugs induce anti-RBC antibody either by binding to the RBC membrane (penicillin, cephalosporins, and others) or by inducing immune complexes (quinidine, sulfonamides, and others). Treatment in all cases involves removing the offending agent(Table 3-12).

"Cold-Type" Immune Hemolytic Anemia. A transient cold-type immune hemolysis is usually associated with infections, especially those caused by *Mycoplasma pneumonia* and Epstein-Barr virus (EBV). The pathologic immunoglobulin is IgM, and its maximal activity is at the range of 4–18°C. IgM activates complement at this temperature, and this occurs in the extremities where the temperature is lower. The complement cascade is completed as the RBCs travel through the warm visceral circulation, resulting in intravascular hemolysis. The direct antiglobulin (Coombs) test usually demonstrates only C3b on the RBC membrane, as the IgM falls off when the RBC warms up during its passage through the circulation. The antibody (cold agglutinin) is polyclonal and is usually directed either against blood group I (in *Mycoplasma pneumoniae* infections) or i (in EBV infections). Patients often develop hemolysis and anemia during the recovery phase of the infection. Treatment is supportive, and the hemolysis is self-limiting.

Chronic cold agglutinin disease is usually seen in older patients, ages 50–80 years, and is often associated with a monoclonal IgM antibody and an underlying lymphoproliferative disorder (chronic lymphocytic leukemia, Waldenstrom's macroglobulinemia). Patients usually have a low-grade anemia but occasionally develop significant intravascular hemolysis and renal failure. Treatment includes avoidance of exposure to the cold, and corticosteroids may benefit some patients. Splenectomy is not recommended, because RBCs coated with C3b are cleared mainly in the liver, not the spleen.

Paroxysmal cold hemoglobinuria is seen in advanced stages of syphilis (Donath-Landsteiner antibody) and as a postviral syndrome. The antibody is an IgG, reactive both in the cold and at 37°C, and is capable of activating complement.

Microangiopathic Hemolytic Anemia

In microangiopathic hemolytic anemia, hemolysis is caused by the traumatic fragmentation of RBCs either during passage through damaged blood vessels or through a prosthetic heart valve. This entity is seen in disseminated intravascular coagulation (Chapter 6), the thrombotic thrombocytopenia purpura/hemolytic uremic syndromes, preeclampsia and eclampsia, the HELLP syndrome of pregnancy (hemolysis, elevated liver enzymes, low platelet count), widely metastatic tumors, and during the administration of some medications (mitomycin C, cyclosporine). The diagnosis may by made by reviewing the peripheral blood smear, which demonstrates fragmented RBCs, also called schistocytes (Table 3-3). Treatment involves controlling the primary process, and is discussed in Chapters 5 and 6.

Hemolysis Associated with Infections

Bacterial toxins and other products can cause direct damage to RBC membranes and hemolysis. This is seen in clostridial sepsis, and sepsis and/or endocarditis from streptococci, staphylococci, and enterococci. Direct RBC infestation by organisms such as plasmodium in malaria, babesia in babesiosis, and bartonella in bartonellosis causes severe intravascular hemolysis. The diagnosis is readily made by demonstrating the parasites in the RBC on peripheral smear (Table 3-3).

EVALUATION OF ERYTHROCYTOSIS

Erythrocytosis is defined as an increase in the red cell mass (generally 36 mL/kg in men and 32 mL/kg in women). This condition is usually suspected by an increase in the hemoglobin concentration and hematocrit. However, these measurements depend on the blood volume. Thus if the patient has a contracted plasma volume, the hemoglobin and hematocrit will increase but the red cell mass remains constant.

A true increase in the red cell mass is caused either by tissue hypoxia, excess secretion of erythropoietin, or autonomous growth and maturation of red cell precursors, independent of the usual regulatory processes (Table 3-13). Tissue hypoxia causing increased erythropoietin secretion is the most common cause of erythrocytosis. In high altitudes with reduced oxygen pressure, improved oxygen-carrying capacity is obtained by an increase in the red cell mass. A similar compensatory mechanism is seen in patients with chronic hypoxemia secondary to lung disease, a right-to-left shunt, and chronic carbon monoxide poisoning. Patients with the sleep apnea syndrome suffer from intermittent nocturnal hypoxemia, resulting in erythrocytosis. The diagnosis is easily missed if it is not sought, because these patients have normal arterial pO_2 during the day. Patients with high-affinity hemoglobins, which release oxygen to the tissues at a lower pO_2 than normal hemoglobin, also develop erythrocytosis because the tissues are hypoxemic.

Inappropriately high erythropoietin levels are seen most commonly in patients with kidney disease, especially with renal cysts and/or hydronephrosis. Up to 15% of patients who have undergone renal transplants develop erythrocytosis secondary to increased erythropoietin secretion. Occasionally, certain tumors may secrete erythropoietin autonomously, and these include renal cell carcinoma, hepatocellular carcinoma, hemangioblastoma of the cerebellum, and tumors of the uterus. Increased erythropoietin levels are also seen in women treated with androgens.

TABLE 3-13. *DIFFERENTIAL DIAGNOSIS OF ERYTHROCYTOSIS*

Spurious Erythrocytosis (reduced plasma volume)
   Dehydration
   Pre-eclampsia
   Hypertension

Increased Red Cell Mass
   Hypoxemia
      High altitude
      Chronic lung disease
      Sleep apnea syndrome
      Right-to-left shunt (congenital heart disease; A-V malformation)
   Kidney diseases
      Hydronephrosis
      Polycystic kidney disease
      Renal transplant
   Tumors
      Renal cell carcinoma
      Hepatocellular carcinoma
      Cerebellar hemangioblastoma
      Other erythropoietin-secreting tumors
   Endocrine disorders
      Thyrotoxicosis
      Androgen therapy
   Familial erythrocytosis
   Myeloproliferative disorders

Polycythemia vera is a myeloproliferative disorder in which red cell precursors divide and mature independently, and do not respond to the usual regulation by erythropoietin. (Erythropoietin levels are typically decreased.) This is a clonal disorder characterized by an increase in all three cell lines, with the increase in hematocrit and hemoglobin being the most prominent (Chapter 9).

Patients with erythrocytosis often have symptoms related to increased blood volume and viscosity, such as headaches, visual disturbances, hypertension, and thrombosis (strokes, ischemic heart disease, and peripheral vascular disease).

A workup for a patient with a high hemoglobin and hematocrit should include a thorough history with regard to recent travel to high altitudes, sleep apnea, smoking, exposure to carbon monoxide (suggested by a faulty furnace at home and symptoms in other family members or a history of heavy smoking), and other affected family members (suggesting familial high-affinity hemoglobins). In the physical examination the patient should be evaluated for evidence of increased blood viscosity. An enlarged spleen supports the diagnosis of polycythemia vera. A murmur or bruit over the heart or lungs may suggest the diagnosis of a right-to-left shunt (Chapter 2).

The diagnosis of erythrocytosis can be established by the measurement of the red cell mass. This test is performed by isotope dilution, and results are expressed in milliliters per kilogram. However, this test is unreliable in many laboratories. Consequently, if the clinical suspicion of erythrocytosis is high, the diagnosis should be entertained despite a normal red cell mass. Evaluation should also include an arterial oxygen pressure, erythropoietin levels, carbon monoxide levels, and hemoglobin electrophoresis. Patients should have imaging studies of their kidneys and workup for sleep apnea syndrome if there are clinical suspicions of renal disease or sleep apnea.

Treatment includes addressing the cause in patients with secondary erythrocytosis, and phlebotomy to reduce the hematocrit to below 45%. The treatment of polycythemia vera is discussed in Chapter 9.

CASE PRESENTATION

A 40-year-old white man comes to see you for a routine checkup. He is a recreational runner who occasionally takes aspirin or nonsteroidal anti-inflammatory drugs for joint aches, especially after 10-km races. His most recent competition was 5 days ago. Your physical examination is not remarkable. However, a sample of stool is not normal. It is brown but it stained weakly for occult blood with the guaiac reagent. His hemoglobin and hematocrit are found to be 13.2 g/dL and 38.1%, respectively.

Question 1. Should you be concerned?

Answer. Yes. Even though the patient may have been taking medications that can lead to blood loss from the gastrointestinal tract and despite the fact that his hemoglobin and hematocrit are only slightly reduced, further evaluation is warranted.

Question 2. What should you do next?

Answer. The patient's peripheral blood smear should be carefully examined and red blood cell (RBC) indices should be obtained.

Examination of the peripheral smear shows that there is some anisocytosis and poikilocytosis of the RBCs and little polychromasia. White blood

cells and platelets are normal in appearance. MCV is 79 fL/RBC, MCH is 26 pg/RBC, and MCHC is 32 g/dL RBC.

Question 3. What clues do you have from the peripheral smear and indexes and what do you do next?

Answer. The lack of polychromasia suggests that despite the patient's anemia there is little response by the bone marrow, which should now be releasing many younger RBCs. On Wright's stain (the usual peripheral blood smear stain) immature RBCs would appear as large cells with no central pallor and a ground-glass gray-purple appearance. You should now request a reticulocyte count, which utilizes another stain (usually new-methylene blue or brilliant cresyl blue), to bring out the polyribosomes and other protein synthetic apparatus that mark cells as reticulocytes.

This is done and the reticulocyte count is 1%. By using the formulas on page 55, it is determined that the corrected reticulocyte count is 0.79% and the reticulocyte production index (RPI) is 0.39%.

These data confirm the suspicion that there was a poor response by the bone marrow to the patient's anemia. One would expect that the RPI would reveal that erythrocytes are being produced at several times the normal rate. Instead, the response is less than one-half the normal rate of 1%. This indicates that despite the stimulus of the patient's anemia, the bone marrow is underproducing RBCs.

Question 4. What should you be thinking now?

Answer. Reasons for the low hematocrit and the underproduction of RBCs should now be considered. At this time the patient has a hypochromic, microcytic anemia with a hypoproliferative bone marrow response. With evidence of blood in the stool (which should be confirmed by more stool testing for occult blood), gastrointestinal blood loss leading to iron deficiency should be thought of first. Iron deficiency would not allow compensatory RBC production by the bone marrow. If RBC were being destroyed (e.g., by spleen-mediated hemolysis) or sequestered (e.g., in an enlarged spleen), iron would be recycled and allow the normal bone marow machinery to produce RBCs. If, on the other hand, the marrow were biochemically impeded in its desire to compensate because of lack of the proper nutrients (iron, folate, B_{12}) or structurally blocked by the presence of inflammation, infection, tumor, lymphoma, fibrosis, granuloma, then a hypoproliferative response would be seen, as it is here.

Question 5. What is the next step in your evaluation?

Answer. More stool samples for occult blood should be obtained and iron studies from serum samples should be analyzed.

These are obtained. The stool is brown but tests positively for occult blood.

> Serum ferritin = 2ng/mL.
> Serum iron = 30 μg/dL.
> Serum total iron binding capacity = 500μg/dL.

Question 6. How do you interpret these data?

Answer. They confirm that severe iron deficiency is present despite the minimally reduced hemoglobin and hematocrit.

Question 7. Should further hematologic testing be performed now (e.g., a bone marrow examination)?

Answer. Although a bone marrow test would help assess the presence or absence of storage iron and allow consideration of other diagnostic possibilities for the poor bone marrow response (e.g., a superimposed megaloblastic state), there is no evidence (e.g., macro-ovalocytes) to suggest a secondary phenomenon now, as judged by the peripheral smear. Also, the data already obtained are characteristic for iron deficiency anemia from gastrointestinal blood loss.

Question 8. What should be done next?

Answer. The patient requires a full gastrointestinal evaluation to discover the site of blood loss. Both upper and lower gastrointestinal regions must be considered.

Follow-up:

The patient underwent gastrointestinal imaging studies and was found to have a cecal adenocarcinoma. He was treated surgically and a good-prognosis lesion was found. He has required no further therapy and remains disease-free after 5 years.

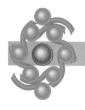

CASE PRESENTATION

A 60-year-old woman was admitted to the hospital with anemia. She had been well previously except for "arthritis" and had been taking naproxen for 17 months for this problem.

One week before admission she found herself to be short of breath while walking up three steps to her front porch. Her next-door neighbor remarked that she looked "yellow in the eyes." When she noticed dark-colored urine she became alarmed and visited a walk-in clinic near her home. The physician there became alarmed when he noted her hematocrit and transferred her to your hospital's emergency room, where you were the first to see her.

The physical examination showed a woman who appeared fatigued and jaundiced. Her sclerae were icteric. The patient demonstrated no other skin or mucous membrane abnormalities. There was no lymphadenopathy. Heart and lung examinations were normal, but the abdominal examination showed the spleen to extend 3 cm below the left costal margin with no other abnormalities in the physical examination.

The hemoglobin was 5 g/dL and the hematocrit 15.3% with a normal white blood count and platelet count.

Question 1. What is the next step?

Answer. Review of the peripheral blood smear. The platelets and WBCs were normal. The RBC series showed marked anisocytosis and poikilocytosis. Spherocytes and blister cells were abundantly present as were cells demonstrating polychromatophilia (polychromasia).

Question 2. What test would you now perform to confirm suspicions that the bone marrow was responding to the low hemoglobin and hematocrit?

Answer. A reticulocyte count (corrected) was 8%.

Question 3. How could you further define the nature of her anemia?

Answer. Coombs testing was performed showing that the direct antibody determination was positive and the indirect component was negative. The cells were found to be coated with an IgG antibody.

Question 4. How would it be best to approach this patient therapeutically given the preceding data?

Answer. It is likely this patient has a warm antibody-associated hemolytic anemia, perhaps associated with an underlying collagen vascular disease or Naproxen. The Naproxen should be discontinued. The patient should receive blood transfusions because she has a profoundly low hematocrit and is symptomatic. Corticosteroids should be given in high doses and should be slowly tapered off after the hematocrit is stabilized.

Follow-up:

The patient continued to have profound hemolysis despite large corticosteroid dosages. Danazol was added to her regimen with no apparent benefit. Splenectomy was considered and the patient was given vaccines against the encapsulated organisms *Haemophilus influenzae, Streptococcus pneumoniae, and Neisseria meningitidis.* She underwent splenectomy with good control of the hemolytic process. Corticosteroids were slowly tapered off postoperatively and there has been continuing remission of the hemolytic anemia.

CASE PRESENTATION

A 39-year-old man was noted to have an elevated hematocrit when blood work was performed in conjunction with an insurance physical examination. He was referred to you for further assessment and advice. He has occasional headaches and has poorly controlled hypertension, although he is taking a diuretic medication. He drinks "an occasional beer" and smokes several packs of cigarettes per day. Your physical examination shows him to be an obese man with a ruddy complexion. His blood pressure is 160/97 but there are no other abnormalities that you can find on thorough physical examination. A complete blood count is drawn and shows the following: White blood cells are 9900/μL with a normal differential count. Platelets are 489,000/μL. Hemoglobin is 18.4 g/dL. Hematocrit is 53.7%.

Question 1. How should you approach this patient?

Answer. The first major diagnostic information should substantiate that there is true or *absolute* erythrocytosis and not *relative* erythrocytosis. This is best established by using nuclear medicine techniques to determine both the red cell mass and plasma volume. It is important in this patient, who has predisposing factors for the development of both *absolute* erythrocytosis (the cigarette smoking, which leads to carbon monoxide binding to hemoglobin, reduced delivery of oxygen to tissues, increased erythropoietin secretion, and subsequent increases in red blood cell production) and *relative* erythrocytosis (the diuretic use, which would reduce plasma volume and thereby create an increase in the hematocrit).

Question 2. This is done, and true or absolute erythrocytosis is found (red cell volume = 39 mL of RBC/kg). What do you do next?

Answer. The causes of true erythrocytosis are many. In designing the best diagnostic approach, clinical urgency, invasiveness, and cost are some of the factors that should be considered. In this patient you have already determined that the increase in hematocrit is real, but he is asymptomatic, so a precise and measured diagnostic approach can be undertaken. His oxygen saturation level determined by pulse oximetry is normal. His carboxyhemoglobin level is (not surprisingly) found to be elevated. He has his home checked for sources of carbon monoxide leaks and finds none. (Even if the carboxyhemoglobin level is normal when you checked it, erythrocytosis could be the only indicator of *intermittent* exposure to this deadly gas.) You ask the patient to discontinue smoking, and to your delight but astonishment he does so. A month later a repeat carboxyhemoglobin level is normal, but his hematocrit is now further elevated at 56%.

Question 3. What do you do next?

Answer. An erythropoietin level is now obtained. (*Note:* Some would have done this test earlier.) It is found to be markedly elevated at 94 units.

Question 4. What does this mean? What should you consider now?

Answer. The diagnosis of polycythemia vera (PCV) becomes less likely now. This entity develops independent of erythropoietin stimulus of erythrocyte stem cells and in PCV, erythropoietin levels are low. Therefore events and diseases that cause an increase in erythropoietin should now be seriously entertained. He has had his home checked for carbon monoxide leaks and found none. Sleep apnea is another intermittent problem that has consequences later in the day. The nocturnal hypoxemia with which it is associated is a cause of erythrocytosis and should be considered in this situation, especially if clues such as apneic spells and snoring are obtained from the patient or family members. The wife reports thunderous snoring from her husband of 25 years, and you schedule a sleep study.

Question 5. The patient undergoes a sleep study, which is normal. Testing for high-affinity hemoglobin showed no abnormalities. Where do you move next?

Answer. Because of the association of erythrocytosis and high levels of erythropoietin with certain tumors, the evaluation for such neoplasms should be undertaken. These include cerebellar hemangioblastomas (unlikely without symptoms here), hepatocellular carcinomas, renal cell carcinomas, and, in women, uterine tumors.

Question 6. What next?

Answer. The patient undergoes CT scan of the abdomen and a renal mass is discovered. A repeat urinalysis shows hematuria. (It showed none a month before.) CT-guided biopsy shows the mass to be a renal cell carcinoma, and it is surgically removed after workup for distant metastases showed none. At operation there is no lymph node involvement or vascular invasion.

Follow-up:

The patient recuperated nicely after surgery. The hematocrit normalized and after 4 years he has shown no evidence of recurrence or metastatic disease.

SELECTED READING

GENERAL STUDIES

Berliner N, Duffy TP, Ablelson HT. Approach to the adult and child with anemia. In: Hoffman RH, et al., eds. *Hematology: Basic Principles and Practice,* 2nd ed. New York: Churchill Livingstone; 1995:468–483.
A practical approach to the etiology of the anemias, complete with tables outlining the different categories grouped by reticulocyte count and MCV.

Beutler E. The common anemias. *JAMA* 1988;259:2433–2437.
A comprehensive and concise description of iron deficiency anemia, thalassemia, and the anemia of chronic disease, including pathogenesis, diagnosis, and treatment.

Tabbara IA. Erythropoietin: biology and clinical applications. *Arch Intern Med* 1993; 153:298–304.
A concise review of the structure and function of erythropoietin and its role in the treatment of anemia of uremia, malignancy, and chronic disease.

IRON DEFICIENCY ANEMIA

Brittenham GM. Disorders of iron metabolism: iron deficiency and overload. In: Hoffman RH, et al., eds. *Hematology: Basic Principles and Practice,* 2nd ed. New York: Churchill Livingstone; 1995:492–522.
A detailed description of iron metabolism, the laboratory evaluation of iron deficiency, and the clinical manifestations and therapy of iron deficiency and overload.

DISORDERS OF HEMOGLOBIN

Bunn HF. Sickle hemoglobin and other hemoglobin mutants. In: Stamatoyannopoulos G, Nienhuis AW, Majerus PW, Varmus H, eds. *The Molecular Basis of Blood Diseases,* 2nd ed. Philadelphia: WB Saunders, 1994:207–256.
A review of the molecular basis and pathophysiology of the hemoglobinopathies.

Bunn HF, Forget BG. *Hemoglobin: Molecular, Genetic and Clinical Aspects.* Philadelphia: WB Saunders; 1986.
Thorough discussions of the structure and function of hemoglobin and the thalassemias, sickle cell disease, and other hemoglobinopathies.

Embury SH, Hebbel RP, Mohandas N, Steinberg MH. *Sickle Cell Disease: Basic Principles and Clinical Practice.* New York: Raven Press; 1994.
A comprehensive text covering all aspects of sickle cell disease, including the molecular basis, pathophysiology, clinical manifestations, and management of the disorder.

Weatherall DJ. The thalassemias. In: Stamatoyannopoulos, G, Nienhuis AW, Majerus PW, Varmus H, eds. *The Molecular Basis of Blood Diseases,* 2nd ed. Philadelphia: WB Saunders; 1994:157–206.
A review of the molecular basis of the thalassemias, with a section on epidemiology, natural history, and management.

HEMOLYTIC ANEMIAS

Benz EJ, Jr. The erythrocyte membrane and cytoskeleton: structure, function, and disorders. In: Stamatoyannopoulos G, Nienhuis AW, Majerus PW, Varmus H, eds. *The Molecular Basis of Blood Diseases,* 2nd ed. Philadelphia: WB Saunders, 1994:257–292.
A review of the structure and function of the erythrocyte membrane lipids and proteins with the corresponding molecular defects.

Paglia DE. Enzymopathies. In: Hoffman RH, et al., eds. *Hematology: Basic Principles and Practice,* 2nd ed. New York: Churchill Livingstone; 1995:656–666.
A concise review of the enzymopathies associated with hemolysis.

Palek J, Kahr KE. Mutations of the red blood cell membrane proteins: from clinical evaluation to detection of the underlying genetic defect. *Blood* 1992;(80):308–330.
An overview of the known molecular defects of the RBC membrane proteins and their clinical correlates.

Schwartz RS, Silberstein LE, Berkman EM. Autoimmune hemolytic anemias. In: Hoffman RH, et al., eds. *Hematology: Basic Principles and Practice,* 2nd ed. New York: Churchill Livingstone; 1995:710–728.
A review of the immunologic mechanisms of RBC destruction, clinical findings in the various types of hemolysis, and their management.

MEGALOBLASTIC ANEMIAS

Anthony AC. Megaloblastic anemias. In: Hoffman RH, et al., eds. *Hematology: Basic Principles and Practice,* 2nd ed. New York: Churchill Livingstone; 1995:552–585.
A thorough discussion of the metabolism of B12 and folic acid and the etiology, pathogenesis, clinical manifestations, and therapy of megaloblastic anemia.

Schilling RF, Williams WJ. Vitamin B_{12} deficiency: underdiagnosed, overtreated? *Hosp Pract* 1995;30(7):47–52.
Emphasizes the need for prompt parenteral therapy in patients with pernicious anemia and neurologic symptoms. Questions the role of therapy in patients with borderline B_{12} levels.

Toh BH, van Driel IR, Gleeson PA. Mechanisms of disease: pernicious anemia. *New Engl J Med* 337:1441–1448, 1997.
An up-to-date review of the pathogenesis, manifestations, and treatment of pernicious anemia.

ERYTHROCYTOSIS

JL Spivak. Erythrocytosis. In: Hoffman RH, et al., eds, *Hematology: Basic Principles and Practice,* 2nd ed. New York: Churchill Livingstone; 1995:484–491.
A discussion of the etiology, differential diagnosis, evaluation and therapy of erythrocytosis.

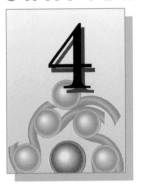

White Blood Cells

Alan G. Rosmarin

White blood cells, or leukocytes, constitute a primary source of the host's defense against invading microorganisms. This diverse group of cells includes the major effectors of the immune and inflammatory responses. Because of their crucial role in initiating and propagating the inflammatory response, leukocytes also play important roles in pathologic states of inflammation such as autoimmune disorders.

The term *leukocyte* reflects their white appearance (*leukos* in Greek) in a centrifuged specimen of blood. Leukocytes constitute a heterogeneous group of cells that can be categorized by their site of origin (myeloid versus lymphoid) and by their functional roles (phagocytes versus immunocytes). In clinical practice, leukocytes are commonly described by nuclear morphology (polymorphonuclear versus mononuclear) and by the presence of cytoplasmic inclusions (granulocytes).

NEUTROPHILS

Neutrophilic granulocytes are the most abundant circulating leukocytes (Fig. 4-1). The term *neutrophil* refers to the appearance of their cytoplasmic granules following Wright-Giemsa staining. Together with eosinophils and basophils, they are classified as granulocytes. Because of the characteristic multilobed nucleus of the neutrophil, this cell is also known as a polymorphonuclear leukocyte (PMN, or "poly" to the clinician). These highly specialized cells migrate to sites of infection, where they recognize, ingest, and kill bacteria. To accomplish these goals, neutrophils have specialized tools for chemotaxis, adhesion, locomotion, and phagocytosis, and they possess the metabolic apparatus to generate toxic substances and enzymes to destroy invading microorganisms.

DEVELOPMENT

Six distinct morphologic stages of neutrophil maturation can be distinguished in the bone marrow. These stages are known sequentially as myeloblast, promyelocyte, myelocyte, metamyelocyte, band form, and polymorphonuclear cell (Fig. 4-2

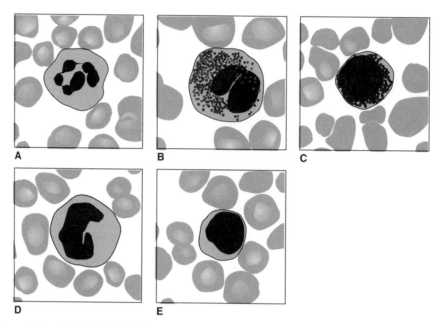

Figure 4-1. White blood cells (leukocytes) seen in peripheral blood. (**A**) Neutrophil (polymorpho-nuclear neutrophil; PMN); (**B**) eosinophil; (**C**) basophil; (**D**) monocyte; (**E**) lymphocyte. (Redrawn from Hoffbrand, AV, Pettit, JE. *Essential Hematology,* 3rd ed. Cambridge, Massachusetts: Blackwell, 1993:169.)

and Appendix 4). Earlier committed neutrophil progenitors (CFU-GM and CFU-G) are also present in the bone marrow but are not morphologically identifiable (Fig. 1-1). The presence of these neutrophil precursors is inferred by the ability of bone marrow to generate committed myeloid colonies *in vitro* and by reconstitution of granulopoiesis following experimental or therapeutic bone marrow transplantation.

Neutrophil maturation is accompanied by a progressive decrease in nuclear size accompanied by condensation of nuclear chromatin and loss of nucleoli. As the neutrophil matures, the nucleus indents and finally assumes its characteristic multi-lobed appearance. Concomitant with these nuclear events are changes in the neutrophil cytoplasm, where the granules that contain compounds crucial for host defense are stored. Primary, or azurophilic, granules are blue-staining inclusions of approximately 0.3 μm that contain elastase and myeloperoxidase. They first appear at the promyelocyte stage, but their number and staining intensity decrease during later neutrophil maturation. Secondary, or specific, granules, which contain lysozyme and other proteases, develop at the myelocyte stage. The staining qualities of these secondary granules account for the characteristic neutrophilic appearance of the cytoplasm (Fig. 4-2 and Appendix 4).

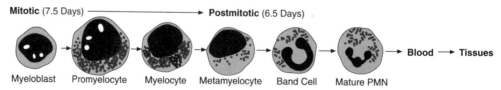

Figure 4-2. Maturation of the neutrophil, showing condensation of nuclear chromatin, loss of nucleoli, and development of primary and secondary granules.

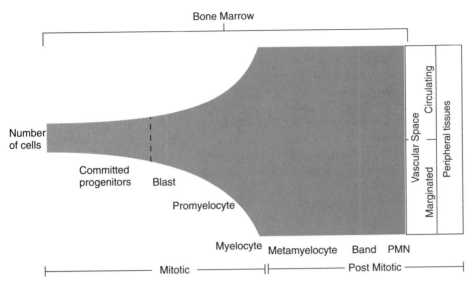

Figure 4-3. Proliferation and differentiation of neutrophil precursors occurs in the bone marrow. Mature neutrophils are available in the bone marrow and vasculature for distribution to peripheral tissues.

PRODUCTION

The turnover of neutrophils as they continually resupply the skin, mucosal surfaces, and other peripheral tissues is on the order of 100 billion cells each day. Neutrophils possess an extraordinary capacity to increase in number at times of great demand, both by expansion of the proliferative pool of cells and by recruitment of mature neutrophils. In contrast to most blood cells, only a small fraction of the neutrophil lifespan is spent in the intravascular space. Therefore the white blood cell count, which largely reflects the level of circulating neutrophils, is an imperfect reflection of the kinetics of neutrophil production (Fig. 4-3).

Most of the 15-day lifespan of the cells destined to become neutrophils is spent in the bone marrow. It is here that the expansion of the pool of neutrophil precursors takes place. The mitotic, or proliferative, pool of cells consists of the committed CFU-GM and CFU-G myeloid progenitors and neutrophil precursors up to the stage of myelocyte. Expansion of this marrow storage pool is strongly enhanced by inflammatory cytokines such as G-CSF and GM-CSF (Fig. 1-1).

En route to peripheral tissues, neutrophils spend approximately 10 hours in the intravascular space. The intravascular compartment is not simply a corridor for granulocytes from bone marrow to peripheral tissues, for only about one-half of intravascular granulocytes circulate at any given time. The balance of neutrophils adhere reversibly to the endothelial surfaces of the microvasculature. These so-called *marginated* cells constitute a storage pool of mature cells that can be recruited as needed in the face of infection or inflammation.

FUNCTION

Neutrophil function is directed toward the protection of the host against infection in a threefold process involving chemotaxis, phagocytosis, and killing. *Chemotaxis* involves the detection of and movement toward microorganisms and sites of inflammation. Neutrophils possess specific receptors for *C5a*, a product generated by the classical or alternative *complement system* pathways, and by proteases released by tissue damage or direct bacterial action. Neutrophils also have receptors for *N-formyl peptides*, which are released by bacteria and damaged mitochondria, and they respond to inflammatory products such as the *leukotriene LTB4* and fibrinopeptides.

Neutrophils move toward sites of inflammation along a chemotactic gradient. Granulocyte locomotion involves complex interactions between cell surface molecules and counterreceptors on endothelial tissues. Neutrophils roll along the endothelial surface to slow their movement from the rapidly flowing current of blood. The rolling of neutrophils is initiated when neutrophil cell surface molecules known as *L-selectins* interact with fucosyl and sulfatidyl moieties expressed on the endothelial cell surface. *P- and E-selectins* are related molecules that are expressed by endothelial cells in response to inflammatory cytokines that bind to neutrophil cell surface molecules. Subsequently, leukocytes express adhesion molecules of the integrin superfamily. In particular, the *β2-integrins*, which are heterodimers of the CD18 molecule and one of three CD11 molecules, bind to counterreceptors on endothelial cells such as ICAM-1 and ICAM-2 (Fig. 4-4A).

A locomoter system that resembles the contractile apparatus of muscle enables the neutrophil to crawl along the endothelial surface toward sites of inflammation. *Actin* filaments interact with the contractile protein *myosin* in a process that consumes ATP. As neutrophils crawl, they extend pseudopods in the direction of the inflammatory chemotaxins. In this process, the protein *gelsolin* catalyzes a gel-to-sol transition of the cytoplasmic actin lattice. Streams of cytoplasmic contents move into the pseudopod, and the nucleus follows as the cell shape changes. Microtubules provide stability during the process of migration.

Neutrophils recognize foreign organisms *via* receptors for *opsonins*, a term derived from Greek, meaning "to prepare for dining." Deposition of serum IgG and complement on bacteria renders them recognizable to granulocytes. The neutrophil possesses receptors for the F_c portion of immunoglobulin molecules and for products of the complement cascade. These receptors initiate the processes of ingestion and adhesion to foreign objects.

Neutrophils engulf opsonized microorganisms within cytoplasmic vesicles known as *phagosomes*. These vesicles move from enfolding pseudopods to fuse with the primary and secondary granules in an energy-dependent process during which phagocytes undergo a burst of glycolysis and glycogenolysis. As the cell degranulates, it empties its granule contents into the phagosome and delivers the degradative enzymes *lysozyme, acid* and *alkaline phosphatases, elastases*, and *lactoferrin* (Fig. 4-4B).

Finally, neutrophils destroy bacteria by metabolizing oxygen to generate reactive products that are toxic to ingested microorganisms. The oxidase apparatus that generates these products is comprised of a flavin- and heme-binding cytochrome b_{558}. These reactions utilize the reducing agent nicotinamide adenine dinucleotide phosphate (NADPH) and are fueled by glucose-6-phosphate dehydrogenase and the hexose monophosphate shunt. The cell thereby generates *superoxide* (O_2) and *hydrogen peroxide* (H_2O_2), which are released into the phagosome to effect bacterial killing. Lactoferrin participates in the generation of free *hydroxyl radicals*, and *myeloperoxidase*, using halides as cofactors, produce *hypochlorous acid* (HOCl) and toxic *chloramines*.

These reactive oxygen products are toxic to the host as well as to the microorganism. Localization of these products in the phagocytic vacuole helps to limit collateral damage to the cell. Other mechanisms to limit damage by these products in-

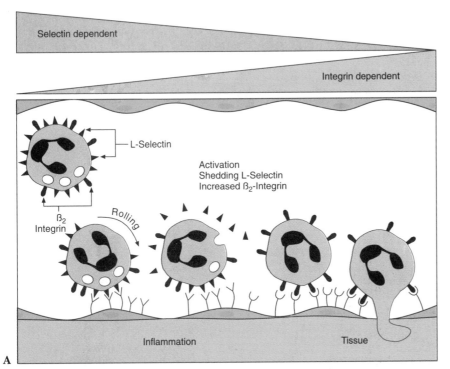

A

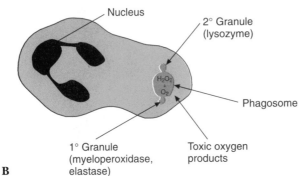

B

Figure 4-4. (**A**)Neutrophil margination and adhesion are mediated by adhesion molecules. Selectins permit initial, loose adhesion to vascular endothelial cells. Firm adherence by β_2 leukocyte integrins permits diapedesis and access to extravascular tissues. (Redrawn from Hillman RA, Ault KA. *Hematology in Clinical Practice.* New York: McGraw–Hill, 1995: 242.) (**B**) Bacterial killing by neutrophils results from the combined effects of proteases in the primary and secondary granules and the destructive effects of toxic oxygen products.

clude *superoxide dismutase,* which converts superoxide to hydrogen peroxide; *catalase,* which destroys hydrogen peroxide; and *reduced glutathione,* which destroys hydrogen peroxide (and thereby regenerates NADPH that can be used for further peroxide production).

The neutrophil possesses other mechanisms for bactericidal action besides the toxic oxygen compounds. The acid pH of the phagosome is detrimental to microorganisms. Lysozyme hydrolyzes the mucopeptide cell wall of some microbial species. Bactericidal proteins such as *defensins* and *perforins* are released into phagosomes and alter the permeability of the target cell membranes.

GRANULOCYTE ABNORMALITIES

A variety of granulocyte abnormalities are morphologically distinct and identifiable (Table 4-1). *Toxic granulations* are prominent azurophilic granules that are

TABLE 4-1. *ABNORMAL WBC*

NAME	MICROSCOPIC APPEARANCE	DESCRIPTION	CLINICAL SIGNIFICANCE
Normal neutrophilic leukocyte (polymorphnuclear leukocyte = PMN)		10–15 μm diameter; two- to five-lobed nucleus; fine pink or violet-pink cytoplasmic granules	Seen in health and in leukocytosis
Toxic granulations		Cytoplasm contains a multitude of dark azurophilic granules whose mucopolyaccharides have not matured.	Seen in infections or inflammatory states. May accompany cytoplasmic vacuoles and Döhle bodies.
Cytoplasmic vacuoles		Cytoplasm contains vacuoles.	Seen with infectious states. May indicate PMN degeneration and accompany toxic granulations or Döhle bodies. Can be seen with Jordan's anomaly–familial vacuolization of leukocytes.
Döhle bodies		Cytoplasm contains light blue cytoplasmic masses of varying size and shape representing RNA from remnants of rough endoplasmic reticulum.	Seen with infectious states and may accompany toxic granulations or cytoplasmic vacuoles.
Alder-Reilly anomaly		Cytoplasm contains numerous dark lilac granules composed of acid mucopolysaccharide deposits.	Seen with the Hurler, Hunter, and Maroteaux-Lamy types of genetic mucopolysaccharidosis.

Name	Image	Description	Disorder
Chédiak-Higashi syndrome		Cytoplasm contains numerous large fused lysosomal granules, some giant and bizarre; lymphocytes and other cells may contain them too.	Rare autosomal recessive disorder featuring leukocyte inclusions, partial oculocutaneous albinism, recurrent infections, and increased bleeding tendency.
May-Hegglin anomaly		Döhle bodies seen are larger, fusiform, bolder staining and lie more centrally in cytoplasm.	A rare autosomal dominant disorder characterized by large abnormal Döhle bodies in granulocytes and monocytes, poorly granulated giant platelets, and thrombocytopenia.
Hereditary giant neutrophilia		1–2% of PMNs are double normal size and nuclei are hypersegmented.	Rare and innocuous autosomal dominant disorder.
Ring-shaped nuclei	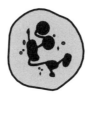	Nucleus is shaped like a ring.	Severe alcoholism.
Hyposegmented PMN Pelger-Huët anomaly	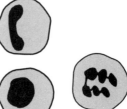	Nucleus is hyposegmented "pince-nez" or peanut-formed in hereditary disorder; rounded or oblong in acquired disorder.	In hereditary form WBC function normally. In acquired form may herald or accompany leukemia, myeloproliferative and myelodysplastic disorders, or drugs or infections.
Hypersegmented PMN		Nucleus has more than five lobes each connected by a thin chromatin strand	Seen in megaloblastic anemia (also rarely in a harmless autosomal dominant disorder).

seen at times of severe infectious or inflammatory stress. *Döhle bodies* are peripherally distributed, gray-blue cytoplasmic inclusion bodies that are also seen at times of severe stress which represent ribosome-containing remnants of the endoplasmic reticulum. *Alder-Reilly* disorder is a hereditary anomaly that does not affect neutrophil function, which is associated with coarse, lilac-staining azurophilic granules that arise from abnormal polysaccharide metabolism. *Chédiak-Higashi* syndrome is a congenital disorder characterized by large azurophilic granules in all myeloid lineages, ocular and skin hypopigmentation, giant melanosomes, and abnormally functioning platelets that lack dense granules. Granulocytes exhibit abnormal lysosome fusion during phagocytosis, and their impaired chemotaxis results in recurrent infections. This syndrome appears to be caused by abnormal microtubular proteins. *May-Hegglin* anomaly is a rare autosomal dominant trait that is manifested by giant platelets and large basophilic bodies in the granulocytes. Some patients exhibit a bleeding tendency with thrombocytopenia with quantitative or qualitative platelet abnormalities.

Normal neutrophils have up to four or five lobes. *Pelger-Huët* anomaly is a congenital abnormality of nuclear segmentation. Mature granulocytes of heterozygotes have only two lobes and are referred to as pince-nez cells because they resemble spectacles; homozygotes have but a single nuclear lobe. This autosomal dominant trait is benign and is seen in one in 6,000 people. More commonly seen is the *pseudo-Pelger-Huët* anomaly, an acquired nuclear abnormality seen in myeloproliferative and myelodysplastic disorders caused by abnormal nuclear maturation.

Excessive hypersegmentation of nuclei is occasionally seen as a benign, autosomal dominant trait. More commonly, acquired hypersegmented neutrophils are seen in megaloblastic anemia. A common rule of thumb is that more than 5% of granulocytes possessing five or more lobes suggests hypersegmentation. This should prompt a search for a cause of megaloblastosis. The hypersegmentation of granulocyte nuclei and abnormal maturation of erythroid nuclei that are caused by deficiencies of folic acid and vitamin B_{12} deficiency are indistinguishable. However, vitamin B_{12} deficiency, but not folate deficiency, is associated with neurologic symptoms caused by degeneration of the posterior columns of the spinal cord (Chapter 3). Granulocyte hypersegmentation may also be seen with chemotherapeutic agents that impair DNA synthesis, such as the antimetabolite hydroxyurea.

FUNCTIONAL NEUTROPHIL DISORDERS

Neutrophils must interact with other cell types and serum factors to defend the host against invading microorganisms (Table 4-2). Because opsonization is required for the identification and destruction of bacteria, antibody deficiency syndromes and disorders of complement disorders may be associated with recurrent bacteremias, meningitis, and pulmonary infections. *Agammaglobulinemia* or *hypogammaglobulinemia* and abnormalities of complement component C3 predispose subjects to infections by encapsulated pathogens such as streptococci, pneumococci, haemophilus, and pseudomonas. Such deficiency states may be congenital or acquired in association with lymphoproliferative disorders, autoimmune diseases, and immune complex states. *Job's syndrome* is a disorder of unknown origin in which recurrent abscesses and pulmonary infections are associated with extremely high levels of immunoglobulin E (IgE).

TABLE 4-2. *NEUTROPHIL FUNCTIONAL DISORDERS*		
FUNCTIONAL DEFECT	**EXAMPLES**	**ORIGIN**
Opsonization	A- or hypogammaglobulinemia	Congenital or acquired
Locomotion/ingestion	Leukocyte adhesion deficiency	Congenital (CD18 deficiency)
	Neutrophil actin dysfunction	Congenital
	Chédiak-Higashi syndrome	Congenital
	Corticosteroids	Cushing syndrome or iatrogenic
Killing	Chronic granulomatous disease	Congenital
	Myeloperoxidase deficiency	Congenital or acquired

DISORDERS OF NEUTROPHIL LOCOMOTION AND INGESTION

Corticosteroids impair the ability of neutrophils to migrate into inflammatory lesions and to ingest microorganisms, but the precise mechanism by which this occurs is unknown. Patients receiving large doses of therapeutic steroids and patients with *Cushing syndrome* are susceptible to pyogenic infection. *Leukocyte adhesion deficiency* is a rare autosomal recessive disorder characterized by delayed healing of the umbilical stump and recurrent bacterial and fungal infections. In this disorder, neutrophils adhere poorly to surfaces and fail to respond adequately to C3-coated bacteria. Multiple molecular defects have been described in leukocyte adhesion deficiency, but all exhibit qualitative or quantitative abnormalities of the leukocyte integrin, CD18. *Neutrophil actin dysfunction* is a rare, autosomal recessive disorder of neutrophil locomotion and ingestion associated with abnormalities of actin polymerization. *Chédiak-Higashi syndrome* is characterized by neutropenia, giant lysosomal granules that fail to fuse normally with phagosomes, and defective chemotaxis. Defects in neutrophil migration are evaluated with a Rebuck skin window, an *in vivo* assay of leukocyte migration.

DISORDERS OF BACTERICIDAL ACTIVITY

Chronic granulomatous disease (CGD) is an X-linked or autosomal recessive disorder in which neutrophils fail to metabolize oxygen to superoxide or hydrogen peroxide. Most cases are caused by abnormalities in the oxidases that generate these toxic oxygen products. Rarely, neutrophils that totally lack G6PD cannot metabolize oxygen because of the lack of NADPH. Affected phagocytes do not kill microorganisms such as staphylococcus, most gram-negative enteric bacteria, and many fungi that express catalase, which destroys hydrogen peroxide. CGD patients suffer recurrent skin, bone, and visceral infections with catalase-positive organisms. Because affected neutrophils do not metabolize oxygen, *hexosemonophosphate* shunt activity is not increased. Reduction of *nitroblue tetrazolium* (NBT) to the blue dye formazan by reactive oxygen products is a clinical laboratory test of phagocyte function that is abnormal in CGD granulocytes.

Myeloperoxidase deficiency is autosomal recessive disorder in which neutrophils lack myeloperoxidase. The phagocytes have a defect in bactericidal activity that is less severe than that of CGD, and patients with this condition are not unduly susceptible to infection.

NEUTROPHILIA

Neutrophilia is generally defined as a neutrophil count of more than 7,500/μL (Table 4-3). Persistent, dramatic neutrophilia, particularly when it is associated with an increase in immature circulating myeloid precursors ("a shift to the left") due to an underlying inflammatory state, may be described as a leukemoid reaction. Neutrophilia is usually caused by stimulation and expansion of the myeloid proliferative compartment by infectious or inflammatory states, tumors, or endocrinopathies. Acute neutrophilia usually involves a shift from the marginated blood pool to the circulating granulocyte pool and recruitment of mature cells from the marrow storage pool. Acute redistribution from the marginated pool may be caused by epinephrine, acute stress, hypoxia, or exercise; mobilization of the marrow pool may be caused by corticosteroids, endotoxin, chemical intoxication, or chronic stress.

TABLE 4-3. *NEUTROPHIL QUANTITATIVE DISORDERS*

Neutrophilia (>7,500/μL)
    Reactive
        Chronic infection or inflammation
    Malignant
        Acute or chronic leukemia

Neutropenia (<1,800/μL) - Selective:
    Congenital
        Kostmann's syndrome
        Cyclical neutropenia
    Benign (e.g., racial)
    Infectious
        Viral (e.g., hepatitis, HIV)
        Bacteria (e.g., miliary tuberculosis)
    Drugs
        Antibiotics
        Anticonvulsants
        Anti-inflammatory agents
        Antithyroid agents
        Phenothiazines
    Autoimmune
        Systemic lupus erythematosis (SLE)
        Felty's syndrome (rheumatoid arthritis)

Neutropenia as part of pancytopenia
    Bone marrow failure
        Leukemia, lymphoma, metastatic cancer
        Aplastic anemia
    Nutritional disorders (e.g., folate or B$_{12}$ deficiency)
    Hypersplenism

Reactive causes of neutrophilia must be distinguished from intrinsic hematopoietic disorders, particularly leukemias. Chronic myelogenous leukemia (CML) is a malignant expansion of myeloid cells that is typically associated with the Philadelphia chromosome, a reciprocal translocations of chromosomes 9 and 22, which generates the chimeric bcr/abl product. CML is often associated with splenomegaly and thrombocytosis, and may be accompanied by decreased leukocyte alkaline phosphatase activity, but distinguishing it from reactive neutrophilia on the blood smear and bone marrow examination may be difficult. Acute nonlymphocytic leukemia (ANLL) is associated with arrested neutrophil maturation in the bone marrow and peripheral blood. The immature myeloid cells, or "blasts," may contain Auer rods—elongated, blue cytoplasmic inclusions that represent granular inclusions (Chapter 9).

NEUTROPENIA

Neutropenia (a neutrophil count of less than $1,800/\mu L$), like neutrophilia, may be caused by transient or chronic shifts in various neutrophil pools and should be confirmed by successive blood counts. Absolute neutrophil counts of more than $500/\mu L$ are generally not associated with a significant defect in host defense. However, severe neutropenia (especially below $200/\mu L$) is regularly associated with an increased risk of infection, particularly when the count falls abruptly. Severe, acute neutropenia may result from a depletion of neutrophil reserves in association with septicemia, high fever, and prostration. Acute severe neutropenia, particularly when associated with fever, demands an aggressive evaluation and early treatment with broad-spectrum antibiotics. Chronic steady-state depletion of neutrophil reserves may be associated with no clinical findings or with malaise, low-grade fever, apthous stomatitis, lymphadenopathy, and recurrent abscesses. Among healthy African-Americans, the lower limit of normal for neutrophil counts is lower $(1,400/\mu L)$ and is not associated with an increased risk of infection.

Numerous medications may cause neutropenia. The most frequently implicated drugs are sulfa-derived antibiotics, phenothiazines, antithyroid medications, and the analgesic phenylbutazone (Table 7-5). Many forms of chemotherapy are associated with a dose-related suppression of granulocyte production, and these agents may be the most common cause of iatrogenic granulocytopenia. Systemic disorders such as rheumatoid arthritis and systemic lupus erythematosis are often associated with decreased granulocyte counts. Some cases are associated with antineutrophil antibodies that mediate intramedullary destruction of maturing neutrophils or affect the survival and proliferation of neutrophil progenitors (Chapter 7). *Pseudo-neutropenia* is caused by increased margination of granulocytes. Such temporary shifts may be caused by hypersensitivity reactions, viremia, hemolysis, or hemodynamic alterations.

Periodic, or *cyclic, neutropenia* is an autosomal dominant disorder of variable penetrance that is first seen in infancy and may persist for decades. Every 3–4 weeks the patient has neutropenia that lasts for 3–6 days and may be associated with fever, mucositis, and skin infections. The bone marrow shows myeloid hypoplasia during the period of neutropenia. Although the cause is unknown, cyclic neutropenia appears to represent dyssynchrony of the feedback loops that regulate granulocyte production and release. Some patients can be successfully treated with GM-CSF or G-CSF. Familial neutropenias include a benign, autosomal dominant *Glänsslen neutropenia.* In contrast, the autosomal recessive *Kostmann's syndrome* exhibits persistently low neutrophil counts, and many patients die of sepsis in childhood. Inborn errors of metabolism, such as *Gaucher disease*, and myelophthisic disorders, such as metastatic cancer, disturb the normal bone marrow architecture and may also be associated with neutropenia (Chapter 7).

EOSINOPHILS

Eosinophils possess a bilobed nucleus and cytoplasm that is filled with distinctive red-colored granules following Wright-Giemsa staining (Fig. 4-1). The basic, or positively charged, proteins in these granules stain red because of their high affinity for the cellular stain, eosin. Eosinophils undergo the same stages of maturation as neutrophils, but their lower abundance in the bone marrow makes eosinophil precursors less apparent except in certain pathologic states. During maturation, eosinophil precursors accumulate large, red-staining granules in their cytoplasm rather than neutrophilic secondary granules, and the nucleus does not become multilobated, as do neutrophils. Eosinophil maturation is promoted by interleukins 3 and 5 (Fig. 1-1).

Eosinophils play a special role in fighting parasites and controlling allergic insults. Because of their low frequency in the peripheral circulation, the role of eosinophils in combatting bacterial infections is uncertain. However, their capabilities for chemotaxis, phagocytosis, and microbicidal activity are similar to those of neutrophils. Eosinophilic granules contain a specialized group of microbicidal proteins, including eosinophilic cationic protein, *Charcot-Leyden crystal* protein, and eosinophil peroxidase.

Eosinophilia is indicated by an absolute eosinophil count of more than $700/\mu L$ and is generally seen when eosinophils constitute more than 10% of the leukocyte differential count. Most cases can be traced to an underlying allergic or atopic condition, parasitic infection, autoimmune or inflammatory state, or malignancy such as Hodgkin's disease. Eosinophilia is often seen, along with basophilia, in chronic myelogenous leukemia. A characteristic syndrome of acute nonlymphocytic leukemia with bizarre eosinophilic precursors is associated with abnormalities of chromosome 16.

Hypereosinophilia (eosinophil count above $1,500/\mu L$), particularly when it persists for many months, can lead to a characteristic pattern of tissue damage. Organ damage may be caused by direct tissue infiltration and the effects of toxic oxygen products and granule proteins. Involved organs typically include endomyocardium and the central nervous system, and therapy usually includes corticosteroids or antimetabolites such as hydroxyurea.

BASOPHILS

Basophils are the least abundant circulating granulocytes, representing less than 1% of leukocytes (Fig. 4-1C and Appendix 4). Their large cytoplasmic granules contain sulfated or carboxylated acidic proteins, such as heparin, that are colored blue with Wright-Giemsa stain. Basophils appear to mediate allergic phenomena, especially those mediated by IgE-dependent mechanisms. They express IgE receptors and release histamine when properly stimulated. Basophils may be related to tissue mast cells, which also release vasoactive substances such as histamine in response to IgE and antigen exposure.

Basophilia is defined as more than 150 basophils per μL; like eosinophilia, it may be associated with acute hypersensitivity reactions such as allergic reactions associated with urticaria. Other causes of basophilia include viral infections such as chickenpox and influenza, chronic infections such as tuberculosis, inflammatory states such as rheumatoid arthritis and ulcerative colitis, iron deficiency, and underlying cancers. Basophilia may be seen in myeloproliferative disorders and may herald blast transformation in chronic myelogenous leukemia. An acute nonlymphocytic leukemia with cells resembling basophils is associated with symptoms attributable to histamine release.

MONOCYTES

Monocytes circulate in the peripheral blood as large cells with blue/gray cytoplasm and a reniform (kidney-shaped) or folded nucleus containing fine reticular chromatin (Fig. 4-1D and Appendix 4). Monocytes are derived from the CFU-GM, a common progenitor to both granulocytes and monocytes, and CFU-M, a progenitor that is restricted to the monocytic lineage. Monocytes spend only about 20 hours in the bloodstream but then enter peripheral tissues, where they are transformed to macrophages of the reticuloendothelial system (RES). These tissue macrophages, or histiocytes, are large cells with eccentric nuclei and vacuolated cytoplasm containing numerous inclusions (Appendix 4).

Monocytes and macrophages are long-lived cells that share many functional features with granulocytes. They are more efficient than granulocytes at ingesting mycobacteria, fungi, and macromolecules; their role in the phagocytosis of pyogenic bacteria is less prominent. In the spleen, macrophages are responsible for clearing sensitized and senescent erythrocytes. Macrophages play critical roles in processing and presenting antigens to lymphocytes in the generation of the cellular and humoral immune responses. Their production of cytokines and interleukins, interferons, and complement components helps to coordinate the complex interplay of the integrated immune response.

Monocytes normally account for 1–10% of circulating leukocytes. Monocytosis is generally defined as more than 1,000 monocytes per μL and may be seen in patients with chronic infections such as tuberculosis or infective endocarditis, or in inflammatory states such as autoimmune diseases or inflammatory bowel disease. Intrinsic disorders of the bone marrow such as chronic leukemias or myeloproliferative states may also be associated with monocytosis. Transient monocytosis often precedes the return of circulating neutrophils by 1 or 2 days following marrow suppression by chemotherapy. Histiocytosis X refers collectively to indolent neoplasms of the monocyte/macrophage system in which bone marrow, skin, lungs, and the central nervous system are infiltrated by these abnormal cells. True histiocytic lymphoma represents a malignancy of monocyte/macrophages and is related to histiocytic medullary reticulosis, which is characterized by phagocytosis of hematopoietic cells by the involved mononuclear cells.

LYMPHOCYTES

Lymphocytes are small, mononuclear cells (Figs. 4-1E and 4-9A) that coordinate and execute the immune response by their production of inflammatory cytokines

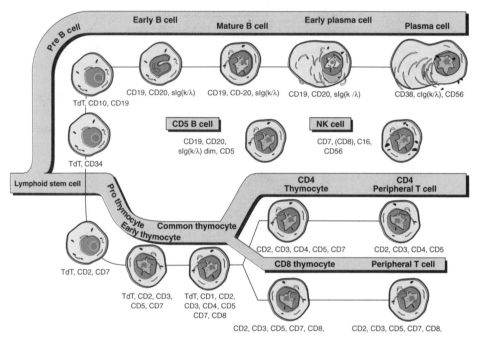

Figure 4-5. Lymphocytes are derived from a common lymphoid stem cell. Maturing B-lymphocytes express the characteristic CD19 and CD20 antigens; they express surface immunoglobulin (sIg) and later cytoplasmic immunoglobulin (cIg). T-lymphocytes express the antigens CD2, CD5, and CD7 throughout development and express TdT while immature. They later acquire T-cell receptor and transiently coexpress CD4 and CD8 prior to committing to either the helper (CD4 positive) or suppressor (CD8) phenotype. The maturation of NK cells is less well understood. (Redrawn from Hillman RA, Ault KA. *Hematology in Clinical Practice.* New York: McGraw–Hill, 1995: 304)

and antigen-specific binding receptors. There are two main categories of lymphocytes, B cells and T cells, and less abundant classes such as natural killer cells. Lymphocyte subsets differ in their sites of production and the effector molecules that they express, but they share the capacity to produce a highly specific response to antigenic challenge (Fig. 4-5).

During fetal development, the yolk sac, liver, and spleen are important lymphopoietic organs (Fig. 1-3). In postnatal life, the bone marrow and thymus are the primary lymphoid organs where lymphocyte division takes place prior to antigen exposure. Secondary, or reactive, lymphoid tissues consist of lymph nodes, the spleen, and lymphoid tissues of the gastrointestinal and respiratory tracts. Lymphocytes travel through the bloodstream and emerge *via* postcapillary venules to reach the spleen, lymph nodes, and other lymphoid tissues (Chapter 1). They return from peripheral tissues *via* an efferent system of lymphatics that ultimately drain into the venous system through the thoracic duct.

B-LYMPHOCYTES

B-lymphocytes express unique antigen receptors—immunoglobulins—and are programmed to produce them in large quantities in response to antigenic stimulation. B cells are derived from stem cells that reside in the bone marrow. The term *B cell* is derived from the bursa of Fabricius, a hindgut organ that is required for

B-cell processing and maturation in birds. No homologous organ has been identified in man, and it appears that B-cell maturation takes place primarily in the bone marrow.

The immune system contains an enormous population of individual clones of B-lymphocytes. Each clone expresses a unique antigen receptor that is essentially identical to the immunoglobulin molecule that it will secrete. Immunoglobulin molecules differ subtly from one another and bind to only a limited number of antigens. The extraordinary number of individual B-lymphocyte clones, each with its unique immunoglobulin molecule, provides the remarkable diversity to antibody production.

B-lymphocytes that emerge from the bone marrow are immunologically immature, for they have not yet been exposed to antigen (Fig. 4-5). The initial maturation steps of B cells are antigen independent. The pre–B cell transiently produces *terminal deoxytransferase (TdT)*, and *common acute leukemia antigen (CALLA*; CD10). It later expresses characteristic B-cell surface antigens such as CD19 and CD20, and produces intracytoplasmic immunoglobulin μ chains. As B cells mature, they express complete antibody molecules on their cell surface (sIg); later these immunoglobulins are secreted. Mature B-lymphocytes are found primarily in germinal centers of the cortex of lymph nodes and in the white pulp of the spleen; fewer than 20% of circulating lymphocytes are B cells.

Subsequent B-cell maturation is antigen dependent. With the aid of helper T cells and specialized macrophages called antigen-presenting cells, B cells whose receptor recognizes the antigen proliferate and mature. The resultant plasma cells produce large quantities of a single immunoglobulin molecule. These cells have a characteristic appearance of an eccentric nucleus with peripherally distributed nuclear chromatin, a strongly basophilic cytoplasm, and a perinuclear clear zone representing their active Golgi complex (Fig. 4-9D). Other stimulated B-lymphocytes become long-lived memory B cells, which perpetuate the memory of a previously encountered antigen and rapidly proliferate and produce large quantities of immunoglobulin upon later antigenic challenge.

ANTIBODY PRODUCTION

There are five major classes of immunoglobulins, or antibodies, which are designated IgG, IgA, IgM, IgD, and IgE. IgG is the most abundant immunoglobulin and is further subclassified as IgG_1, IgG_2, IgG_3, and IgG_4. IgA is the predominant antibody in gastrointestinal and respiratory secretions and has two subcategories. IgD and IgE are minor immunoglobulin categories that are predominantly involved in allergic and delayed hypersensitivity reactions. IgM multimerizes to form large pentameric structures when secreted by mature B cells (Table 4-4).

IgM is the first antibody produced by B-lymphocytes in response to antigen, but as B cells mature they may switch to expression of either IgG, IgA, IgD, or IgE. The conversion of antibody production from IgM to one of the other categories is known as class or *isotype switching*. In switching to another heavy-chain isotype, there is retention of the variable region of the antibody, which is largely responsible for the specificity of antigen recognition.

The classes of immunoglobulin share a common structure of two heavy chains that are linked by disulfide bonds to two light chains (Table 4-4). The heavy chains are called gamma (γ) in IgG, alpha (α) in IgA, mu (μ) in IgM, delta (δ) in IgD, and

TABLE 4-4. *PROPERTIES OF IMMUNOGLOBIN MOLECULES*			
	IgG	**IgA**	**IgM**
Molecular weight (kD)	150,000	150,000 300,000 400,000	950,000
Sedimentation constant	7S	7S	19S
Normal serum level (g/dL)	0.8–1.5	0.09–0.325	0.045–0.150
Present in	Serum and extracellular fluid	Serum and other body fluids (e.g., of bronchi and gut)	Serum only
Complement fixation	Usual	Yes (alternative pathway)	Usual and very efficient
Placental transfer	Yes	No	No
Heavy chain	(γ_{1-4})	α $(\alpha_1$ or $_2)$	μ
Secretory form	Monomer	Variable	Pentamer

From Hoffbrand AV, Pettit JE. *Essential Haematology, 3rd ed.* Cambridge, Massachusetts.: Blackwell Scientific Publication, 1993:168.

epsilon (ϵ) in IgE. The light chains in any single molecule are either kappa (κ) or lambda (λ). Light chains and heavy chains each have constant regions that are nearly identical among antibodies of a class. Each light and heavy chain also has highly variable regions that provide the specificity of antibody recognition. Antibodies can be digested by proteases into the Fc fragment containing the constant region and the highly variable Fab fragment (Fig. 4-6).

The generation of antibody diversity involves a complex pattern of somatic gene rearrangements and acquired mutations. Immunoglobulin heavy-chain and κ and λ light chains are encoded on chromosomes 14, 2, and 22, respectively. In the germ line (unrearranged) state, each of these genes contains multiple copies of regions designated as variable (V), diversity (D), joining (J), and constant (C) regions. In all tissues except B-lymphocytes, these genes remain in the germ line configuration. However, early in B-cell development, gene rearrangements take place that combine one each of the V, D, and J regions with the adjacent C region. The rearrangements are catalyzed by recombinases that are active only in immune cells, and the intervening gene segments are excised (Fig. 4-7).

Recombination among the library of immunoglobulin gene segments can theoretically generate thousands of possible antibodies. Further antibody diversity is contributed by terminal deoxytransferase. In contrast to most DNA polymerases, TdT incorporates variable numbers of nucleotides into the sites of recombining immunoglobulin gene segments without requiring a DNA template. The added nucleotides further alter the sequence encoding the immunoglobulin and contributes to molecular heterogeneity. In each cell, a similar process of rearrangement takes place with either the κ or λ light chain. The rearrangements bring a promoter region upstream of the V region under the influence of a transcriptional enhancer located between the J and C regions. The resultant rearranged genes are transcribed and spliced to form mRNA, and later translated to generate functional immunoglobulin molecules.

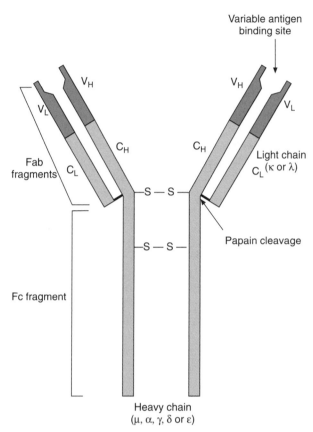

Figure 4-6. Immunoglobulin molecules are heterotetramers that consist of two light chains and two heavy chains linked by disulfide bonds. The variable regions determine antigen specificity and the F_c regions define the Ig subclass (IgA, IgD, IgE, IgG, or IgM). (Redrawn from Hoffbrand AV, Pettit JE. *Essential Haematology.* Cambridge, Massachusetts: Blackwell, 1993: 167.)

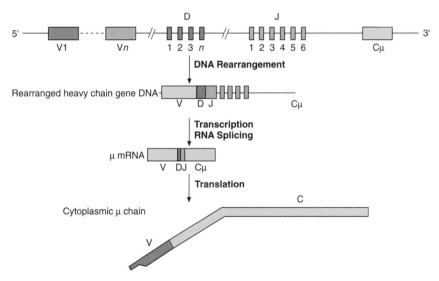

Figure 4-7. Rearrangements of genomic DNA link individual exons from the V, D, J, and C regions. The resulting spliced mRNA transcript is translated to produce the actual Ig protein molecule.

Because the recombinations that encode antibody molecules take place in the genomic DNA, all progeny of a rearranged lymphocyte share characteristic genomic rearrangements that can be detected in the laboratory. Amplification of the rearranged gene *via* polymerase chain reaction, or identification of a specific gene rearrangement by Southern blotting, can be used to characterize a particular clone of B-lymphocytes. These techniques can distinguish a polyclonal proliferation of lymphocytes from a monoclonal (and presumably malignant) clone of cells. If a large population of lymphocytes contains the same immunoglobulin rearrangement, the cells likely represent a B-cell malignancy.

Immunoglobulins play an important role in defending the host against invading microorganisms, but abnormal antibody production is characteristic of certain disorders of lymphoid cells. Multiple myeloma is a malignant proliferation of B-lymphocytes in which the clonal myeloma cells secrete the same immunoglobulin, usually IgG, IgA, or IgM (Chapter 9). The level of antibody expressed by the myeloma cells can be used as tumor marker. Multiple myeloma patients may be immunodeficient because the malignant lymphoid cells produce large amounts of a single immunoglobulin molecule but restrict the broad range of antibodies seen in the normal host. Because of the propensity of IgM to multimerize, B-cell malignancies that secrete this immunoglobulin isotype may make the blood hyperviscous and cause central nervous system or circulatory problems. Some types of myeloma produce incomplete immunoglobulin in the form of light-chain fragments; when these proteins are found in the urine, they are described as Bence-Jones proteins. Lymphomas and autoimmune diseases are often associated with aberrant immunoglobulin production, and antibodies that react with antigens present on blood cells may cause immune cytopenias.

T-LYMPHOCYTES

T-lymphocytes play the predominant role in cellular immunity. Sensitized T cells mediate delayed hypersensitivity, allograft rejection, graft-versus-host disease, contact allergy, and immunity to tumors and intracellular parasites. Cell-mediated immunity involves direct cellular killing by cytotoxic T cells and is enhanced by cytokines that are elaborated following complex interactions between T cells and macrophages. T-lymphocytes are also intimately and crucially involved in the regulation of B-cell proliferation and immunoglobulin production.

T cells are derived from bone marrow stem cells, but they must undergo further processing in the thymus to generate mature, fully functional T cells (Chapter 1). Immature prothymocytes migrate from the bone marrow and populate the subcapsular cortex of the spleen. In the thymus, T-lymphocytes mature and acquire characteristic antigen expression and functions associated with mature T cells. They express the antigens CD2 (sheep red blood cell receptor), CD3, CD4, CD7, CD8, and T-cell receptor. Later, as they become either helper cells or suppressor cells, they switch to expression of either CD4 or CD8, respectively. A crucial function of the spleen in T-cell development is the elimination of self-reactive T cells that have the potential to recognize host antigens. Thymic selection eliminates these cells through a complex series of events that result in *apoptosis,* or programmed cell death.

T-lymphocytes express on their surface an antigen-recognizing structure called the T-cell receptor (TCR). The TCR shares structural homology with immunoglobulin molecules and is similarly composed of two distinct subunits. Most

TCRs are composed of α and β chains, but a small minority instead contain γ and δ chains. The α, β, γ, and δ chains of TCR each include V, D, J, and C regions that undergo somatic rearrangements *via* recombinases and TdT in processes analogous to those in B cells. The TCR is affixed to the plasma membrane of the T cell, but unlike immunoglobulin molecules it is not secreted (Fig. 4-8).

Antigen presenting cells (APC), such as macrophages, are required to fully activate T-lymphocytes. APCs process antigens to make them more immunogenic and present them to T cells in the context of receptors of the major histocompatibility complex (MHC). MHC receptors vary substantially from person to person based on inheritance of the encoding genes, but unlike immunoglobulin and TCR, MHC variability is not the result of gene rearrangements. MHC receptors were first recognized as being responsible for rejection of blood transfusions or tissue grafts in patients who had been exposed to foreign tissues, or in women with numerous pregnancies. These so-called human lymphocyte antigens (HLA) can predict immune responsiveness to certain antigens and susceptibility to autoimmune diseases.

Because T cells do not bind antigens free in solution, activation of T cells depends on TCR recognition of antigen in the context of self-MHC. There are two classes of MHC proteins. Class I MHC proteins (HLA-A, -B, and -C) mediate recognition of intracellular antigens resulting from processes such as viral infections. Class I molecules, which stabilize the interaction of APCs with T cells, are bound by CD8 molecules, which are expressed on suppressor T cells. Class II MHC proteins (HLA-DP, -DQ, and -DR) are recognized by CD4 antigen-expressing helper T cells; they are particularly important for the response to extracellular antigens such as bacterial proteins. Both classes of MHC molecules possess a pocket in which they display fragments of antigens that have been processed by APCs. Class I expression is constitutive, but class II expression by B cells and mononuclear phagocytes increases following exposure to gamma interferon and other cytokines. The interaction between APCs and T cells is further stabilized by the CD3 complex and other leukocyte adhesion molecules and counterreceptors. Not all antigens require MHC molecules for activation of T cells. Notably, superantigens such as some viral products and bacterial toxins directly activate T cells, probably via the TCR β subunit.

T cells are activated by binding antigen to TCR in the context of MHC molecules and CD3 molecules. T-cell activation is associated with tyrosine phosphorylation events, signaling by second messengers such as diacylglycerol and inositol triphosphate, and activation of protein kinase C. These events culminate in cell proliferation and expression of interleukin 2 (IL-2) and other characteristic genes.

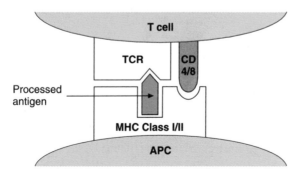

Figure 4-8. T-lymphocytes possess antigen specificity that results from the particular T-cell receptor that they express. T cells recognize antigens that are presented by macrophages and other antigen-presenting cell in the context of MHC molecules and either the CD4 or CD8 counterreceptor.

IL-2 is prominently involved in an autocrine loop of T-cell activation, but other cytokines—including IL-3, IL-4, IL-6, and IL-7—also have important roles.

Helper cells, which are characterized by expression of the CD4 antigen, constitute the majority of circulating lymphocytes. Their proliferation and expression of IL-2, following interactions of CD4 with MHC class II molecules, greatly enhance immunoglobulin expression by B cells. Helper cells also strengthen the response of suppressor T cells following the interaction of CD8 with antigen presented in the context of MHC class I molecules by APCs. CD8-expressing cells comprise the majority of suppressor and cytotoxic T cells. They kill their prey by inducing pores in cell membranes by insertion of perforins and other toxic molecules.

Wright-stained lymphocytes cannot be distinguished as either B or T cells. Lymphocytes range in size from one to three times the diameter of an erythrocyte and have blue or gray cytoplasm and clumped chromatin. Cells with small amounts of cytoplasm are described as mature or small lymphocytes; those with large amounts of cytoplasm are called large lymphocytes. Variant or atypical lymphocytes are commonly seen in viral illnesses such as infectious mononucleosis. These reactive cells have monocytoid nuclei, often with nucleoli, and abundant blue-gray cytoplasm that appears to drape over adjacent erythrocytes. Large, granular lymphocytes have abundant cytoplasm with distinct reddish granules (Fig. 4-9C).

Less abundant categories of lymphocytes include null cells, so called because they do not express the antigens characteristic of either B or T cells. Null cells include immature lymphocytes that have not yet committed to either the B- or T-cell lineage, and they express TdT, the DNA polymerase involved in antigen receptor rearrangement.

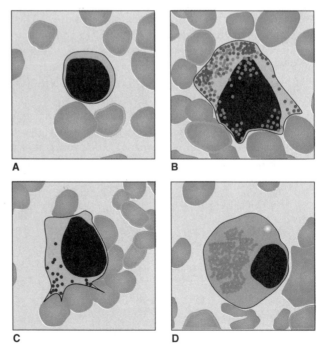

Figure 4-9. Lymphocytes. (**A**) Small lymphocyte; (**B**) activated lymphocyte; (**C**) large granular lymphocyte; (**D**) Plasma cell. (Redrawn from Hoffbrand AV, Pettit JE. *Essential Hematology.* Cambridge, Mass.: Blackwell, 1993:161.)

Natural killer (NK) cells, unlike other categories of lymphocytes, are capable of cytotoxicity in the absence of prior antigenic sensitization. Their ability to kill is not restricted by MHC antigens, does not require TCR or Ig rearrangement, and is markedly enhanced by interferons. NK cells express the cell surface antigen CD16 and appear morphologically as large granular lymphocytes. They attack abnormal cells such as damaged, virus-infected, or cancerous cells by release of the cytolytic granules. NK cells can kill directly or via antibody-dependent cell-mediated cytotoxicity (ADCC), in which antibody bound to a target attracts NK cells through their receptors for the F_c portion of immunoglobulin.

LYMPHOCYTE DISORDERS

Lymphocytosis ($>5,000/\mu L$) is seen in response to acute viral infections and in chronic infections such as tuberculosis and syphilis, and is associated with endocrinopathies such as thyrotoxicosis. Chronic lymphocytic leukemia causes lymphadenopathy, hepatosplenomegaly, and lymphocytosis, and the blood smear frequently contains fragile *smudge cells.* Acute lymphocytic leukemia, certain non-Hodgkin's lymphomas, and hairy cell leukemia also cause lymphocytosis (Chapter 9).

Infectious mononucleosis is a clinical syndrome characterized by fever, pharyngitis, lymphadenopathy, splenomegaly, and atypical lymphocytosis. It is caused by Epstein-Barr virus (EBV) a double-stranded DNA virus of the herpes family. EBV infects B cells *via* the CD21 cell surface antigen and drives them to proliferate. CD8-expressing T cells and NK cells respond to these infected cells and flood the circulation and lymph tissues with large lymphocytes. A similar atypical lymphocytosis can be seen with infections by most viruses, mycoplasma, tuberculosis, and hypersensitivity reactions to drugs.

A large number of inherited or acquired abnormalities of lymphocytes cause immunodeficiencies (Table 4-5). Patients with *X-linked agammaglobulinemia* have normal T-cell function, such as graft rejection and hypersensitivity reactions, but B-cell dysfunction leads to recurrent pyogenic infections. Other disorders of B-cell function include *common variable immune deficiency* and selective IgA or IgG deficiencies. DiGeorge's syndrome is associated with thymic aplasia and deficient T-cell function. Consequently, such patients have restricted cell-mediated immunity and are unusually susceptible to infection by viruses, mycobacteria, and fungi. In *severe combined immunodeficiency (SCID)* both B and T cells are absent because of abnormalities of adenosine deaminase or other disorders. Patients generally require bone marrow transplantation to survive the recurrent viral, bacterial, and fungal infections. Other rare disorders that lead to variable B- and T-cell dysfunction include *Bloom's syndrome, ataxia-telangiectasia,* and *Wiskott-Aldrich syndrome.*

Lymphopenia (fewer than $1,000/\mu L$) is seen with severe bone marrow failure and following marrow suppression by radiation or chemotherapy. Abnormal immune function may persist for years after bone marrow transplantation and causes a high incidence of infections with cytomegalovirus and herpes zoster (Chapter 8). Corticosteroids are lympholytic, and their therapeutic use is associated with lymphocyte dysfunction and increased susceptibility to infection.

Acquired immunodeficiency syndrome (AIDS) is caused by infection with *human immunodeficiency virus (HIV)* (Chapter 10). HIV is a CD4 lymphotropic retrovirus that is transmitted via intimate exposure to blood, tissue, or secretions that contain

TABLE 4-5.	*CLASSIFICATION OF IMMUNE DEFICIENCIES*	
Primary	B-cell (antibody deficiency)	X-linked agammaglobulinemia, acquired common variable hypogammaglobulinemia, selective IgA or IgG subclass deficiencies
	T-cell	Thymic aplasia, purine nucleoside phosphorylase (PNP) deficiency
	Mixed B- and T-cell	Severe combined immune deficiency (SCID, due to adenosine deaminase deficiency [ADA] or other causes) Bloom's syndrome Ataxia-telangiectasia Wiskott-Aldrich syndrome
Secondary	B-cell (antibody deficiency)	Myeloma Nephrotic syndrome, protein losing enteropathy
	T-cell	AIDS Hodgkin's disease, non-Hodgkin's lymphoma Drugs: steroids, cyclosporine, azathioprine, etc.
	T- and B-cell	Chronic lymphocytic leukemia, post–bone marrow transplantation and postchemotherapy/radiotherapy

From Hoffbrand AV, Pettit JE: Essential Haematology. Cambridge, Mass.: Blackwell Scientific Publication; 1993: 178.

the virus. The most common modes of transmission include sexual contact, intravenous drug abuse, exposure to contaminated blood, or maternal–fetal transmission in the perinatal period. Initial infection by HIV results in a mild, influenza-like illness. Over time a progressive destruction of host defenses takes place, most notably by attrition of CD4-bearing cells. AIDS is associated with cytopenias of all hematopoietic lineages and results in a profound immunodeficiency. The cytopenias are compounded by the effects of many of the antiretroviral agents and antibiotics used to treat the patients. Ultimately, patients succumb to infection by opportunistic infectious agents such as *Pneumocystis carinii* or atypical mycobacteria, AIDS encephalopathy, Kaposi's sarcoma, high-grade non-Hodgkin's lymphomas, or a wasting syndrome.

CASE PRESENTATION

A 65-year-old woman comes to the emergency room because of fever and a sore throat. Four months earlier, an "overactive" thyroid gland was diagnosed by her primary care physician, whom she saw because of a rapid heartbeat. She treated her with digoxin and propylthiouracil 300 mg/day. She took this medication quite faithfully and white blood cell counts were dutifully checked each month by her internist. The most recent check was 2 weeks earlier and was reported to be normal. Thyroid function tests were normal as well. For 3 days prior to admission she noted a raw feeling in her mouth and throat as well as chills; her temperature has been as high as 39.1°C po. Your examination reveals an oral temperature of 39.4°C. Pulse rate is 120/min and regular. The mouth and pharynx are erythematous. There are several 0.5-cm ulcers in the oral mucosa, some with thick exudate over their bases. The remainder of the examination gives no further clues about the reason for the fever.

The blood count is surprising. It shows a normal hemoglobin and hematocrit with a normal platelet count. However, the white blood cells were markedly reduced. There were 980/μL, and the differential count showed 5% neutrophils, 2% band forms, 79% lymphocytes, 10% monocytes, and 4% eosinophils.

Question 1. What should happen now?

Answer. The patient should have a full evaluation for the source of infection (with culture of blood and oropharyngeal lesions especially), but broad-spectrum antibiotic should be started without delay.

Question 2. What about the medications she was taking?

Answer. On a statistical basis, the propylthiouracil is the culprit here for the profound leukopenia. Other causes should be considered, but while you are ruminating, no further PTU should be administered. The digoxin is low on the likelihood list for causing neutropenia, and the patient may well need this medication to keep the presumed atrial fibrillation under control.

Question 3. What else should be done now?

Answer. Granulocyte colony stimulating factor (G—CSF) shortens the length of the neutropenic period but does not lessen the nadir in chemotherapy-induced neutropenic states. There is an evolving literature on its use in situations such as this where there may be an immune as well as a toxic component. The patient was given G—CSF.

Question 4. Once the neutropenia has resolved, should PTU be resumed but at a lower dosage?

Answer. NO! Neither PTU nor similar drugs (such as methemazole) should be given, since they may provoke the same or a worse neutropenic response.

Question 5. Could the patient's physician have provided closer surveillance with CBCs and therefore avoided development of neutropenia here?

Answer. No. In fact, some authorities believe that the onset of neutropenia may be too sudden, so that even frequent testing is not effective. The risk factors for development of neutropenia for patients on methemazole are known. They include female sex, age over 40, and more than 40 mg of methemazole per day. All patients should be alerted to report sore throats or mouth pain (frequent symptoms in leukopenic patients) as well as fever to their physician immediately.

Follow up. This patient defervesced after 3 days, although there was never any growth from bacteriologic/viral or fungal cultures. The white blood cell count remained low for 1 week but then rose sharply and returned to normal. The patient's symptoms cleared in synchrony with the rising white count. For continuing treatment of her hyperthyroidism she was given I^{131} therapy and has done well since then.

SELECTED READING

Clark EA, Ledbetter JA. How B and T cells talk to each other. *Nature* 1994;367:425–428.
A summary of the molecular mechanisms that underlie the dialog between B- and T-lymphocytes during the immune response.

Cline MJ. Histiocytes and histiocytosis. *Blood* 1994;84(9):2840–2853.
A review of the ontogeny of histiocytes and the clinical disorders that are associated with their dysfunction.

Miller RA, Britigan BE. The formation and biologic significance of phagocyte-derived oxidants. *J Invest Med* 1995;43(1):39–49.
A description of the generation of toxic oxidants of phagocytes and their importance in the host defense.

Moore MAS. Expansion of myeloid stem cells in culture. *Semin Hematol* 1995;32: 183–200.
A thorough review of myeloid stem cell characteristics, cytokines that stimulate them, and culture systems for their growth.

Orkin SH. Transcription factors and hematopoietic development. *J Biol Chem* 1995;270: 4955–4958.
A review of the role of transcription factors in hematopoiesis and how they influence lineage selection and commitment.

Rosen FS, Cooper MD, Wedgewood RJP. The primary immunodeficiencies. *New Engl J Med* 1995;333(7):431–440.
An introduction to the clinical manifestations of immune disorders of lymphoid cells and recent advances in our understanding of their molecular basis.

Schwartz RS. Jumping genes and the immunoglobulin V gene system. *New Engl J Med* 1995;333(7):42–44.
A brief, illustrated introduction to the complexity that underlies immunoglobulin rearrangement and the mechanisms that generate antibody diversity.

Spits H, Lanier LL, Phillips JH. Development of human T and natural killer cells. *Blood* 1995;85(10):2654–2670.
A thorough review of the ontogeny of NK and T lymphocytes.

Stossel TP. The machinery of blood cell movements. *Blood* 1994;84(2):367–379.
A comprehensive description of the the molecular basis for the remarkable ability of neutrophils to crawl.

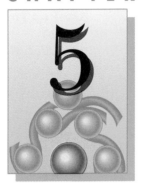

Platelets

Eric M. Mazur

Normal hemostasis is generally believed to be achieved by the cooperation and interaction of two separate coagulation systems, the soluble system (which consists of procoagulant proteins) (Chapter 6) and the cellular system (comprised of platelets). The end result of activation of the soluble coagulation system is the formation of a fibrin clot or red thrombus, whereas platelet stimulation accompanied by adhesion and aggregation results in the formation of a platelet plug or white thrombus. Although these two coagulation systems are typically considered separately, it is important to recognize that in life, their functions are intricately interwoven. Soluble coagulation factors (e.g., fibrinogen and von Willebrand factor) are essential for normal platelet function, and conversely, platelets are both important suppliers of procoagulant proteins and indispensable catalysts of several reactions in the soluble coagulation cascade. Therefore, although this chapter focuses on platelets, it does not ignore their integrated functions in the entire coagulation and tissue repair systems.

Unstimulated platelets are small (3.6 ± 0.7 μm in diameter), disk-shaped, anucleate fragments of megakaryocyte cytoplasm that circulate in the peripheral blood at a normal concentration of $150,000-400,000/\mu$L. Platelets participate in an important way in the inflammatory response and in tissue repair, and they may play a significant role in atherogenesis. The ready availability of normal platelets has resulted in their use in experimental models for cellular biological functions as diverse as transmembrane signal transduction, prostaglandin synthesis, and uptake and secretion of neurotransmitters. Clinically, the use of platelet transfusions is growing at a disproportionately rapid rate, stimulated by the increasing use of high-dose, cytotoxic chemotherapy and bone marrow transplantation for malignant disease. The recent discovery and cloning of thrombopoietin, the physiologic regulator of platelet production, promises to help ameliorate the demand for platelet transfusion as well as to aid scientists to further elucidate the normal regulatory biology of this smallest of all blood cells.

PLATELET PRODUCTION AND KINETICS

CELLULAR BIOLOGY OF MEGAKARYOCYTOPOIESIS

Platelets, the smallest of the formed elements of the peripheral blood, are derived from the largest of bone marrow cells, the megakaryocyte. Megakaryocytes have been shown to originate from the same pluripotent hematopoietic stem cell that gives rise to red cells, neutrophils, and monocytes (Chapter 1). Once the stem cell begins irrevocably to develop along the megakaryocytic hematopoietic lineage, it is said to be committed. Committed megakaryocyte stem cell development is characterized by four nearly sequential stages: (1) the exponential expansion of committed stem cell numbers by mitotic cell division, (2) serial nuclear replication without cell division (i.e., endoreduplication or polyploidization), (3) megakaryocyte cytoplasmic maturation, and (4) platelet shedding or release.

Each of these four processes may affect the rate of platelet production and delivery from the bone marrow to the peripheral blood. Therefore each is a potential focus for the homeostatic regulatory system that controls circulating platelet numbers. The extent of mitotic expansion of the committed stem cell is the determinant of the number of megakaryocytes derived from that stem cell. Since the number of committed megakaryocyte stem cells does not appear to change with varying peripheral blood demand for platelets, the number of mitotic divisions of this stem cell most likely determines the frequency with which mature megakaryocytes develop in the bone marrow. Endoreduplication is initiated only when the developing megakaryocyte loses its capacity for cell division. The nucleus continues to replicate without accompanying cell division, and this proceeds for a variable number of cycles, resulting in a final megakaryocyte population exhibiting heterogeneous ploidy values. The total number of endomitotic cycles typically varies between three and six, corresponding to megakaryocyte ploidy values ranging from 8 to 64 N. Although the teleology of megakaryocyte endoreduplication is not understood, it is clear that there is a direct relationship between the ploidy of a megakaryocyte and the number of platelets it can produce. Therefore by increasing the extent of endoreduplication, the megakaryocyte compartment can rapidly augment its output of platelets. In experimental animals and patients, the ploidy distribution of megakaryoctes has been observed to shift to higher values (representing approximately one extra endomitotic cycle) in the presence of significantly accelerated platelet demand. In addition, ploidy increases have been shown to be an early adaptive response to accelerated platelet demand, a logical observation because an extra cycle of endoreduplication, occurring relatively late in the process of megakaryocyte development, can augment platelet production more rapidly than increases in mitotic stem cell expansion.

Although developing megakaryocytes acquire some characteristic membrane glycoproteins and begin to synthesize small amounts of α-granule proteins during endoreduplication, most cytoplasmic development occurs after endomitosis has been completed. At its earliest postendomitotic stage, the immature megakaryocyte is recognizable by light microscopy as a large, 6–24-μm cell with a tightly packed, multilobulated nucleus surrounded by a thin rim of deep blue cytoplasm. By electron microscopy, a Golgi apparatus is present accompanied by a rudimentary demarcation membrane system and rare α-granule. (See later.) Further maturation is characterized on light microscopy by progressively increasing cytoplasmic acidophilia, granularity, and volume. Ultrastructurally, while expanding dramatically in volume, the cytoplasm becomes filled with α-granules, dense granules, and an extensive, interwoven network of membrane channels and tubules known as the demarcation membrane system (DMS). Fully mature megakaryocytes range widely in size from 20 to 50 μm and comprise approximately 0.04% of nucleated bone marrow cells. These cells are characterized by voluminous, highly granular pink cytoplasm and an eccentrically located, compact, lobulated nucleus.

The process of platelet shedding is only poorly understood. One hypothesis is that the mature DMS segregates the megakaryocyte cytoplasm into platelet fields and that individual platelets are produced by the dissolution of the megakaryocyte cytoplasm along the defined planes of demarcation. More recent evidence suggests that platelet formation from megakaryocytes is a more dynamic process. In response to an undefined signal, megakaryocytes have been observed to transform into spiderlike cells projecting outward large numbers of long, filamentous cytoplasmic processes marked by regular foci of constriction. These sausaged processes, called proplatelets, are believed to project into marrow sinusoids (Fig. 1-3) and there fragment into platelets, possibly because of the shear force of flowing blood. Although platelet shedding is restricted to only the most mature megakaryocytes, it does appear to be a regulated process. Following an acute increase in the peripheral demand for platelets, the most immediate detectable response is an increase in platelet volume, reflecting a change in the mechanism of platelet formation.

HUMORAL REGULATION OF PLATELET PRODUCTION

Under steady-state conditions, the circulating platelet count is maintained within a tightly controlled, narrow range. However, in those pathologic states that result in accelerated platelet consumption, platelet production by the bone marrow may increase up to eight times normal. This increase is accomplished by the stimulation of an increased number of megakaryocytes as well as by stimulated increases in average megakaryocyte ploidy, size, and rate of maturation. In fact when thombocytopenia (a decrease in circulating platelets) is evaluated, an important clue to its pathogenesis can be found in the bone marrow. If increased numbers of bone marrow megakaryocytes are noted, then the thrombocytopenia can be presumed to be due to consumption of platelets in peripheral blood or reticuloendothelial system (or sequestration by the spleen), and generally no additional clinical studies need be performed.

Despite the long-standing clinical belief that platelet production was closely regulated, the specific mechanism responsible for this regulation has been elusive. More than 30 years ago, physicians began to speculate that platelet production was controlled by a circulating plasma factor, subsequently termed *thrombopoietin*, which increased in response to thrombocytopenia. However, the identification of thrombopoietin as a specific, defined hematopoietic regulatory cytokine was not accomplished until 1994, when its amino acid sequence was determined and its gene cloned simultaneously by four groups of investigators. Successful cloning was greatly facilitated by the recognition that thrombopoietin is the ligand for the hematopoietic receptor c-Mpl, the normal homolog of a viral oncogene demonstrated to induce a myeloproliferative leukemic state in mice.

It is now known that thrombopoietin is a lineage-specific, stimulatory regulator of megakaryocyte development and platelet production that acts at both the level of the committed megakaryocyte stem cell and that of the developing megakaryocyte (Fig. 1-1). Thrombopoietin (also called TPO, Mpl-ligand, megakaryocyte growth and development factor, and megapoietin) is produced primarily by the liver, with only trace amounts of its mRNA detected in the kidney. Unlike other hematopoietic cytokines, thrombopoietin does not appear to be regulated at the level of gene transcription. In fact, despite the experimental induction of severe thrombocytopenia, caused by either accelerated platelet consumption or decreased platelet production, hepatic mRNA levels do not vary significantly from baseline. It has been proposed that thrombopoietin is produced constitutively by the liver (at a constant rate) and that its stimulatory effect results only from that proportion that is not bound to circulating platelet thrombopoietin-receptors. Such a model requires confirmation but would explain the clinical observation that thrombocytopenia induced by splenic pooling, in which the platelet mass is constant, does not result in a compensatory stimulation of thrombopoiesis.

A number of other hematopoietic cytokines have been shown to stimulate platelet production, but none to the degree or with the lineage specificity of thrombopoietin. Interleukin 3 (IL-3), a multilineage hematopoietic growth factor, stimulates mitotic expansion and early development of the megakaryocytic committed stem cell, but it has little effect on megakaryocytic endoreduplication and cytoplasmic maturation. Conversely, both IL-6 and IL-11 exert thrombocytopoietic effects by modestly stimulating the postmitotic phases of megakaryocyte development. Preliminary data suggest that IL-6 may mediate the reactive thrombocytosis associated *in vivo* with some instances of systemic inflammatory disease (e.g., rheumatoid arthritis). All three of these cytokines have shown some activity in stimulating platelet production in a variety of experimental systems. However, the degree of the maximal platelet stimulatory activity for these cytokines *in vivo* has been modest (platelet counts rising only two- to threefold above baseline), and there has been significant associated toxicity. There are no data to suggest that either IL-3, IL-6, or IL-11 has a physiologic role in the regulation of the megakaryocytopoiesis and the circulating platelet count. Only plasma thrombopoietin activity has been demonstrated to vary inversely with the platelet count in a physiologically coherent manner. Because of its significantly greater maximal activity, its lineage specificity, and its initially favorable toxicity profile, it is also likely that only thrombopoietin will emerge as a clinically significant therapeutic for the management of thrombocytopenia.

PLATELET STRUCTURE

At rest, the platelet is a small, disc-shaped cell with a smooth plasma membrane supported by a ring of microtubulin. The plasma membrane invaginates to connect with a complex network of redundant membrane channels, the open canalicular system (OCS), which weaves throughout the platelet interior. It has been demonstrated that the central channels of the OCS are contiguous with the extracellular space of the platelet, and the OCS expresses the same membrane glycoproteins as the plasma membrane. A second internal membrane system, the dense tubular system, is thought to be derived from the endoplasmic reticulum of the megakaryocyte, is independent of the OCS, and does not connect with the extracellular milieu. Contractile microfilaments extend from the submembranous space throughout the platelet cytoplasm and are responsible for the dramatic shape change that accompanies platelet activation. Four types of granules can be found in the cytoplasm of inactivated platelets: α-granules, dense granules, lysosomes, and peroxisomes (Fig. 5-1). α-Granules, the most abundant platelet granule, contain both platelet-specific

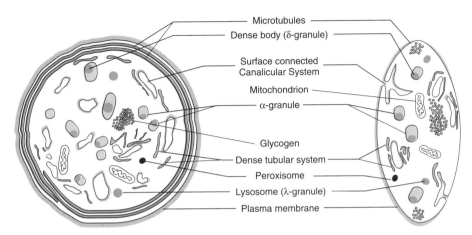

Figure 5-1. Schematic diagram of a human platelet. The figure on the right is a cross section of that on the left. (From Bentfeld-Barker ME, Bainton DF. Identification of primary lysosomes in human megakaryocytes and platelets. *Blood,* 59:472–481, 1982.)

and platelet-nonspecific peptides that contribute to and modulate coagulation, inflammation, immunity, and tissue repair. Dense granules, so named because of their electron-dense appearance on electron microscopy, are rich repositories of ADP and serotonin, substances that promote platelet aggregation, the antiaggregant ATP, and Ca^{2+}, an essential coagulation cofactor. Lysosomal granules contain hydrolytic enzymes, and peroxisomes contain catalase (Table 5-1).

The external plasma membrane and the OCS are studded with glycoproteins that play essential roles in platelet adhesion and aggregation (Table 5-2). These molecules consist of both external domains acting as receptors that bind to extracellular adhesive glycoproteins (such as fibrinogen, collagen, and von Willebrand factor) and transmembrane peptides that anchor the glycoproteins and transduce the processes of platelet activation and shape change (see later). Most of the platelet glycoproteins, with the exception of the glycoprotein Ib–IX complex, are members

TABLE 5-1. *PLATELET ALPHA GRANULE CONTENTS AND THEIR PROPOSED FUNCTIONS*

ALPHA GRANULE COMPONENT	FUNCTION
Platelet-derived growth factor (PDGF)	Fibroblast mitogen-tissue repair
Transforming growth factor β (TGF-β)	Tissue repair
Platelet factor 4 (PF-4)	Heparan neutralization, inflammation
β-thromboglobulin (β-TG)	Inflammation, tissue repair
von Willebrand factor (vWf)	Coagulation, platelet adhesion
Fibrinogen	Coagulation, platelet aggregation
Factor V	Coagulation
Protein S	Anticoagulant
Albumin	Hormone/toxin/drug binding
Immunoglobulin	Immunity

TABLE 5-2. *PLATELET GLYCOPROTEINS AND THEIR LIGANDS*

GLYCOPROTEIN	LIGANDS	
	Primary	Secondary
GP IIb–IIIa	Fibrinogen	vWf, fibronectin vitronectin
GP Ib-IX	vWf	Thrombin
GP Ia-IIa	Collagen	
GP Ic-IIa	Fibronectin	Laminin
α_6/IIa	Laminin	
Vitronectin receptor	Vitronectin	Thrombospondin

of the integrin gene family. Platelet membranes exhibit receptors for the physiologic mediators of platelet activation—including ADP, epinephrine, serotonin, and thromboxane A_2—and for the Fc portion of immunoglobulins. Platelet membranes also display HLA class I (but not class II) antigens.

PLATELET FUNCTION

Platelets serve a variety of functions *in vivo*, including (1) the promotion of immediate hemostasis by platelet adhesion and platelet aggregation, resulting in the formation of a platelet plug; (2) the local release of vasoconstrictors to decrease blood flow to the injured area; (3) catalysis of reactions of the soluble coagulation cascade leading to fibrin clot formation; (4) initiation of the tissue repair process; and (5) regulation of local inflammation and immunity. Unstimulated platelets circulate as smooth, disc-shaped cells that exhibit little, if any, metabolic activity. Such platelets do not interact meaningfully with the other formed elements of the peripheral blood or with the endothelial cell monolayer that lines the endovascular space.

Physiologic activation of platelets begins only when the vascular endothelium is damaged, thus exposing the subendothelial extracellular matrix. Damage to the endothelium exposes collagen, other extracellular matrix proteins, and microfibrils anchoring large multimers of von Willebrand factor (which are synthesized and secreted by the endothelial cells). The platelet membrane glycoprotein Ib (GPIb) receptor binds specifically to exposed von Willebrand factor (vWf), with secondary vWf binding to platelet membrane GPIIb/IIIa. Exposed subendothelial collagen binds to the membrane GPIa receptor. Platelet adhesion, while providing a marginal degree of hemostasis in and of itself, initiates the process of platelet activation, which results in a dramatic change in platelet shape, the irreversible secretion of dense and α-granule contents, and platelet aggregation with the formation of a hemostatic platelet plug.

Shape change is an early, and reversible, manifestation of platelet activation that is mediated by the platelet's intracellular contractile microfilament system. The platelet membrane ruffles and projects out a large number of short, filamentous pseudopodia or filopods, drawing on redundant membrane of the open canalicular system. This process substantially increases the platelet membrane surface area available to catalyze soluble coagulation reactions and may stabilize subsequent platelet aggregates (Figs. 6-2, 6-4, 6-6, and 6-11). Platelet activation also leads to a conformational change in GP IIb/IIIa that permits fibrinogen binding to the platelet membrane, a prerequisite for platelet aggregation. With the initiation of platelet activation, the intracellular organelles are gathered to the center of the cell by contraction of the microtubular ring, which is followed by fusion of the membranes of the dense and the α-granules with each other, the platelet plasma membrane, and the membrane of the open canalicular system. These fusion events result in exocytosis of the granular contents into the external microenvironment, because the interior channels of the OCS are contiguous with the extracellular space. Exocytosis also translocates the platelet α-granule membrane protein P-selectin (also called GMP-140 and PADGEM) from the interior surface of the granule to the OCS and external plasma membrane. Biochemical reactions stimulated by platelet activation include both the synthesis of thromboxane A_2 by arachidonate released from membrane of the dense tubular system and the synthesis of platelet-activating factor (PAF), a complex lipid molecule. Thromboxane A_2, an unstable member of the prostaglandin family, is a potent proaggregant and vasoconstrictor, whereas PAF appears to amplify the platelet aggregation reaction and is a powerful activator of neutrophils. With the initial phase of platelet activation, secreted ADP, serotonin, and thromboxane A_2 activate nearby platelets, and this self-amplifying cascade of platelet activation, thromboxane A_2, synthesis, and granule release results in the formation of a platelet aggregate, cross-linked by fibrinogen that bridges the GP IIb/IIIa receptors on adjacent platelet membranes. The fibrinogen bridging is further stabilized by thrombospondin, another α-granule constituent released with platelet activation. The generation of thrombin as a product of the soluble coagulation cascade further amplifies platelet aggregation, because thrombin is another potent agonist of platelet aggregation (Fig. 6-15).

Not only does thrombin activate platelets, but platelets contribute meaningfully to the generation of thrombin by catalyzing and providing factors for the reactions of the soluble coagulation cascade (Figs. 6-2, 6-4, 6-6, and 6-11). Megakaryocytes are known to synthesize and store in platelet α-granules the coagulation factors V, VIII, XIII, vWf, and fibrinogen. These clotting factors are discharged to the microenvironment, with platelet activation and exocytosis raising their local concentrations. The extracellular adhesive glycoproteins fibronectin, osteonectin, and vitronectin are also stored in platelet α-granules and released with platelet activation.

The platelet membrane also plays an essential role in promoting specific coagulation reactions. A platelet membrane lipoprotein, so-called platelet factor 3, is an important catalyst in the activation of factor X by factors IXa and VIII and in the formation of prothrombinase by the interaction between factors Xa and V (Figs. 6-4, and 6-6). The platelet membrane may also play an important role in the assembly of other soluble coagulation factors for optimal reactivity. Conversely, the activated platelet also appears to limit the coagulation cascade. Activated platelet membrane binds thrombin and thrombomodulin, an α-granule constituent, which together activate the anticoagulant protein C (Fig. 6-11). α-Granules also supply tissue plasminogen activator to the microenvironment.

The functioning of platelets in the inflammatory process and tissue repair is less well defined. However, it is clear that platelet α-granules deliver the powerful cytokines platelet-derived growth factor (PDGF) and transforming growth factor-β (TGF-β) to the site of tissue injury. PDGF is a potent stimulator of the proliferation of fibroblasts and smooth muscle cells, whereas TGF-β exhibits both growth-stimulatory and growth-inhibitory properties. Platelet factor 4 and β-thromboglobulin are two other platelet-specific α-granule proteins that are members of the small inducible gene family and that appear to have roles in coagulation, the inflammatory response, and cell growth. Finally, platelets also interface with the system of humoral immunity. As described earlier, platelet membranes have receptors for the Fc portion of the IgG molecule and will bind immune complexes and aggregated IgG. It has also been demonstrated that resting platelets take up plasma immunoglobulin by endocytosis and store it in the α-granule for later secretion by exocytosis.

LABORATORY EVALUATION

PLATELET COUNT

The platelet counts of normal individuals are normally quite stable in any single person, but among individuals they range fairly widely, between 150,000 and 400,000/μL. Since the mean platelet volume (MPV) varies inversely with the platelet count, the platelet mass in the circulation across individuals is more constant than the platelet counts would otherwise suggest. In the modern laboratory, peripheral blood platelet counts are determined by automated particle counting of blood samples that have been diluted and in which the red cells have been lysed. Since this method quantitates only particles of given size and does not specifically differentiate platelets, an abnormal platelet count should always be confirmed by an examination of the peripheral smear. The average number of platelets per 1,000 magnification microscopic oil immersion lens field $\times$12,000–15,000 should equal the platelet count per microliter. Artifactually low platelet counts may result from EDTA-induced platelet clumping (so-called pseudothrombocytopenia) or satellitism, the adherence of platelets to the plasma membranes of neutrophils as a result of IgG or IgM platelet agglutinins. Conversely, artifactually high platelet counts may be seen when the peripheral blood is contaminated with small, nonplatelet cell fragments (e.g., in acute leukemia in which circulating blasts may release small, cytoplasmic blebs and when red cells exhibit microspherocytosis). If there is any uncertainty about the automated platelet count, a manual platelet count should be obtained. The peripheral blood smear should always be examined to confirm the data obtained by laboratory testing (Chapter 2).

PLATELET VOLUME MEASUREMENT

The routine application of automated particle counting has resulted in the widespread availability of the MPV, a measure of mean circulating platelet size. There is substantial evidence that platelet volume correlates directly with mean megakaryocyte ploidy and that MPV is increased in the clinical context of accelerated platelet production. The presence of significant numbers of large platelets or megathrombocytes on the peripheral smears from patients with thrombocytopenia has been proposed as a diagnostic discriminator of those patients whose thrombocytopenia has a consumptive pathogenesis. However, the automated determination of MPV is affected by the nonclinical variables of specimen temperature, storage time, and anticoagulant. Therefore MPV has proven to be a difficult measurement to standardize and, when available, should be interpreted with caution.

BLEEDING TIME

Platelet-associated hemostasis is a function of two variables, platelet number and platelet function. Although determination of platelet number is straightforward, the assessment of platelet function is quite difficult, and complex clinical variables affect test interpretation. Despite the heterogeneity of potential mechanisms and clinical manifestations of platelet dysfunction, there is only one widely available clinical test of platelet function, the bleeding time (BT). The BT measures the time interval between the placement of a small, standard, superficial wound on the forearm and the formation of a stable platelet plug, evidenced clinically by the cessation of bleeding. The modified Ivy BT is that in most widespread use and employs a spring-loaded blade that is used to create a 1-cm-long, 1-mm-deep wound on the volar forearm with a blood pressure cuff inflated on the ipsilateral upper arm to 40 mmHg. Blood is blotted from the edge of the wound with filter paper every 30 seconds, with care being taken not to disturb the developing platelet plug in the center until the bleeding ceases. Using this technique, the normal BT is 3-8 minutes; using the so-called template BT, it is 2-7 minutes..

Despite its crude simplicity and its modest discomfort, the BT is the test of choice when platelet dysfunction is clinically suspected. A properly performed BT generally will be abnormal under only three circumstances: (1) thrombocytopenia of less than 100,000/μL, (2) qualitative platelet dysfunction of any type, and rarely, (3) abnormalities of the microvasculature (i.e., amyloidosis). With normal platelet function and between platelet counts of 10,000/μL and 100,000/μL, the BT varies linearly with the platelet count according to the empirically determined equation: BT (in minutes) = 30.5 − (platelet count per μL)/3,850 (Fig. 5-2). In thrombocytopenic states due to platelet consumption (i.e., immune thrombocytopenia), the BT will often be shorter than predicted by this equation because of the exuberant phospholipid content of the younger, larger platelets in this condition. Conversely, in certain instances of productive thrombocytopenia in which megakaryocyte and platelet maturation are disordered (e.g., myelodysplasia), the BT will be longer than predicted. The ingestion of a single tablet of aspirin will predictably prolong a normal BT to 8–10 minutes. However, it may disproportionately prolong the BT in pa-

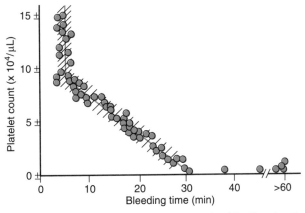

Figure 5-2. Relationship between the platelet count and template bleeding time for normal platelets. Note the bleeding time is insensitive to the platelet count for platelets ≥ 100,000/μL and varies linearly with the platelet count for platelets <100,000/μL and >10,000/μL. (From Harker LA. Philadelphia: FA Davis; *Hemostasis Manual.*; 1974:8.)

tients with mild qualitative platelet dysfunction and thus uncover a mild qualitative platelet disorder. This so-called aspirin tolerance test should be used with caution in patients suspected of having a bleeding disorder, because aspirin will exacerbate the bleeding tendency in such patients. Aspirin irreversibly acetylates platelet cyclo-oxygenase and will therefore affect platelets over their entire lifespan of approximately 8–10 days. (Compare this with nonsteroidal anti-inflammatory drugs that bind this enzyme reversibly and thus inhibit platelet function only as long as plasma levels of these drugs are maintained.)

PLATELET AGGREGOMETRY

Formal testing of platelet aggregometry permits the separation of qualitative platelet disorders into discrete etiologic categories. Platelet aggregometry is a conceptually simple laboratory test in which the conglomeration of single platelets into clumps or aggregates of increasing size is quantified by the extent of light transmission through the platelet-containing plasma. The platelet aggregometer (Fig. 5-3) consists of a small, transparent cuvette containing the patient's concentrated platelets at a standard concentration across which a calibrated light source shines into a photoelectric cell. The photoelectric cell is linked to a strip recorder that measures light transmission (or optical density) over time. When the platelets exist as a single cell suspension (i.e., prior to aggregation), the light transmission is at its lowest. With increasing aggregation, the platelet-containing plasma becomes progressively clearer and light transmission increases. Although this phenomenon may not at first appear intuitive, it can be reconciled by considering the differing clarities of

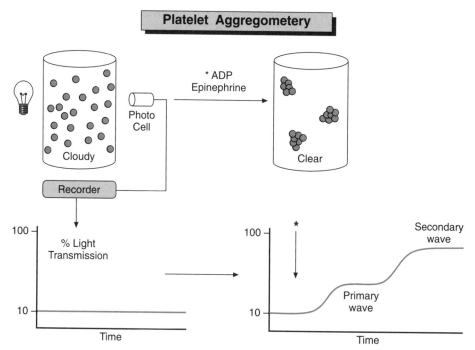

Figure 5-3. Platelet aggregometry testing process. At the *, a platelet aggregation agonist such as ADP or epinephrine is added to the system. The formation of platelet aggregates from single platelets transforms the cloudy platelet-rich plasma to relatively clear plasma.

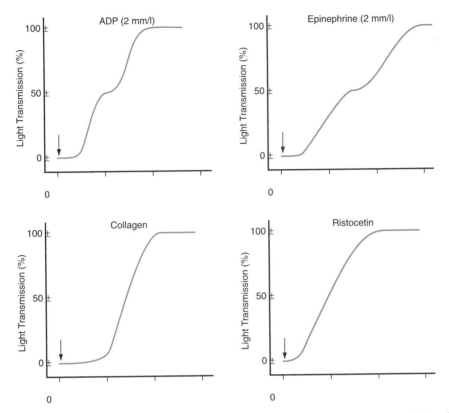

Figure 5-4. Normal patterns of platelet aggregation using the aggregometry apparatus depicted in Fig. 5-3: Response to selected concentrations of ADP, epinephrine, collagen, and ristocetin are illustrated (added at the arrow).

liquid suspensions containing either large numbers of fine particles of clay or the same mass of clay consolidated into only a few pebbles.

In vitro platelet aggregation may be initiated by adding a variety of exogenous agents to the aggregometry cuvette, the most common of which are ADP, epinephrine, collagen, thrombin, arachidonic acid, and ristocetin. ADP, epinephrine, and thrombin are unique in their capacity to induce platelet aggregation by themselves, without requiring platelet degranulation and exocytosis. Therefore at low concentrations, these agents will stimulate only a reversible primary wave of platelet aggregation, which begins as soon as these substances are added to the aggregometer. At slightly higher concentrations of ADP, epinephrine, and thrombin, platelets become fully activated and the release of granule contents, along with the synthesis of thromboxane A_2 results in a slightly delayed but amplified secondary wave of platelet aggregation (Fig. 5-4). At even higher concentrations, the primary wave of aggregation is buried in the secondary wave, and only a single, complete wave of aggregation is seen.

Although collagen binds to platelet membrane glycoprotein Ia, it does not aggregate platelets in and of itself. However, after a lag, collagen does induce complete platelet aggregation as a result of intrinsic platelet activation. The capacity of arachidonic acid to stimulate platelet aggregation depends upon the functioning of the enzyme cyclo-oxygenase in the prostaglandin synthesis pathway. The synthesis of thromboxane A$_2$ from arachidonic acid results in complete platelet activation, exocytosis, and aggregation.

Ristocetin is unique in its mechanism of aggregation in that such aggregation does not require platelet metabolism. In fact, ristocetin-induced platelet aggregation can be achieved using formalin-fixed platelets. Ristocetin is thought to support platelet aggregation by associating with platelet membrane GP Ib, thus rendering it active as a primary binding site for vWf. Therefore in the presence of ristocetin, vWf serves to cross-link platelets into large aggregates. If the platelets are viable, ristocetin aggregation will also result in platelet activation and endogenous granule release. In the absence of vWf, activation does not occur.

QUALITATIVE PLATELET DISORDERS

INTRODUCTION AND CLINICAL FEATURES

Clinical disorders of platelet function or qualitative platelet disorders may be congenital in origin or acquired as a result of drug exposure or systemic disease (Table 5-3). Regardless, platelet dysfunction per se is not usually associated with a severe spontaneous bleeding diathesis. Significant bleeding occurs in such patients almost exclusively in association with surgery, parturition, trauma, dental extraction, and other major hemostatic stress. Otherwise, patients with qualitative platelet dysfunction typically present with easy bruising and intermittent mucosal bleeding (e.g., epistaxis, gingival bleeding with teeth brushing, and occult gastrointestinal blood loss). Hemarthroses and deep soft-tissue bleeding are characteristic of a severe deficiency of one of the soluble coagulation factors and are not usually platelet related. Qualitative platelet dysfunction should be suspected in the patient with a suggestive history when the BT is abnormal with a normal aPTT, PT, thrombin time, and platelet count. The formal testing of platelet aggregometry in such patients usually defines the specific diagnosis. In a patient with a suggestive history but a normal BT, an exaggerated prolongation of the BT after a standard dose of oral aspirin, the so-called aspirin tolerance test, may identify those patients appropriate for further testing with platelet aggregometry. Patients who exhibit both a prolonged BT and PTT should be suspected of having von Willebrand disease. (See later.)

CONGENITAL DISORDERS OF PLATELET ADHESION AND THE PLATELET MEMBRANE

Von Willebrand Disease. Von Willebrand disease (vWD) is the most common inherited bleeding disorder in man, with prevalence figures in different populations ranging from 1% to more than 2%. Since vWD is caused by a deficiency or qualitative abnormality in the von Willebrand factor/factor VIII protein complex, it is technically a defect in the soluble coagulation system and is therefore discussed in greater detail in the following chapter. However, normal concentration and function of von Willebrand factor (vWf) is also essential in supporting normal platelet function; thus vWD is also considered a disorder of platelet function. As discussed earlier, vWf is present in the plasma and subendothelial extracellular matrix and binds specifically to the platelet membrane glycoprotein GP Ib with secondary bind-

TABLE 5-3. *CLASSIFICATION AND ETIOLOGIES OF QUALITATIVE PLATELET DISORDERS*

I. Congenital disorders
  A. Membrane glycoprotein defects/deficiency
    1. Glanzmann's thrombasthenia
    2. Bernard–Soulier syndrome
  B. Congenital plasma protein abnormalities
    1. Von Willebrand disease
    2. Hereditary afibrinogenemia
  C. Storage pool diseases
    1. Dense granule deficiencies
    2. Alpha storage pool deficiency (gray platelet syndrome)
    3. Primary granule release defects
      a. Cyclo-oxygenase deficiency
      b. Thromboxane synthetase deficiency

II. Acquired disorders
  A. Secondary granule release defects
    1. Drug related
      a. Aspirin and NSAIDs
      b. Ticlopidine
      c. Dipyridamole
      d. Carbenicillin and other β-lactam antibiotics
      e. Omega-3 fatty acids
    2. Uremia
    3. Cyanotic congenital heart disease
  B. Storage pool diseases
    1. Due to stem cell dysfunction
      a. Myeloproliferative disorders
      b. Myelodysplastic syndromes
      c. Acute leukemia
    2. Due to partial activation
      a. Disseminated intravascular coagulation (DIC)
      b. Severe valvular heart disease
      c. Extracorporeal circulation
  C. Disordered interaction between the platelet membrane and extracellular matrix proteins
    1. Paraproteinemia
    2. DIC
    3. ITP (occasional cases)

ing to GP IIb/IIIa. vWf is crucial for the initial adhesion of platelets to collagen and other extracellular matrix proteins exposed by damaged subendothelial surfaces. vWD can result from two principal types of molecular defects in vWf production: (1) quantitatively low-level synthesis of functionally normal vWf protein and (2) quantitatively normal synthesis of functionally defective vWf. These two classes of defects are called type I vWD and type IIA vWD and account for more than 70% and 10–15% of cases of vWD, respectively (Tables 6-5 and 6-6). Functional deficiency of vWf can be detected in the laboratory as a diminished capacity of patient plasma to support ristocetin-induced platelet aggregation *in vitro* (Fig. 5-4). This capacity is called *ristocetin cofactor activity* and is characteristically decreased in types I and IIA vWD (Tables 6-5 and 6-6). A third and rare variant of vWD, type IIB, is characterized by an increased affinity of defective high-molecular-weight vWf multimers for platelet GP Ib, resulting in specific adsorption of these multimers to the platelet membrane, a resultant circulating deficiency of high-molecular-weight vWf, and thrombocytopenia, presumably due to intravascular platelet aggregation. In this rare variant, ristocetin—induced platelet aggregation (with low doses of ristocetin) is paradoxically increased. (Table 6-5, Figs., 6-20B, C)

vWf multimer subunits are coded by an approximately 180-kilobase gene at the tip of the short arm of chromosome 12 (Fig. 6-23). Therefore vWD is inherited in an autosomal dominant pattern. However, penetrance can vary because circulating vWf levels are affected by a number of unrelated variables. These include exogenous estrogen therapy, pregnancy, blood group type, and even stress. These factors can also result in significant clinical heterogeneity among affected individuals with vWD, even within single kindreds. A single patient may also exhibit variable bleeding tendency due to intervening clinical and environmental factors.

Since vWf binds to, stabilizes, and prevents catabolism of circulating factor VIII, both quantitative and qualitative abnormalities in vWf may result in decreased levels of factor VIII procoagulant activity. Factor VIII levels below 30–40% will affect the aPTT and begin to compromise normal hemostasis. Thus patients with vWD may have clinically significant defects in both the soluble coagulation system and platelet function. This explains the concurrent prolongation of both the aPTT and the BT in patients with vWD. However, factor VIII levels rarely are as low as those observed in even mild hemophilia A.

The clinical manifestations of vWD are extremely variable. Easy bruising, mucosal bleeding, and menorrhagia are common. The bleeding tendency may be greatly exacerbated by the ingestion of aspirin or other nonsteroidal anti-inflammatory agents. Spontaneous hemarthroses and soft-tissue bleeding are distinctly uncommon, but vWD patients may be at significant risk for bleeding with invasive surgical and dental procedures. Therapy is directed at raising the circulating levels of vWf by either the infusion of exogenous, blood product–derived vWf or the mobilization of endogenous vWf from cellular storage sites. Exogenous vWf can be administered in the form of fresh-frozen plasma, cryoprecipitate, and some commercial preparations of factor VIII concentrate. Since the amount of vWf in commercial factor VIII concentrates varies with the isolation process, each brand must be individually assessed for its adequacy to replace vWf. Blood product exposure may be eliminated by the use of desmopressin (DDAVP), which variably mobilizes endogenous vWf from endothelial storage sites. Desmopressin, a synthetic analog of vasopressin that can be administered either intravenously or intranasally, is particularly effective in patients with type I vWD, is less effective in patients with type IIA, and is contraindicated in patients with the rare type IIB vWD (Chapter 6). Since the therapeutic effect of desmopressin in any single individual cannot be predicted, a therapeutic trial is recommended (with postdesmopressin measurements of the aPTT, BT, and levels of factor VIII, vWf, and ristocetin cofactor) before it is employed for preoperative prophylaxis. In some instances, particularly dental work, administration of an antifibrinolytic agent, ε-aminocaproic acid (EACA), or tranexamic acid, may be sufficient to prevent serious bleeding.

Bernard-Soulier Syndrome. The Bernard-Soulier syndrome is a rare, inherited qualitative platelet disorder in which there is a molecular defect in platelet membrane GP Ib. Since GP Ib is the primary receptor for vWf, these patients exhibit a clinical picture similar to moderately severe vWD and generally present in infancy or early childhood. Functionally, like vWD, platelet adhesion to vascular subendothelial matrix is significantly impaired. Although platelet aggregation is normal with the standard platelet agonists, ristocetin-induced aggregation is significantly impaired or absent and is not corrected by the addition of normal vWf (Fig. 6-19). Other characteristic clinical features include mild to moderate thrombocytopenia and an increase in circulating platelet size. The hemorrhagic tendency may be sufficiently severe to cause death in some patients, whereas in others, disease severity diminishes over time.

Glanzmann's Thrombasthenia. Glanzmann's thrombasthenia is a rare but illustrative congenital qualitative platelet disorder that results from the absence or dysfunction of the platelet membrane fibrinogen receptor and glycoprotein complex IIb/IIIa. Like the Bernard-Soulier syndrome, Glanzmann's thrombasthenia usually presents in infancy or early childhood and is characterized by menorrhagia, easy bruising, epistaxis, and gingival bleeding. The BT is abnormal, as are all tests of platelet aggregation except ristocetin. This profound platelet dysfunction arises from the failure of fibrinogen binding to the platelet membrane and the resulting absence of the fibrinogen cross-linking required for platelet aggregation. Only ristocetin-induced aggregation, which is independent of fibrinogen and depends exclusively upon vWf and membrane GP Ib, is preserved in these patients (Fig. 6-19).

CONGENITAL STORAGE POOL DISEASES

The congenital platelet storage pool diseases represent a heterogeneous group of disorders characterized by a prolonged BT, easy bruising and a mild to moderate tendency to bleed with trauma, surgery, and dental work (Table 5-3). Conventionally, the storage pool diseases have been divided into two groups, those with an absolute deficiency of pro-aggregatory storage granules (i.e., the dense granules containing ADP, ATP, calcium, and serotonin) and those with normal platelet granular content but a malfunction in the granule secretory mechanism, the so-called aspirin-like defect (see later). In both instances, platelet adhesion and primary waves of *in vitro* aggregation to ADP, epinephrine, and thrombin remain intact. However, there is an absence or diminished secondary wave of aggregation because of the failure of the platelets to release adequate quantities of endogenous ADP and other pro-aggregatory substances with platelet activation. There is also an absent or diminished *in vitro* response to collagen, since collagen-induced aggregation also requires the active secretion of dense granules (Fig. 5-1).

Congenital dense granule deficiency can exist as an isolated disorder of variable penetrance and variable clinical severity. An autosomal dominant pattern of familial inheritance may be observed. Kindreds have been described exhibiting an autosomal dominant pattern of both dense granule deficiency and albinism, this constellation termed the **Hermansky-Pudlak syndrome.** Since dense granule-deficient platelets lack granular ADP, an increased ratio of whole-platelet ATP:ADP may be useful in diagnosis.

Alpha storage pool deficiency, or the **gray platelet syndrome,** is characterized clinically by a mild bleeding diathesis, moderate thrombocytopenia of 60,000–100,000/μL, and large circulating platelets. The disorder is believed to arise from the defective packaging of the synthetic products of developing megakaryocytes into nascent α-granules. This postulate is supported by the observed increases in circulating thromboglobulin and platelet factor 4 as well as the presence of reticulin fibrosis of the bone marrow, presumably resulting from leakage of PDGF and transforming growth factor-β into the marrow microenvironment.

Congenital defects in the platelet granule release process present a clinical picture similar to that of absolute storage pool deficiency states. In such patients, the stimulus–response coupling between platelet activation and granule secretion appears to be defective. With platelet aggregometry testing, besides an absent or deficient secondary wave, these patients may exhibit an impaired response to arachidonic acid (the metabolic precursor of the potent pro-aggregatory prostaglandin endoperoxides and thromboxane A_2). The pattern of inheritance of this heterogeneous group of disorders is unknown. Aspirin, which will greatly exaggerate the BT abnormality in these patients, may also greatly exacerbate the bleeding tendency. The aspirin tolerance test may be useful for diagnosis in the patient with a suggestive history.

The treatment of the congenital storage pool disorders is generally nonspecific. Platelet transfusions may transiently correct the bleeding diathesis but are not often warranted because of the risk of transfusion-related disease. DDAVP improves platelet function by an as yet undefined mechanism and is the treatment of choice in most situations where prophylaxis or therapy for bleeding is required. Cryoprecipitate, which also carries the risk of blood-borne disease transmission, may also be salutary in some clinical situations.

ACQUIRED QUALITATIVE PLATELET DISORDERS

Medications. There are a number of etiologies for acquired qualitative platelet dysfunction (see Table 5-3). The most common cause encountered in clinical practice is the ingestion of aspirin or other nonsteroidal anti-inflammatory drug (NSAID). Aspirin irreversibly binds and inactivates cyclo-oxygenase, a pivotal enzyme in the prostaglandin biosynthetic pathway. This uncouples the platelet's intrinsic stimulus–response mechanism, resulting in an inability to secrete the platelet granules and thus an acquired defect in the release reaction process. Once a platelet's cyclo-oxygenase has been inactivated by aspirin, it remains permanently disabled until the platelet is finally removed from the circulation. Since approximately 100,000–150,000 platelets/μL are replaced every 5 days and because a concentration of 100,000 platelets/μL results in normal hemostasis, the aspirin defect requires 5 days from the most recent ingestion until it can be considered negligible. The clinical corollary to this observation is that elective surgery and other invasive procedures should be postponed until at least 5 days after any aspirin exposure. NSAIDs exert their antiplatelet effect by a similar inhibitory effect on cyclo-oxygenase. However, with nonaspirin NSAIDs, the inhibitory effect is reversible and dissipates as soon as the circulating NSAID plasma levels fall to near zero. Although this time varies from one NSAID to another based upon their plasma half-lives, platelet function generally returns to normal well within 24 hours. Should surgery be absolutely necessary in the context of recent aspirin or NSAID exposure, DDAVP may transiently improve platelet function. Platelet transfusions are reserved for severe bleeding in DDAVP-unresponsive patients.

Uremia. Uremia is associated with a variable and diverse set of qualitative platelet defects. Although the BT and tests of platelet aggregation are frequently abnormal, neither the presence nor the degree of abnormality predicts the risk for clinical bleeding. It is generally believed that uremia-induced platelet functional defects result from the accumulation of toxic metabolites in the uremic plasma. Platelet function improves with aggressive dialysis, and this is a preferred method of treatment. Platelet dysfunction is also believed to result from the significant anemia characteristic of uremic patients. The decrease in mass of circulating red cells permits the streaming of platelets in the central cross-sectional area of the blood vessel, thus reducing random platelet interactions with the blood vessel walls. (In health, platelets serve to plug normally occurring gaps between endothelial cells.) Raising the hematocrit to more than 30 by red cell transfusion or erythropoietin therapy will significantly improve the platelet functional abnormality. Other measures that have been shown to improve platelet function in uremia include DDAVP administration, estrogen therapy, and cryoprecipitate. Platelet transfusions are relatively contraindicated because the transfused platelets will acquire the uremic defect after exposure to the patient's uremic plasma.

Cardiopulmonary Bypass. Patients undergoing cardiopulmonary bypass develop a complex coagulopathy of which qualitative platelet dysfunction is a component. This dysfunction is thought to arise from platelet interaction with the artificial surfaces of the bypass machinery, resulting in partial platelet activation and granule release. Platelets and platelet membranes are also damaged mechanically by shear stress within the bypass circuit. The partially activated and/or damaged platelets are returned to the circulation, where they exhibit multiple abnormalities, including a release reaction defect. The platelet functional abnormality usually resolves within hours. For clinically significant bleeding, platelet transfusions and the administration of DDAVP have been shown to be beneficial.

Paraproteinemias. Approximately one-third of patients with IgA myeloma and Waldenström's macroglobulinemia (Chapter 9) exhibit an accompanying qualitative platelet defect. Although the pathogenesis of this defect is unclear, in some instances the defect is thought to arise from interactions between the paraprotein and the platelet surface membrane glycoproteins, which interfere with fibrinogen and vWf binding. The defect can be improved with plasmapheresis and other measures directed at reducing the plasma paraprotein concentration.

Disseminated Intravascular Coagulation. Disseminated intravascular coagulation (DIC) may also be accompanied by qualitative platelet dysfunction. This results from partial platelet activation by circulating thrombin and from the increase in fibrin/fibrinogen degradation products that compete with fibrinogen for the GP IIb/IIIa receptor on the platelet membrane (Chapter 6).

Myeloproliferative and Myelodysplastic Disorders. Intrinsic qualitative platelet defects have been reported in patients with one of the myeloproliferative disorders or with a myelodysplastic syndrome. Since these disorders arise in the hematopoietic stem cell, the platelet dysfunction is believed to result from disordered megakaryocyte and platelet development.

THROMBOCYTOPENIA

INTRODUCTION

General. Thrombocytopenia is technically defined as a platelet count below the normal range of 150,000–400,000/μL. However, satisfactory surgical hemostasis is achieved with a platelet count of 50,000/μL, and spontaneous hemorrhage is rare until platelet counts fall below 10,000–20,000/μL. The clinical hallmarks of thrombocytopenia, generally manifest only when the platelet count is less than 50,000/μL, are easy bruising, gingival bleeding, menorrhagia, and petechiae in dependent areas. A more severe hemostatic defect is indicated by epistaxis, gastrointestinal bleeding, and hemorrhagic mucosal bullae (wet purpura).

Pseudothrombocytopenia. Any laboratory report of thrombocytopenia requires the immediate evaluation of the peripheral blood smear. Although such examination is important to help determine the pathogenesis of the thrombocytopenia, it is also necessary to rule out the laboratory artifact of pseudothrombocytopenia. In the presence of EDTA, the standard blood collection anticoagulant, platelets may clump into aggregates too large to be enumerated as platelets by the automated particle counter. In other instances in which there are platelet autoantibodies or high levels of platelet-associated IgG, platelets may either clump or form rosettes around circulating neutrophils *in vitro*. These platelets are also missed by automated platelet counting devices. Pseudothrombocytopenia can be confirmed by repeating the blood collection into a tube anticoagulated with heparin and then repeating the platelet count.

Distributional and Dilutional Thrombocytopenia. Once true thrombocytopenia is established, it is essential to establish its etiology. This can best be approached by assigning the thrombocytopenia into one of four major categories based upon pathogenesis (Table 5-4). Assignment to either of two of these categories, distributional and dilutional, is usually obvious based upon the clinical situation and the physical examination. Dilutional thrombocytopenia develops in the clinical context of substantial hemorrhage with replacement by crystalloid, plasma, and red cell transfusions. Blood loss of 5–10 U with replacement as described can result in platelet counts falling to 25–50% of baseline. Distributional thrombocytopenia reflects the extent to which platelets are sequestered in an enlarged spleen. Normally, approximately 70% of the platelet mass exists as circulating platelets in the peripheral blood. The other 30% is sequestered in the spleen and forms the splenic platelet pool (Chapter 1). Splenomegaly results in an increasing proportion of the platelet mass sequestered in the splenic pool. In instances of massive splenomegaly, the splenic pool may comprise up to 90% of the total platelet mass. Since the thrombopoietic regulatory system appears to control platelet mass rather than concentration (see earlier), massive splenomegaly and splenic sequestration can result in significant circulating thrombocytopenia. Although the splenomegaly contributing to modest thrombocytopenia may not be clinically obvious, that associated with severe thrombocytopenia should be evident to even the most casual observer. It should be noted that immune thrombocytopenic purpura (see later) is associated with a spleen of normal size.

Consumptive Versus Productive Thrombocytopenia. Once it is clear that thrombocytopenia is neither dilutional nor distributional in origin, the clinician must distinguish between productive and consumptive etiologies for the throm-

TABLE 5-4. *CLASSIFICATION OF THROMBOCYTOPENIC DISORDERS BY PATHOGENESIS*

Productive
  Aplastic anemia
  TAR syndrome
  Acquired amegakaryocytic thrombocytopenia
  Myelodysplastic syndromes
  Acute leukemia
  Myelophthisis
  Cytotoxic chemotherapy
  Radiotherapy
  Drugs (estrogens, thiazides)
  Alcohol
  B_{12} and folate deficiency
  Cyclic thrombocytopenia
  Paroxysmal nocturnal hemoglobinuria
  Viral infection (rare)

Dilutional
  Massive hemorrhage

Distributional
  Splenomegaly

Consumptive
  Adult immune thrombocytopenic purpura
  Childhood immune thrombocytopenic purpura
  Drugs (quinidine, gold, heparin)
  Posttransfusion purpura
  Neonatal alloimmune thrombocytopenia
  Thrombotic thrombocytopenic purpura/hemolytic uremic syndrome
  Disseminated intravascular coagulation
  Eclampsia/pre-eclampsia/HELLP syndrome
  Malignancy

bocytopenia. Consumptive thrombocytopenia results from accelerated platelet utilization and a shortened circulating half-life in which there is not adequate compensation by the bone marrow. Since the bone marrow can increase platelet production eight- to twelvefold, accelerated platelet turnover will not necessarily result in thrombocytopenia unless this compensatory capacity is exceeded. Most consumptive thrombocytopenias result from either immune-mediated platelet destruction, intravascular activation of the coagulation system, or widespread endothelial damage (Table 5-4). Productive thrombocytopenia develops when the bone marrow fails to keep up with the supply necessary for normal platelet turnover. (Since the normal platelet circulating lifespan is 8–10 days, the bone marrow must replace an average of 10–13% of the platelet mass daily.) Productive thrombocytopenia generally results from hematopoietic stem cell failure resulting from neoplasia or nutritional deficiency or from myelophthisis, the replacement of the bone marrow with non-blood-forming tissue (Table 5-4).

In response to accelerated peripheral platelet demand, healthy bone marrow responds with an increase in megakaryocyte number, size, ploidy, and rate of maturation. Platelets produced in the context of accelerated demand, so-called stress platelets, are often larger and exhibit greater hemostatic efficacy than normal platelets. This explains the clinical observation that patients with consumptive thrombocytopenia, in the absence of other complicating factors, do not usually develop life-threatening hemorrhage. In approaching a patient with thrombocytopenia, several clinical clues suggest a consumptive etiology. These include the following:

1. The presence of large platelets or megathrombocytes on the peripheral smear;
2. The absence of significant hemorrhage;
3. For platelet counts between $10,000/\mu L$ and $100,000/\mu L$, a BT that is shorter than that predicted by Fig. 5-2;
4. Associated microangiopathic hemolytic anemia (suggesting specifically DIC, thrombotic thrombocytopenic purpura [TTP], or metastatic malignancy involving the pulmonary microvasculature);
5. Associated autoimmune disease or thrombocytopenia in a young adult female;
6. An underlying lymphoproliferative disease, especially chronic lymphocytic leukemia (CLL), without evidence of myelophthisis by the neoplastic lymphocytes;
7. In children, a preceding viral infection;
8. HIV positivity.

Conversely, clinical clues suggestive of a productive etiology for thrombocytopenia include the following:

1. Normal sized platelets, significant associated hemorrhage, and a BT equal to or exceeding that predicted by Figure 5-2;
2. A leukoerythroblastic peripheral blood smear (teardrop and nucleated RBCs, early white blood cell [WBC] precursors), suggesting a myelophthisic process;
3. Circulating blasts indicative of acute leukemia;
4. Other cytopenias, with or without mild red cell macrocytosis, suggesting stem cell dysfunction (e.g., aplastic anemia, a myelodysplastic syndrome, or amegakaryocytic thrombocytopenia);
5. Neutrophil hypersegmentation with marked red cell macrocytosis indicative of B_{12} or folate deficiency.

Bone Marrow Examination. Although clinical clues and findings on the peripheral smear may suggest either a consumptive or a productive process, a bone marrow examination is generally required to absolutely distinguish between the two. The presence of normal or increased numbers of megakaryocytes in the marrow is a reliable indication that any thrombocytopenia is at least in part consumptive. The only significant exception to this rule arises in B_{12} and folate deficiency in which megakaryocytopoiesis is ineffective and intramedullary megakaryocyte death may occur prior to platelet release. In this instance, apparent bone marrow megakaryocytic hyperplasia and productive thrombocytopenia occur concurrently. However, the diagnosis is usually obvious because of megaloblastic changes in the other cell lineages. In some cases of accelerated platelet demand, bone marrow megakaryocytes may exhibit a larger population of more immature forms because of the rapid platelet release from and apoptosis of fully mature megakaryocytes. Such a shift to immaturity is often and inappropriately referred to as a maturation arrest, which should not be misinterpreted as suggesting a disorder of platelet production. In productive thrombocytopenia, there is usually an absence or markedly decreased number of normal megakaryocytes. Dysplastic megakaryocytes may be observed with stem cell dysfunction (e.g., myelodysplasia, acute leukemia, and aplastic anemia). In such instances, diagnostic morphologic abnormalities are usually detectable in the other hematopoietic cell lineages.

PRODUCTIVE THROMBOCYTOPENIA

Chemotherapy and Radiotherapy. Chemotherapy and radiotherapy damage both dividing and maturing cells by their effect on DNA replication and translation, respectively. Since in the absence of ongoing platelet production, the peripheral platelet count decays linearly, a nadir platelet count is generally reached 7–10 days after significant chemotherapy exposure. For radiotherapy, usually delivered incrementally over periods of weeks, the timing of the nadir platelet count is less predictable. Chemotherapy doses are typically limited by neutropenia, not thrombocytopenia. Exceptions include carboplatin, which has a disproportionate and dose-limiting effect on platelets; nitrosoureas, which may produce thrombocytopenia 3–6 weeks after exposure (even after the WBC has recovered); and busulfan, which in large doses may produce a significant thrombocytopenia lasting weeks or months.

Myelophthisis. Bone marrow infiltration by malignant neoplasm, fibrosis, or granulomata may decrease platelet production by crowding megakaryocytes out of their normal hematopoietic niche. This process, known as myelophthisis (weak marrow), is typically associated with leukoerythroblastic changes in the peripheral blood (see earlier) and may also be associated with splenomegaly. In addition to thrombocytopenia, there are usually abnormalities in other circulating blood counts—anemia and either leukopenia or leukocytosis. When myelophthisis is due to solid tumors, carcinomas of the lung, prostate, breast, stomach, and colon are the most common.

Hematopoietic Stem Cell Dysfunction. Hematopoietic stem cells are functionally characterized by their ability to replicate and to differentiate or mature. Both processes are necessary for the continued production of mature blood cells for the circulation. Disruption of either of these processes can result in inadequate blood cell production, of which thrombocytopenia may be a part. However, isolated thrombocytopenia due to stem cell malfunction is rare, manifested clinically as the disease amegakaryocytic thrombocytopenia. Much more commonly, thrombocytopenia is only one of several hematologic abnormalities present in hematopoietic stem cell disease, reflecting the multilineage capacity of such stem cells (Chapter 7).

Diseases of the hematopoietic stem cell can be categorized based upon the mechanism of stem cell dysfunction (Table 5-5). The complete failure of hematopoietic stem cell replication results in aplastic anemia. Replication without maturation results in acute myeloid leukemia, and replication with *disordered* maturation results in one of the myelodysplastic syndromes. Amegakaryocytic thrombocytopenia appears to be related to the myelodysplastic syndromes because there is frequently associated red blood cell macrocytosis (a finding unrelated to megaloblastic anemia here but associated with myelodysplasia), and evolution to acute

TABLE 5-5. *CLASSIFICATION OF HEMATOLOGIC DISEASES BASED UPON THE MECHANISMS OF STEM CELL DYSFUNCTION*

STEM CELL FUNCTION		
Proliferation	Differentiation	DISORDER
Absent	—	Aplastic anemia
Normal	Absent	Acute myeloid leukemia
Normal	Disordered	Myelodysplastic syndromes
Increased	Normal	Myeloproliferative disease

myeloid leukemia is not uncommon. Other diseases of stem cell dysfunction causing thrombocytopenia include paroxysmal nocturnal hemoglobinuria (PNH), cyclic thrombocytopenia, and congenital megakaryocytic hypoplasia (thrombocytopenia and absent radius syndrome). Additional rare, congenital thrombocytopenias exist that are associated with multiple nonhematologic abnormalities (e.g., Wiskott-Aldrich syndrome, Alport's syndrome). The bleeding diathesis associated with the thrombocytopenia due to stem cell dysfunction may by exacerbated by either an associated qualitative platelet functional defect resulting from defective megakaryocyte maturation or the concurrent presence of DIC, observed especially in the promyelocytic variant of acute myelogenous leukemia. PNH, conversely, is associated with hypercoagulability and unprovoked arterial and venous thromboses.

Infection-Related Thrombocytopenia. Although most viral infections cause thrombocytopenia by a consumptive mechanism (see later), some viruses exhibit direct bone marrow and megakaryocyte cytotoxicity, resulting in productive thrombocytopenia. HIV-related thrombocytopenia is now believed to be at least in part productive (Chapter 10). The evidence for this includes the following: HIV has been shown to infect megakaryocytes directly, dysplastic megakaryocyte maturation is frequently observed in bone marrow examinations from HIV-infected persons, and kinetic studies have directly demonstrated decreased platelet production in such individuals. B19 parvovirus, although primarily trophic for developing erythroid cells, may rarely be associated with total marrow suppression and pancytopenia. Similarly, hepatitis C and Epstein-Barr viral infections have been reported to cause productive thrombocytopenia in the context of virus-induced aplastic anemia.

Megaloblastic Anemias. As discussed previously, vitamin B_{12} or folate deficiency, with associated ineffective hematopoiesis and specifically ineffective megakaryocytopoiesis, may result in severe thrombocytopenia. In fact, thrombocytopenic bleeding may rarely dominate the clinical presentation. The diagnosis is usually obvious with peripheral blood and bone marrow examination. In the marrow, megakaryocytes are usually large and hyperlobated. Nutritional repletion will correct the thrombocytopenia within 1–2 weeks.

Drug- and Alcohol-Related Selective Suppression of Megakaryocytopoiesis. Although megakaryocytes are necessarily affected by any agent that damages the pluripotent hematopoietic stem cell, some agents appear to have a selective effect on the developing megakaryocyte. The most common of these agents is alcohol. Chronic alcohol ingestion is often associated with a mild to moderate thrombocytopenia that is multifactorial in origin. Elements of hypersplenism, decreased thrombopoietin production from a damaged liver, and direct toxicity of the alcohol on platelets and megakaryocytes are all likely to be contributory. However, very heavy alcohol intake may be accompanied by moderately severe thrombocytopenia and decreased numbers of bone marrow megakaryocytes, indicative of a suppressive effect on megakaryocytopoiesis. One investigation suggests that alcohol selectively arrests developing megakaryocytes at the postmitotic but pre-endomitotic stage of development (i.e., when the cells are 2N, exhibit platelet membrane glycoproteins, but have as yet developed essentially no platelet specific organelles). Withdrawal of alcohol exposure results in recovery of the platelet count within 1—2 weeks, often accompanied by a period of rebound thrombocytosis.

Thiazide diuretics and estrogens also have been reported to exert a selective, albeit variable suppressive effect on platelet production in some patients. Thiazide effects are usually mild, affect up to 25% of patients taking the drug, and are evident 2–3 weeks after drug initiation. Even with continued administration, the thrombocytopenia generally remains stable. Recovery to normal is usual 2–3 weeks after drug withdrawal. The thrombocytopenic effect of estrogens is less well documented in humans. However, a few patients have been reported to develop amegakaryocytic thrombocytopenia after prolonged exposure to diethylstilbestrol.

PLATELET TRANSFUSION

The administration of allogeneic platelets will generally stop bleeding in patients in whom hemorrhage is due solely to thrombocytopenia. Although platelet transfusions are also effective in correcting qualitative platelet defects, other, less risky therapeutic alternatives (i.e., DDAVP) are preferred in such circumstances. A Consensus Conference in 1987 suggested that platelet transfusion for qualitative dysfunction not even be considered unless the BT is twice the upper limit of normal. Platelet transfusions are generally administered in two clinical contexts: (1) therapeutically, for patients who are both thrombocytopenic and bleeding dangerously and (2) prophylactically, for patients who are stable but at high risk for thrombocytopenic bleeding. There are no absolute rules that can be established for either indication, but general guidelines do exist.

For any patient with a platelet count of less than 50,000/μL who is *actively bleeding*, therapeutic platelet transfusion should be considered. However, if the platelet count is more than 50,000/μL, it is unlikely that the thrombocytopenia alone is contributing significantly to the process. For some neurosurgical procedures, maintenance of a platelet count of in excess of 100,000/μL has been advocated, but even in those situations, circulating platelet concentrations of more than 50,000/μL are probably adequate. Thrombocytopenia may be accompanied by qualitative platelet dysfunction (e.g., in the thrombocytopenia of cardiopulmonary bypass or in thrombocytopenic patients who have recently ingested aspirin). In such instances, a more liberal threshold for platelet transfusion can be entertained.

Prophylactic platelet transfusion has traditionally been advocated for patients with productive thrombocytopenia and platelet counts less than 20,000/μL. However, a more recent critical review of the clinical literature suggests that a threshold of 5,000–10,000/μL is more appropriate. The 5,000/μL threshold should apply to clinically stable, afebrile patients; the 10,000/μL, to patients with accompanying risk factors for hemorrhage. Such risk factors include a falling platelet count, fever and sepsis, exposure to antiplatelet drugs, and leukemia-associated thrombocytopenia.

Platelet transfusion is only rarely considered in the clinical context of consumptive thrombocytopenia. Platelets produced in response to accelerated consumption are typically hyperfunctional, and thus very low platelet counts can be tolerated clinically with minimal hemorrhagic sequelae. Furthermore, because of the short circulating platelet half-life in such patients, transfused platelets have only a very short salutary effect. Only when there is active bleeding or reason to suspect accompanying qualitative platelet dysfunction should platelets be transfused for consumptive thrombocytopenia (see later).

By definition, a unit of platelets is that quantity obtained from a single unit of whole blood, approximately 7×10^{11} platelets. A typical dose of platelets is approximately 6 U, which can be expected to raise the circulating platelet count by 30,000–50,000/μL, a number usually sufficient to attain hemostasis. A platelet count should be obtained between 10 minutes and 1 hour after the completion of the platelet transfusion and then daily to assess the patient for alloimmunization and platelet survival, respectively. Transfused platelets generally survive for 2–4 days in the circulation, after which repeat platelet transfusion may be necessary. Between 20% and 70% of patients receiving repeated platelet transfusion will become alloimmunized, at which time they will fail to exhibit an immediate posttransfusion rise in the platelet count. For such patients HLA-matched single-donor platelet transfusions are often useful.

CONSUMPTIVE THROMBOCYTOPENIA

Consumptive thrombocytopenia results from accelerated peripheral platelet utilization with inadequate bone marrow compensation. Although such patients typically present with dependent petechiae and purpura, in the absence of an accompanying qualitative platelet functional defect, severe hemorrhage is unusual. Relative protection from life-threatening hemorrhage results from the greater hemostatic efficacy of platelets produced under "stress conditions" (i.e., increased peripheral platelet demand). Therefore consumptive thrombocytopenia, regardless of its numerical severity, is rarely life threatening. Therapy of the consumptive thrombocytopenias is most effectively directed at reducing platelet consumption by the reticuloendothelial system and at reversing the underlying disease process. Platelet transfusions are rarely indicated and are needed only when a very transient rise in the platelet count is essential to reverse serious clinical bleeding. As described earlier, increased circulating platelet volume may be a clue to the existence of a consumptive pathogenic mechanism. However, a bone marrow aspirate and biopsy demonstrating normal or increased numbers of megakaryocytes are generally required for accurate categorization. Examination of the peripheral blood smear is essential for *all* patients who present with thrombocytopenia, both to help define the underlying diagnosis and to rule out associated microangiopathic red blood cell changes. Microangiopathic red cell changes are a marker of thrombotic thrombocytopenic purpura, a potentially life-threatening disease process for which effective, specific, disease-directed therapy exists (see later).

IMMUNE CONSUMPTIVE THROMBOCYTOPENIA

Adult Immune Thrombocytopenic Purpura (Chronic ITP). Autoimmune thrombocytopenia is the most common form of consumptive thrombocytopenia in adults, and ITP is the most common form of autoimmune thrombocytopenia. Typically affecting women in their 20s and 30s (female:male = 3:1), ITP most often presents as isolated moderate to severe thrombocytopenia. However, if other hematologic abnormalities are present, a systemic illness of which ITP may be a component should be considered. ITP is not uncommonly associated with systemic autoimmune disease (e.g., systemic lupus erythematosus and lymphoproliferative disorders, especially chronic lymphocytic leukemia and Hodgkin disease). When ITP presents in tandem with autoimmune hemolytic anemia, it is called Evans' syndrome and an underlying lymphoproliferative disorder should be sought.

As is typical of patients with thrombocytopenia, patients with ITP most often present with petechiae, purpura, gingival bleeding, and, because of the population most commonly affected, menorrhagia. The onset of symptoms may be acute to subacute. Characteristically, in contrast to childhood ITP (see later), there is no history of viral infection. Hemorrhagic mucosal bullae, epistaxis, and gastrointestinal bleeding are less common and may portend a more serious risk of major bleeding for the individual patient. The spleen has a voracious appetite for antibody-coated platelets, but splenomegaly is not part of the ITP disease spectrum, and its presence should alert the clinician to consider alternative diagnoses.

ITP results from platelet sensitization by autoreactive antibodies, usually IgG, directed at components of the platelet plasma membrane. The most commonly affected membrane epitope appears to be the glycoprotein IIb/IIIa complex, although a variety of other membrane glycoproteins may be affected. Clinically, platelet sensitization by autoantibodies may be confirmed in up to 90% of ITP patients by detecting increased amounts of platelet-associated IgG. However, the clinical measurement of platelet-associated IgG is fraught with uncertainty and prone to technical artifact, resulting in inadequate specificity to be of routine utility in diagnosis. Contributing to artifact and uncertainty are the observations that platelet-associated IgG is increased nonspecifically in proportion to both the level of circulating plasma immunoglobulins and the platelet volume. Platelet-associated IgG is also increased in the presence of circulating immune complexes.

Platelet sensitization by IgG leads to a markedly shortened survival as a result of Fc receptor-mediated platelet phagocytosis by splenic macrophages. IgG reactivity with the membrane of developing megakaryocytes may also result in relative impairment of megakaryocytopoiesis and thus in up to 50% of ITP patients, a less than maximal thrombopoietic response to the accelerated platelet consumption. In addition to its role in ITP as the principal site of platelet removal, the spleen is believed to be the major source of platelet autoantibody production.

Hospitalization of adult patients presenting with ITP is reserved for those patients who are actively bleeding or those with platelet counts of less than 10,000–20,000/μL. A bone marrow aspiration and biopsy will rapidly confirm the suspected diagnosis, and treatment can be initiated. For most patients, the administration of oral prednisone at moderate daily doses is satisfactory. However, for patients with existing hemorrhage or believed to be at significantly increased risk for hemorrhage, intravenous immunoglobulin, intravenous high-dose methylprednisolone, or both may result in a more rapid clinical response than oral steroids. For serious hemorrhage, platelet transfusion should be considered as part of the emergent therapy (see earlier).

Corticosteroids are believed to function acutely by inhibiting the interaction of the IgG-coated platelets with the Fc receptors of splenic macrophages and thus impairing phagocytosis. Over the longer term, corticosteroids are thought to suppress platelet autoantibody production. Intravenous immunoglobulin, by saturating splenic macrophage Fc receptors, also works acutely by reducing the rate of platelet phagocytosis.

Patients generally respond to either of these two measures from within days to 1–3 weeks. For nonresponding patients, alternative therapy such as splenectomy will need to be considered. The responses to intravenous immunoglobulin tend to be transient, and in virtually all instances, chronic therapy with oral prednisone is required to maintain an adequate platelet count. Steroids are routinely continued for 2–3 months at tapering doses, at levels necessary to maintain adequate platelet counts (i.e., 30,000–50,000/μL). After this time period, steroids are tapered and discontinued in those 10–20% of patients who have achieved a spontaneous remission. Even moderate chronic thrombocytopenia may be acceptable off steroids if the patient is asymptomatic and the platelet function is normal. Unfortunately, approximately 80% of adult ITP patients relapse on tapering steroid doses and ultimately require splenectomy for control. Prior response to corticosteroids and perhaps to intravenous immunoglobulin is predictive of a good response to splenectomy (Fig. 5-5). For splenectomy failures there is no established therapeutic protocol. However, one should always consider the possibility of residual splenic tissue in the form of splenosis or an accessory spleen. This may be suggested by the *absence* of Howell-Jolly bodies on the peripheral blood smear and can be confirmed by ^{99m}Tc sulfur

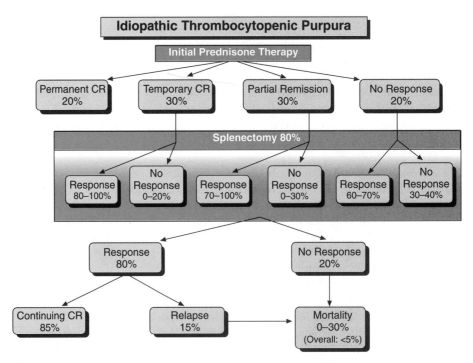

Figure 5-5. Outcome of adults with chronic idiopathic thrombocytopenic purpura stratified by their responses to prednisone therapy and splenectomy. (CR, complete response)

colloid scanning (Chapter 3). Chronic low-dose or alternate-day steroids and intermittent intravenous immunoglobulin therapy have each been used with success in a minority of refractory ITP patients. Other therapies used sporadically in refractory cases include danazol, vinca alkaloids, α-interferon, and the immunosuppressive agents cyclophosphamide, azathioprine, and cyclosporine. Despite the frustration incurred in treating refractory ITP, extended follow-up suggests that most of these patients do well over the long term.

Childhood Immune Thrombocytopenic Purpura (Acute ITP). Although the clinical presentation of ITP in children is similar to that in adults, it differs substantially both in pathogenesis and in clinical course, resulting in a significantly different approach to management. Acute ITP typically affects children between the ages of 2 and 9, peaking between the ages of 3 and 5. Males and females are affected equally, and the disorder commonly follows a viral infection by 1–3 weeks. Children generally feel well and are brought to medical attention by the sudden onset of petechiae and purpura. Like adults, children with ITP should manifest a CBC that is remarkable only for thrombocytopenia with no other cytopenias or abnormal circulating cells. Furthermore, neither lymphadenopathy nor hepatosplenomegaly should be present on physical examination. The differential diagnosis of isolated thrombocytopenia is much more limited in children than in adults; more than 95% of such pediatric patients have ITP. Thus the necessity of bone marrow examination for confirmation of the diagnosis is debated. Other considerations in the child with thrombocytopenia include HIV infection, systemic lupus erythematosus, and congenital humoral immunodeficiency (especially IgA). However, in the absence of clinical suspicion, routine blood testing is potentially justifiable only for humoral immunodeficiency.

Unlike adult ITP, in which the development of platelet *auto*antibodies is the primary pathogenic process, acute ITP of childhood is believed to result from antibodies directed against viral protein antigens produced during the recent systemic viral infection. Circulating platelets are sensitized by adsorption onto the platelet membrane of either the viral antigens (with secondary antiviral antibody binding) or complete virus/antibody immune complexes. Since viral antigens are ultimately cleared, acute ITP tends to be a self-limited illness that resolves spontaneously in 80% of individuals within 2 months. Splenectomy is rarely indicated because up to 95% of affected children will ultimately achieve acceptable platelet counts over a period of several months. Intracranial hemorrhage, often without other signs of bleeding, occurs slightly more frequently in children and justifies treatment of virtually all children presenting with platelet counts of less than 20,000/μL. Therapy with both high-dose parenteral steroids and/or intravenous immunoglobulin has been recommended. Because of the high risk of postsplenectomy sepsis in the pediatric population, splenectomy should be considered only the treatment of last resort and the procedure should be delayed as long as possible.

Drug-Induced Immune Thrombocytopenia. Drug-induced immune thrombocytopenia is produced by interaction among a drug, a drug-dependent antibody, and the platelet membrane, which results in platelet opsonization and/or activation. Therefore drug-induced thrombocytopenia typically develops 2–3 weeks after primary exposure to a drug, a time sufficient to mount a measurable humoral antibody response. Thrombocytopenia with repeat drug exposure may develop much more rapidly because of the presence of pre-existing antidrug antibodies or the generation of a brisk amnestic antidrug antibody response. Since antibody binding to the platelet membrane is drug dependent, the time course for resolution of drug-induced thrombocytopenia will reflect the kinetics of drug clearance from the body. However, for most drugs, resolution usually occurs within days after the offending drug is removed.

Heparin is the most common cause of drug-induced thrombocytopenia, developing in 3–5% of patients receiving therapeutic doses of heparin. Usually, the thrombocytopenia is mild to moderate, with a mean platelet count of $50,000/\mu L$ in affected patients. However, in a small minority of patients, the platelet count may fall to less than $20,000/\mu L$. In an even smaller minority, heparin-induced thrombocytopenia may presage and lead to catastrophic venous and arterial thrombi. Although the exact risk of heparin-associated thrombosis is unclear, it is evident that virtually all patients who develop this devastating complication will first manifest thrombocytopenia. Therefore because of the severe morbidity and mortality resulting from the heparin-associated thrombocytopenia/thrombosis syndrome, it is recommended that platelet counts be monitored closely in all patients receiving heparin and that heparin be immediately discontinued if heparin-associated thrombocytopenia develops.

The mechanism of heparin-associated thrombocytopenia appears to require specific antibody binding to a complex of heparin and a platelet component, which recent work suggests is platelet factor 4. Antibody binding to this complex approximates the Fc portion of the IgG molecule to the platelet membrane Fc receptor, which in turn leads to platelet activation, aggregation, and the generation of procoagulant activity. Aggregated platelets may be removed by the reticuloendothelial system, resulting in thrombocytopenia. However, if the magnitude of platelet activation and aggregation is sufficient, then thrombosis may ensue. Laboratory confirmation of heparin-associated thrombocytopenia requires that antibody in the patient's plasma activate normal platelets in the presence of therapeutic concentrations of heparin (Chapter 6).

Other drugs appear to cause thrombocytopenia by leading to drug-dependent platelet membrane binding of specific antibody, usually IgG. Although the exact mechanism is unclear, the development of thrombocytopenia requires an interaction between the drug and a component of the platelet membrane, in most instances one of the glycoproteins, which renders either the glycoprotein, the drug, or the drug/glycoprotein complex immunogenic. Subsequent specific antibody binding to the platelet membrane in the presence of drug either opsonizes the platelet for removal by the reticuloendothelial system or leads to activation of complement with intravascular platelet lysis. In virtually all instances of drug-induced thrombocytopenia, there are very significantly elevated levels of platelet-associated IgG. Drug-dependent platelet antibody binding may also be demonstrable in some patients. However, because the inciting agent is often a drug metabolite, specific antibodies are often not detectable.

Quinine and quinidine are prototypical drugs responsible for thrombocytopenia with an estimated risk of one in 1,000 individuals exposed to either of these related compounds. The clinical onset of quinine-induced thrombocytopenia may be abrupt, and the thrombocytopenia may be severe. Because of the ubiquitous presence of quinine-containing compounds, a careful history may be necessary to differentiate quinine-induced thrombocytopenia from ITP. Gold-induced thrombocytopenia is also relatively common, affecting approximately 2% of treated patients. There appears to be a genetic predisposition for this complication as most patients with gold-induced thrombocytopenia exhibit the HLA-DR3 histocompatibility antigen. Resolution of gold-induced thrombocytopenia tends to be sluggish and to require several weeks, probably because of the prolonged systemic half-life of gold as well as the possibility that gold exposure stimulates a population of true platelet autoantibodies. Other drugs known to be associated with immune thrombocytopenia include digoxin, rifampin, and the sulfonamides.

The treatment of drug-induced thrombocytopenia usually focuses on identification and withdrawal of the offending agent. In complex patients on large numbers of drugs, an effort should be made to discontinue or change all but the most essential medications. Greatest suspicion should be directed toward those drugs known to most commonly produce thrombocytopenia. Although of unproven benefit (and with the exception of heparin), the treatment of severe drug-induced thrombocytopenia with moderate doses of corticosteroids is favored by most clinicians. Intravenous immunoglobulin therapy represents another rational alternative. Platelet transfusion should not be used in heparin-induced thrombocytopenia.

Other Causes of Immune Thrombocytopenia. The entity of **posttransfusion purpura** is a rare but dramatic immune thrombocytopenia resulting from alloimmunization. This disorder typically develops 1 week after a routine blood transfusion and presents explosively with severe, refractory thrombocytopenia and bleeding. There is significant mortality due to intracranial hemorrhage associated with this disorder; consequently, early diagnosis and appropriate therapy are essential. Affected patients characteristically either are multiparous females or have been previously exposed to blood products. This infrequent disorder arises in those patients who lack the platelet antigen Pl^{A1} (approximately 2% of the population) who receive blood products that are Pl^{A1} positive. Endogenous antibodies directed against the Pl^{A1} antigen are induced that destroy not only the allogeneic platelets but the patient's own Pl^{A1} negative platelets. The reason for the autoreactivity of these anti-Pl^{A1} antibodies remains an enigma. The early treatment of the affected patient with intravenous immunoglobulin has recently been shown to be an effective therapy and may be life-saving.

Neonatal alloimmune thrombocytopenia may develop in infants because of the transplacental transfer of maternal antibodies reactive with fetal platelets. The most common underlying pathogenesis is the immunization of a Pl^{A1}-negative mother by platelets from a Pl^{A1}-positive fetus. Other platelet antigen mismatches have been implicated in this disorder as well. Unlike posttransfusion purpura, the mother is usually unaffected in this process. The fetus is mildly thrombocytopenic at birth and worsens during the first 1–2 weeks of life. The disorder then usually resolves by 4 weeks of age. Treatment is reserved only for the most severely affected infants and consists of the transfusion of washed maternal platelets and/or the administration of intravenous immunoglobulin.

NONIMMUNE CONSUMPTIVE THROMBOCYTOPENIA

Thrombotic Thrombocytopenic Purpura and the Hemolytic Uremic Syndrome (HUS). Thrombotic thrombocytopenic purpura (TTP) and the hemolytic uremic syndrome (HUS) are potentially fatal acute thrombocytopenic disorders of obscure etiology. Both are characterized clinically by the acute onset of the dyad of severe, nonimmune consumptive thrombocytopenia and microangiopathic hemolytic anemia (MAHA, or fragmentation hemolysis). Because of the potential for a rapidly fatal outcome in these disorders (and the availability of relatively simple, life-saving therapy), the peripheral blood smears from all patients with thrombocytopenia should be reviewed at presentation for microangiopathic hemolysis (Fig. 3-3). If both consumptive thrombocytopenia and microangiopathic hemolytic anemia are present, the patient should be assumed to have TTP or HUS until proven otherwise.

Pathologically, both TTP and HUS are characterized by the deposition of hyaline platelet thrombi in terminal arterioles and capillaries. Such thrombi are believed to develop from spontaneous platelet aggregation and vascular occlusion. Although these thrombi may contain some fibrin polymers, there is *no* generalized activation of the soluble coagulation system; thus this syndrome is distinct and easily distinguishable from disseminated intravascular coagulation (see later and Chapter 6). In TTP, which principally affects adults, the deposition of platelet thrombi is systemically widespread, resulting in multiorgan dysfunction from the microvascular ischemia and dysfunction. The characteristic clinical pentad of TTP includes consumptive thrombocytopenia, microangiopathic hemolytic anemia, fever, fluctuating neurologic symptoms, and renal insufficiency. However, all these features need not be present in any individual patient. In HUS, a disease primarily of children, the platelet thrombi develop predominantly, but not exclusively, in the kidney, resulting in acute renal failure as the major clinical manifestation. TTP and HUS are not always clinically distinct from one another and are therefore best considered ends of the spectrum of a single disease entity. TTP and HUS are clinical diagnoses in which pathologic confirmation is generally not required. However, biopsies of the bone marrow, kidney, or gingiva may demonstrate characteristic but not pathognomonic platelet hyaline thrombi.

Although the primary pathogenic event in TTP/HUS appears to be platelet aggregation and microvascular occlusion, the precipitant of such platelet aggregation is unknown. Some have suggested that vascular endothelial cell injury with the resultant release of unusually large vWf multimers into the circulation is the primary initiating event. These multimers, it is postulated, bind spontaneously to platelet membrane GP Ib/IX and GP IIb/IIIa, leading to spontaneous platelet aggregation and microvascular occlusion. Others have suggested that platelet aggregation is stimulated by the introduction of other, nonendothelial cell–derived platelet-aggregating proteins.

Occasionally, a viral illness, bacterial illness, or immunization may precede the development of TTP. TTP is also reported at an increased frequency among patients with HIV infection (Chapter 10). Other reported associations include pregnancy, oral contraceptive use, the administration of certain antineoplastic chemotherapeutic agents, and connective tissue disease. Rarely, TTP has been reported as a hereditary disorder. However, in most instances, TTP occurs sporadically and without antecedent. In contrast, 90% of HUS occurs in children and is preceded by bloody diarrhea caused by *Shigella dysenteriae* or enterotoxigenic *Escherichia coli* of the serotype O157:H7. Both of these organisms are believed to precipitate HUS by producing toxins that damage specifically renal capillary endothelial cells, leading to the intravascular release of unusually large vWf multimers and subsequent platelet aggregation.

As mentioned earlier, the diagnosis of TTP/HUS should be entertained whenever consumptive thrombocytopenia occurs in association with microangiopathic hemolytic anemia. The consumptive character of the thrombocytopenia can be confirmed by a bone marrow aspirate that demonstrates normal to increased numbers of megakaryocytes. MAHA is a diagnosis based upon characteristic red cell changes on the peripheral smear and is supported by the presence of very high serum levels of lactate dehydrogenase (LDH), an intracellular red cell enzyme, as well as other evidence of intravascular hemolysis (e.g., increased reticulocytes, unconjugated bilirubin and serum iron, and decreased haptoglobin). Disseminated intravascular coagulation can be ruled out by normal PT, aPTT, fibrinogen, and fibrin degradation product levels, and malignant hypertension can be excluded by a normal or near normal blood pressure. A systemic vasculitis may be more difficult to differentiate rapidly from TTP, but final diagnosis should not delay definitive therapy for presumptive TTP.

In the past, most patients with TTP died. However, with the advent of plasma infusion and plasma exchange therapy, most patients can be expected to survive the acute episode. Plasma exchange or plasma infusion therapy, replacing one to two plasma volumes (3–4 L) daily, should be initiated immediately when TTP/HUS is suspected. Therapy should be continued until there is a clinical response manifested by improved symptoms, a falling LDH, and a rising platelet count. Therapy may need to be continued for several weeks, and relapses are common when the plasma exchanges are reduced or discontinued. Some physicians also add corticosteroids to the therapy of TTP/HUS, and splenectomy is occasionally performed in refractory cases. There does not appear to be any meaningful therapeutic role for antiplatelet agents, and platelet transfusions should be reserved only for active hemorrhage (in fact, they may be dangerous).

Disseminated Intravascular Coagulation (DIC). (See also Chapter 6.) Certain systemic disorders can trigger the activation of the soluble coagulation system, resulting in intravascular clot formation and the consumption of factors V and VIII, fibrinogen, and platelets. Concomitant activation of fibrinolytic enzymes invariably results in the production of fibrin and fibrinogen degradation products (FDPs), which can be detected in the plasma and may interfere with fibrin polymerization and platelet function. DIC may be precipitated by severe bacterial infections, tissue death, and ischemia caused by trauma or hypoperfusion, obstetric complications, and certain tumors. In severe instances, the intravascular deposition of fibrin may result in MAHA of varying severity.

The diagnosis of DIC should be suspected in the appropriate clinical setting when there is evidence of thrombosis or bleeding (or both), a prolongation of the PT, and a falling platelet count. The aPTT in DIC is more variable but is also generally prolonged. DIC may be confirmed by a low fibrinogen level and increased levels of FDPs. Since DIC is a dynamic process, evidence of a falling platelet count and fibrinogen level may be more important than their absolute levels in establishing the diagnosis of DIC. Rarely, quantitation of factors V and/or VIII may be necessary to pin down the diagnosis.

Therapy for DIC is generally directed at controlling or eliminating the precipitating disease process, and it is the underlying disease that ultimately determines morbidity and mortality. In the acute setting, red cell, fresh-frozen plasma, and platelet transfusions are provided as necessary. Some clinicians recommend heparin anticoagulation therapy for patients in whom thrombosis is the dominant clinical manifestation of DIC or for whom transfusion therapy alone is inadequate to maintain hemostasis. Heparin may also be of use in obstetric emergencies. For the chronic DIC associated with some malignancies, chronic anticoagulation with sub-cutaneous heparin may be required (Chapter 6).

Consumptive Thrombocytopenia Caused by Microvascular Disease. Any damage to the vascular endothelium will result in platelet adhesion to subendo-thelial collagen, vWf multimers, and other adhesive glycoproteins of the extracellu-lar matrix. (See earlier.) When the microvascular damage is widespread, the rate of platelet deposition may exceed the compensatory capacity of the bone marrow and result in a nonimmune form of consumptive thrombocytopenia. Such widespread damage may occur in the clinical context of malignant hypertension, systemic small-vessel vasculitis, and renal allograft rejection. Therapy is directed at the underlying disease, and thrombocytopenia generally resolves as disease control is achieved.

A peculiar form of consumptive thrombocytopenia may occur in the context of **malignancy** with widespread microscopic, subendothelial metastases to the pul-monary microvasculature. The pulmonary microvascular disruption results in mi-croangiopathic hemolytic anemia, often accompanied by thrombocytopenia, with-out evidence of DIC. This syndrome must be differentiated from DIC and occurs most often with metastatic adenocarcinoma of the stomach, although it may occur in association with other metastatic adenocarcinomas, particularly those of the breast, lung, and unknown primary.

Thrombocytopenia is commonly associated with the **obstetric complications** of **eclampsia** and **pre-eclampsia**. Twenty percent of pre-eclamptic and 40% of eclamp-tic patients have been reported to develop thrombocytopenia. Although the mech-anism of such thrombocytopenia is not entirely clear, systemic and placental mi-crovascular damage has been implicated by some investigators. In most instances, there is minimal, if any, evidence for activation of the soluble coagulation system. Delivery of the fetus results in resolution of the thrombocytopenia. Aggressive anti-hypertensive therapy or antiplatelet therapy with aspirin may also lead to improve-ment of the thrombocytopenia.

In a clinical variant of pre-eclampsia, the thrombocytopenia may be associated with microangiopathic hemolysis and elevated liver function tests (the so-called **HELLP** [**H**emolytic anemia, **E**levated **L**iver tests, **L**ow **P**latelets] **syndrome**). This clinical constellation may precede the development of hypertension and protein-uria but is otherwise not clinically distinct from pre-eclampsia. Although the HELLP syndrome must be discriminated from TTP, it otherwise is treated as pre-eclampsia with delivery of the fetus.

THROMBOCYTOPENIA AND PREGNANCY

Mild thrombocytopenia, with platelet counts of 70,000–150,000/μL, develops in approximately 6% of otherwise healthy pregnant women. Such thrombocytope-nia should be considered incidental, because platelet counts are sufficient for ma-ternal hemostasis and the frequency of thrombocytopenic infants born to such women is not different from normal. Therefore no additional diagnostic testing or therapeutic intervention is warranted. Occasionally, women may develop *de novo* ITP while they are pregnant, or women with a history of ITP may become pregnant. Because of the theoretical risk that maternal antiplatelet IgG antibody may cross the placenta and induce severe thrombocytopenia in the fetus, there has been consid-erable controversy as to how to manage such patients. As in nonpregnant patients, pregnant women with ITP and potentially symptomatic thrombocytopenia (i.e., less than $50,000/\mu L$) should be treated with either systemic corticosteroids or intravenous immunoglobulin until a satisfactory platelet count is obtained. However, more commonly the mothers are in remission (often as a result of splenectomy) at the time of their pregnancy. Although 10–30% of mothers with a known history of ITP may deliver infants with platelet counts of less than $50,000/\mu L$, clinically significant complications in the infant, specifically intracranial hemorrhage, are rare. Some clinicians recommend fetal scalp or umbilical vein platelet count determinations to identify those infants who would benefit from delivery by Caesarean section. Others have suggested that high levels of maternal platelet-associated IgG serve to identify the neonatal population at greatest risk for symptomatic thrombocytopenia. Still others recommend the empiric administration of prednisone to all mothers with ITP for the final 3–4 weeks of pregnancy. However, because the risk of severe neonatal thrombocytopenia is extremely low, even in mothers with a history of ITP, none of the preceding approaches has yet proven sufficiently accurate, efficacious, and cost effective to achieve universal acceptance.

THROMBOCYTOSIS

Although thrombocytosis may be broadly defined as a platelet count above the normal range (i.e., more than $400,000\text{-}450,000/\mu L$), mild elevations of the platelet count may accompany a variety of disease states and are clinically inconsequential. For the purposes of this discussion, thrombocytosis will be defined as a platelet count in excess of $600,000/\mu L$, a number with potentially greater diagnostic utility. Thrombocytosis may be categorized pathogenetically into one of two groups: reactive thrombocytosis and primary thrombocytosis. Reactive thrombocytosis develops as a consequence of a disease process not believed to primarily affect the hematopoietic stem cell. As such, in reactive thrombocytosis, the regulatory mechanisms controlling thrombocytopoiesis and stem cell development remain normal and intact. In contrast, primary thrombocytosis develops as a consequence of a fundamental defect in the hematopoietic stem cell, which results, at least in part, in autonomous hematopoiesis and disordered stem cell development. Thus primary thrombocytosis develops almost exclusively as a complication of one of the myeloproliferative disorders, clonal hematopoietic stem cell diseases, which are characterized by excessive proliferation.

REACTIVE THROMBOCYTOSIS

The potential causes of reactive thrombocytosis are protean and are listed in Table 5-6. The pathogenetic mechanisms causing reactive thrombocytosis appear heterogeneous and are often obscure. Postsplenectomy thrombocytosis is believed to result in part from the loss of the splenic platelet pool, which normally sequesters approximately one-third of the total mature platelet numbers. With removal of the spleen, the platelet mass remains unchanged but the intravascular platelet numbers are increased by those normally present but not counted in the splenic pool. However, postsplenectomy thrombocytosis often is delayed, peaking 1–3 weeks following surgery, and the magnitude of postsplenectomy thrombocytosis often exceeds that predicted simply by mobilization of the splenic pool. Therefore it is likely that other mechanisms also contribute to thrombocytosis following splenectomy. Many of the

TABLE 5-6. *ETIOLOGIES OF REACTIVE THROMBOCYTOSIS*

Splenectomy

Iron deficiency anemia

Acute hemorrhage

Chronic inflammatory disorders
  Especially rheumatoid arthritis, inflammatory bowel disease

Acute and chronic infections
  Especially chronic pulmonary

Malignancy
  Especially lung, pancreas, Hodgkin's disease

Alcohol withdrawal

Hemolytic anemia

Drugs (vincristine, epinephrine)

Recovery from thrombocytopenia
  Therapy for B_{12} and folate deficiency

other instances of reactive thrombocytosis are associated with systemic inflammatory diseases and are believed to result from the release of immunomodulatory cytokines that stimulate platelet production as a secondary effect. This model has been best substantiated in rheumatoid arthritis in which serum levels of interleukin 6 (IL-6) correlate directly with the degree of thrombocytosis. IL-6 is a known inflammatory cytokine that also stimulates megakaryocyte polyploidization and platelet production.

Reactive thrombocytosis should be considered a benign disorder. Platelets, although increased in number, generally exhibit normal morphology and function. In fact, normal platelet function on formal platelet aggregometry testing may be useful in distinguishing a reactive from a primary thrombocytotic process. In reactive thrombocytosis, the circulating platelet count rarely exceeds 1 million per microliter, and significantly higher values strongly suggest a primary disorder. There is no clear linkage between the presence of reactive thrombocytosis and the development of thrombotic or hemorrhagic clinical events. Therefore therapy with inhibitors of platelet function or treatment directed at lowering the platelet count is almost never indicated.

PRIMARY THROMBOCYTOSIS

Primary thrombocytosis is defined as thrombocytosis occurring in the context of a clonal defect involving the hematopoietic stem cell. For the overwhelming majority of patients, primary thrombocytosis develops in the context of one of the myeloproliferative disorders, such as chronic myelogenous leukemia, polycythemia vera, essential thrombocythemia, or idiopathic myelofibrosis (Chapter 9). Primary thrombocytosis may also rarely occur in association with one of the myelodysplastic syndromes, especially the 5q-syndrome and occasional cases of idiopathic ringed sideroblastic anemia.

The range of the platelet count among patients with primary thrombocytosis is quite wide, extending from just above normal to several million per microliter. Platelet morphology is also highly variable. Unusually large platelets and even fragments of megakaryocyte cytoplasm on the peripheral blood smear are indicative of a primary thrombocytotic process, although such changes are not uniformly present. Since primary thrombocytosis results from a defect affecting the pluripotent hematopoietic stem cell, abnormalities in the hematocrit and/or the WBC are also typically seen. Splenomegaly is an additional clinical clue that a thrombocytotic process is primary. The BT is variable among patients with primary thrombocytosis; it may be short, normal, or prolonged. However, some abnormality of platelet function, most commonly the aggregatory response to epinephrine, is detectable in most patients.

The clinical manifestations of primary thrombocytosis relate, to a large extent, to the underlying disease process. However, both thrombosis and bleeding have been ascribed to primary thrombocytosis itself. Particularly noteworthy complications are thromboses of vessels in unusual anatomic sites (e.g., the mesenteric veins, hepatic vein, and digital arteries). Digital arterial ischemia results in the distinctive clinical syndrome of erythromelalgia, painful erythema, and swelling of the fingers. Transient ischemic attacks and cardiac ischemia are also not uncommon complications in older individuals. Hemorrhagic complications are at least twice as frequent as thrombotic events and most commonly involve the gastrointestinal tract. As a general rule, there does not appear to be a clear relationship between the height of the platelet count and the risk of thrombotic or hemorrhagic complications. However, should thrombosis or hemorrhage occur in the context of a primary thrombocytotic disorder, most clinicians believe that the risk of subsequent complications can be reduced substantially by lowering the platelet count.

Since many patients may remain asymptomatic for years, not all patients need to receive specific therapy directed at reducing their platelet counts. Only age, duration of the thrombocytosis, and a history of prior thrombotic events have been demonstrated to identify patients prospectively at greater risk for thrombosis. Platelet counts may be lowered by a variety of cytotoxic alkylating agents, including busulfan, melphalan, and uracil mustard. All these agents are leukemogenic and therefore must be employed with great care, especially in the younger patient. Hydroxyurea, an antimetabolite, may be safer in such individuals. Possibly safer still is the specific platelet-lowering agent anagrelide, which exerts its thrombocytopenic effect by disrupting megakaryocyte maturation. Interferon-α has also been used successfully to control primary thrombocytosis in some individuals. A recent prospective clinical investigation indicates that the administration of hydroxyurea to high-risk patients with essential thrombocythemia significantly reduces the frequency of thrombotic events, including TIAs, peripheral artery occlusions, and both superficial and deep-vein thrombophlebitis. Therapeutic agents that interfere with platelet function should *not* be routinely employed in patients with primary thrombocytosis. Routine use may exacerbate the tendency such patients have for gastrointestinal bleeding. However, for those patients whose clinical course has been complicated only by pure thrombotic episodes, aspirin or other antiplatelet agents are indicated.

CASE PRESENTATION

A 21-year-old woman comes to see her physician because of malaise and low-grade fever. One week ago, she believed that she had recovered from an up-

per respiratory infection. However, since that time, she has developed shortness of breath on mild exertion, some dizziness, fatigue, and low-grade fever. On physical examination she has a rectal temperature of 37.9°C. Other vital signs are normal, and the remainder of the physical exam is not remarkable, but at times the patient seemed slightly confused. The white blood cell count is 14,300/μL; the differential count shows 82% neutrophils; 3% bands, 15% lymphocytes. Hemoglobin is 5.2 g/dL; hematocrit is 16%; platelet count is 8,000/μL; serum chemistry tests show BUN of 32 mg % and creatinine of 1.7 mg %. PT and aPTT are within normal limits. LDH is 6,700 U.

Question 1. What is your concern at this time?

Answer. The patient presents with fever, slight confusion, anemia, thrombocytopenia, and mild azotemia. These are all consistent with a diagnosis of thrombotic thrombocytopenic purpura (TTP). Because there are specific therapies that can be life-saving and time is of the essence in successfully treating this disorder, immediate steps must be taken to make the diagnosis.

Question 2. What should be done next?

Answer. The peripheral blood smear should be reviewed. In this case the white cell series appears to be fine. However, the platelets are reduced markedly in amount and are somewhat enlarged. The red cell series shows dramatic changes. There are many cells that look like helmets or tri-cornered hats, and smaller fragments are seen as well. Such schistocytes are seen in microangiopathic hemolytic anemias (Table 3-3).

Question 3. What is in the differential diagnosis of a microangiopathic hemolytic anemia?

Answer. Major diagnostic entities to consider besides TTP (or a variant called hemolytic uremic syndrome) include (a) Abnormalities of the heart and large blood vessels that can affect flowing blood and destroy cells because of gross mechanical trauma. This is exemplified by the so-called Waring—Blender syndrome, in which red blood cells are squashed by malfunctioning ball and cage prosthetic heart valves. (b) Microvascular abnormalities such as congenital blood vessel tangles. (c) Immune mediated problems associated with small vessels such as those associated with acute glomerulonephritis, hypertension, or malignancy. These may be accompanied by local intravascular coagulation and fluid phase activated procoagulant problems. (d) Other such microangiopathic processes include those associated with abruptio placenta, promyelocytic leukemia, or snake bite. (e) In addition, inflammatory processes such as sepsis, pancreatitis, heat stroke, or transfusion reactions may all be associated with a microangiopathic anemia with disseminated intravascular coagulation.

To help make a definitive diagnosis, hyaline thrombi (composed of aggregated platelets in a fibrinogen and vWf mesh) could be sought for in terminal arterioles or capillaries. A gum or bone marrow biopsy could be done that might reveal such changes in blood vessels. In this situation, given the patient's historical and physical examination data, thrombocytopenia anemia, normal PT and aPTT, TTP is the most compelling diagnosis and the one that demands immediate attention if therapeutic interventions are to be most effective.

Question 4. What should you do now?

Answer. Plasmapheresis with infusion of fresh-frozen plasma to replace the plasma removed is the therapy of choice. The pathogenesis of TTP is felt by some to involve the release of unusual forms of vWf into the circulation by injured endothelial cells. These multimers are more effective than other vWf forms in flowing systems to bind to platelet surface glycoprotein complexes. This binding would induce exaggerated platelet aggregation and mechanically damage red cells as they pass through this gauntlet. Infused fresh-frozen plasma provides a substance (thought to be a limited disulfide reductase) that helps the body to clear the ultralarge vWf complexes that have been released by damaged endothelial cells.

Follow-up. This patient did well with intensive therapy. Plasma exchange using plasmapheresis and plasma infusion with normal fresh-frozen platelet-poor plasma in the amount of 3–4 L/day succeeded in reversing the hemolytic anemia and thrombocytopenia. The patient's LDH fell and her fever, neurologic changes, and renal failure normalized.

CASE PRESENTATION

A 31-year-old woman who has been healthy in the past except for joint aches has come to an emergency room where you are working. She complains of red spots on her ankles and "blood blisters" in her mouth. Her menstrual period began a week before it was expected. Physical findings of importance are hemorrhagic bullae in the oral mucosa, petechiae over ankles and thighs, no lymphadenopathy or hepatosplenomegaly, and bleeding from the cervical os. The CBC showed a WBC of 11,200/μL, normal differential count, Hb = 11.7 g/dL, Hct = 35%. Platelet count was 2,000/μL.

Question 1. What is the next step?

Answer. Examination of the peripheral smear. This showed normal RBC and WBC morphology, but platelets were few in number and large in size. This picture was consistent with accelerated production of platelets, many of which were younger and larger but were being actively consumed after they reached the peripheral bloodstream.

Question 2. What needs to be done further from a diagnostic viewpoint?

Answer. A bone marrow aspirate was performed. It showed normal maturation of all cell lines, but megakaryocytes were numerous and basophilic (young). Platelet-associated antibodies will not be diagnostically useful. Because of the patient's joint symptoms a workup for rheumatologic/collagen vascular disease should be considered when she is more stable.

Question 3. What is appropriate therapy now?

Answer. Because you find hemorrhagic bullae (wet purpura) on oral mucosa membrane surfaces and she is actively bleeding from the vagina, therapy needs to be started immediately. Most clinicians would begin with high dose, oral prednisone but IV corticosteroids might also be used. IV immunoglobulin could be given as well. Although platelet transfusions might not lead to demonstrable increment in platelet count, her bleeding could be immediately stanched, and life-threatening could be hemorrhage prevented by such infusions. There would be no agreement among hematologists about the need for all three therapeutic modalities at this point.

Question 4. The patient's bleeding is halted by your therapeutic maneuvers. Her corticosteroids are tapered, but as this is done over several months, her platelet count falls once again to a dangerously low level. Despite two more attempts to sustain adequate platelet counts with high-dose prednisone and slow tapers, platelets dropped to $<1,000/\mu L$ with more hemorrhagic bullae in oral mucosa and this time, lower gastrointestinal bleeding. What therapeutic modalities should be considered next?

Answer. Splenectomy would be the convevtional approach, but first immunization with vaccines against *Streptococcus pneumoniae*, *Neisseria meningitidis*, meningococci, and *Haemophilus influenzae* should be done. Some might try danazol or other immunosuppressive agents or chemotherapy, but these medications are usually reserved for postsplenectomy failures.

Follow-up:

The patient responded well to splenectomy and remains in sustained remission with good platelet counts.

SELECTED READING

Ballem PJ, Belzberg A, Devine DV, et al. Kinetic studies of the mechanism of thrombocytopenia in patients with human immunodeficiency virus infection. *New Engl J Med* 1992;327:1779–1784.
Interesting investigation demonstrating that the thrombocytopenia in patients with HIV results from both decreased platelet production and accelerated platelet consumption. Zidovudine therapy improves thrombocytopenia by accelerating platelet production.

Beutler E. Platelet transfusions: the 20,000/μL trigger. *Blood* 1993;81:1411–1413.
A very important editorial questioning the evidence for administering prophylactic platelet transfusions at platelet counts below 20,000/μL. Beutler proposes that a platelet count of 5,000–10,000/μL is a more appropriate trigger for prophylactic platelet transfusion.

Burrows RF, Kelton JG. Incidentally detected thrombocytopenia in healthy mothers and their infants. *N Engl J Med* 1988;319:142–145.
Prospective evaluation of the frequency and outcome of thrombocytopenia developing in otherwise healthy pregnant women.

Choi ES, Nichol JL, Hokom MM, Hornkohl AC, Hunt P. Platelets generated *in vitro* from proplatelet-displaying human megakaryocytes are functional. *Blood* 1995;85:402–413.
Interesting in vitro investigation suggesting that platelets develop from megakaryocytes via intermediary filamentous cytoplasmic projections termed proplatelets.

Consensus Conference. Platelet transfusion therapy. *JAMA* 1987;257:1777–1780.
Somewhat old but still relevant guidelines for the use of platelet transfusional therapy.

Cortelazzo S, Finazzi G, Ruggeri M, et al. Hydroxyurea for patients with essential thrombocythemia and a high risk of thrombosis. *New Engl J Med* 1995;332:1132–1136.
Important prospective study demonstrating that cytotoxic therapy with oral hydroxarea reduces thrombotic complications in patients with essential thrombocythemia and a high risk of thrombosis. High-risk patients were defined as those with prior thrombotic episodes and/or age greater than 60 years.

Cortelazzo S, Viero P, Finazzi G, d'Emilio A, Rodeghiero F, Barbui T. Incidence and risk factors for thrombotic complications in a historical cohort of 100 patients with essential thrombocythemia. *J Clin Oncol* 1990;8:556–562.
Retrospective evaluation of risk factors for thrombotic complications in patients with essential thrombocythemia. Age, prior thrombosis, and a long history of preceding thrombocytosis were identified as independent risk factors.

George JN, Caen JP, Nurden AT. Glanzmann's thrombasthenia: the spectrum of clinical disease. *Blood* 1990;75:1383–1395.
Comprehensive recent review of a rare disorder.

George JN, et al. Idiopathic thrombocytopenia purpura: a practice guideline developed by explicit methods for the American Society of Hematology. *Blood* 88:3-40, 1996.
An authoritative, comprehensive overview of the diagnosis and treatment of ITP. See also accompanying editorial by A. Lichtin which explains the process by which guidelines were developed.

Gernsheimer T, Stratton J, Ballem PJ, Slichter SJ. Mechanisms of response to treatment in autoimmune thrombocytopenic purpura. *N Engl J Med* 1989;320:974–980.
Important research investigation examining the mechanism of thrombocytopenia in patients with ITP. This article suggests that platelet autoantibody, in addition to accelerating platelet consumption in the spleen, also damages marrow megakaryocytes resulting in decreased platelet production. Kinetics vary from patient to patient.

Gewirtz AM, Hoffman R. Transitory hypomegakaryocytic thrombocytopenia: aetiological association with ethanol abuse and implications regarding regulation of human megakaryocytopoiesis. *Br J Haematol* 1986;62:333–344.
One of very few studies evaluating the mechanism of alcohol-induced thrombocytopenia. This investigation suggests that alcohol induces an arrest of megakaryocyte development at the mitotic/endomitotic interface.

Harker LA. *Hemostasis Manual.* Philadelphia: FA Davis; 1974.
Somewhat dated but wonderful manual that briefly but elegantly reviews the kinetics of megakaryocytopoiesis and platelet production.

Kelton JG, Smith JW, Warkentin TE, Hayward CPM, Denomme GA, Horsewood P. Immunoglobulin G from patients with heparin induced thrombocytopenia binds to a complex of heparin and platelet factor 4. *Blood* 1994;83:3232–3239.
Important article indentifying the probable antigenic target of pathologic antibodies in patients with heparin-induced thrombocytopenia.

Kuter DJ, Beeler DL, Rosenberg RD. The purification of megapoietin: a physiological regulator of megakaryocyte growth and platelet production. *Proc Nat Acad Sci USA* 1994;91:11104–11108.
Report from one of several groups successful in the cloning of thrombopoietin (here called megapoietin). This article also proposes a thrombopoietic regulatory system governed by the concentration of free thrombopoietin (i.e., that which is not bound to thrombopoietin receptors on platelets and megakaryocytes).

Mazur, EM. Megakaryocytes and megakaryocytopoiesis. In: Loscalzo J, Schafer AI, eds. *Thrombosis and Hemorrhage.* Cambridge, Mass.: Blackwell Scientific Publishing; 1994: 161–194.
Comprehensive review of the biochemistry and cellular biology of megakaryocytes and megakaryocytopoiesis. The discussion concerning megakaryocytopoietic regulation is partially outdated as a result of the cloning of thrombopoietin.

Metcalf D. Thrombopoietin—at last. *Nature* 1994;369:519–520.
Brief description of the background, difficulties, and final success in the discovery and cloning of thrombopoietin.

Picozzi VJ, Roeske WR, Creger WP. Fate of therapy failures in adult idiopathic thrombocytopenic purpura. *Am J Med* 1980;69:690–694.
Fascinating retrospective evaluation of patients with ITP who failed initial therapy. Remarkably, several years later, most patients are doing extremely well.

Souyri M, Vigon I, Penciolelli JF, Heard JM, Tambourin P, Wendling F. A putative trun-
cated receptor gene transduced by the myeloproliferative leukemia virus immor-
talizes hematopoietic progenitors. *Cell* 1990;63:1137–1147.
*Seminal investigation that identified the MPL oncogene that later turned out to be the throm-
bopoietin receptor and directly resulted in the successful cloning of thrombopoietin.*

Stoll DB, Blum S, Pasquale D, Murphy S. Thrombocytopenia with decreased megakaryocytes. Evaluation and prognosis. *Ann Intern Med* 1981;94:170–175.
Important, retrospective description of the clinical entity termed amegakaryocytic thrombocytopenia.

Zucker-Franklin D, Cao Y. Megakaryocytes of human immunodeficiency virus-infected
individuals express viral RNA. *Proc Natl Acad Sci USA* 1989;86:5595–5599.
*First experimental demonstration, using in situ hybridization, that HIV directly infects human
megakaryocytes. This important finding could explain the suppressed platelet production observed in HIV patients. This observation is disputed by some investigators.*

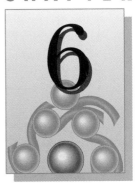

Hemostasis and Thrombosis

Angelina C. A. Carvalho

NORMAL HEMOSTASIS

The hemostatic process begins with a vascular break or injury. It culminates in the formation of a platelet–fibrin meshwork (hemostatic plug). This serves as both a mechanical seal that prevents further blood loss and the nidus for tissue repair. The hemostatic mechanism function involves interactions among the vessel wall, the platelets, the blood coagulation proteins, and the fibrinolytic system (Fig. 6-15). Rapid localization of hemostasis within a fluid medium is not without risk. Imbalance in one direction may lead to excessive bleeding; imbalance in the other may lead to thrombus formation.

THE VASCULAR ENDOTHELIUM

Blood loss from intact vessels is prevented by the maintenance of vessel wall integrity. The structural and functional integrity of the vessel wall depends upon the characteristics of its cellular components and on the composition and organization of the extracellular matrix, which the cells synthesize. The platelets also exert a nurturing effect on the endothelium. Although all components of vessel wall (endothelium, subendothelium, media, and adventitia) are involved in the response to injury, the endothelium deserves special mention because of its active participation in hemostasis.

Endothelial cells (ECs) form a monolayer resting on a continuous basement membrane, which constitutes the first barrier of defense against multiple processes, including hemostasis and thrombosis (Fig. 6-1). The ECs provide the following to the subendothelium: the basement membrane, collagen, elastin, lamilin, proteases, protease inhibitors, thrombospondin, mucopolysaccharides, vitronectin, fi-

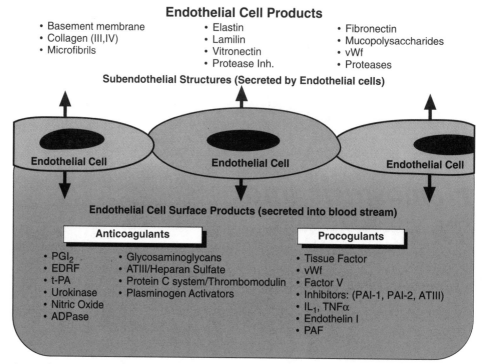

Figure 6-1. Endothelial cell products secreted into the subendothelial region and into the blood vessel lumen. See text for abbreviations.

bronectin, and von Willebrand factor (vWf). These proteins are essential for cell-to-cell interaction and formation of a diffusion barrier to prevent blood escape from intra- to extravascular spaces. In addition, ECs provide a diversity of physiologic functions, including regulation of platelet reactivity, control of white cell efflux and trafficking, regulation of growth factor activities, and regulation of blood fluidity. The EC also produces substances that are secreted into the vascular lumen that promote the fluidity of blood. These are the glycosaminoglycans, the heparin (heparan-sulfate)–antithrombin III system, the thrombin–thrombomodulin–protein C system, and the plasminogen–plasmin activator system. The ECs also produce prostacyclin (PGI₂) and endothelium-derived relaxing factor (EDRF), two potent inhibitors of platelet adhesion and aggregation. These substances are also vasodilators and act synergistically.

Primarily, the normal endothelium acts as a potent *anticoagulant surface,* which neither activates blood coagulation proteins nor attracts the cellular components of blood. Upon stimulation or injury, however, the endothelium transforms into a potent *procoagulant surface.* This is accomplished by synthesis, release, or availability of many procoagulant substances, including tissue factor (TF), von Willebrand factor (vWf), factor V, plasminogen activator inhibitors (PAI—1 and PAI-2), interleukin 1 (IL-1), tissue necrosis factor (TNF), and endothelin-1 (a vasoconstrictor) (Fig. 6-1).

The immediate response of the vascular endothelium to injury is vasoconstriction. Vasoconstriction is transient, lasting less than 60 seconds, but it reduces blood flow, which allows better interaction among platelets, blood coagulation factors, and the site of injury. Vasoconstriction in response to minor injury alone can arrest the bleeding, but in widespread injury it only slows down blood loss to prevent exsanguination.

PLATELETS

Exposure of subendothelial structures, as a result of endothelial cell injury, causes platelet shape change and adherence. The platelet adhesion is mediated by vWf, which bridges platelet membrane glycoprotein Ib to the exposed collagen structures at the site of injury. Collagen (types I, II, and III) of the subendothelium and thrombin formed locally cause the adherent platelets to secrete their granule contents. Both the collagen and thrombin also stimulate platelet membrane phospholipases to free arachidonic acid (AA) from platelet membrane phospholipids. The AA is converted by platelet cyclo-oxygenase to prostaglandins H_2 and G_2 (PGH$_2$ and PGG$_2$). The PGH$_2$ and PGG$_2$ are converted by platelet thromboxane synthetase to thromboxane α_2 (TxA$_2$) and other hydroxyfatty acids. The intracellular TxA$_2$ contracts the platelet tubular system, which moves the granules to the center of the cell and facilitates their release. TxA$_2$ is also a potent vasoconstrictor and inducer of platelet aggregation. Together with ADP released by the platelets, TxA$_2$ stimulates the platelets in circulation to aggregate and add on to the platelet-plug to seal the area of injury. At the periphery of the platelet-plug, the platelets tend to disaggregate, because of the release of antiaggregant substances, such as prostacyclin (PGI$_2$), nitric oxides (NO), adenosinediphosphatases (ADPases) and other enzymes, produced by the intact adjacent endothelial cells. This primary platelet-plug is usually sufficient to initiate hemostasis and to stop bleeding in the first minute, but alone it cannot sustain hemostasis (Chapter 5.).

BLOOD COAGULATION

The permanent hemostatic plug is formed when thrombin is generated via blood coagulation activation. Thrombin plays an essential role in the initiation, growth, and localization of the permanent hemostatic plug. It causes irreversible platelet aggregation and the deposition of fibrin on the platelet aggregates formed at the site of vascular injury. The fibrin–platelet meshwork forms the structural barrier to prevent further escape of blood and initiates the process of tissue repair.

The blood coagulation system (Fig. 6-2) is composed of a series of linked proteolytic enzyme reactions. At each stage of this biological amplification system, a proenzyme (parent zymogen) is converted to a corresponding serine protease, which catalyzes a subsequent zymogen–serine protease transition. The serine proteases hydrolyze peptide bonds at the amino acid serine center (the active serine center). Thirteen of these proteins (the blood coagulation factors) comprise the coagulation system; seven are activated to serine proteases (factors XII, XI, IX, X, II, VII, and prekallikrein), three are cofactors for these transitions (factors V, VIII, and high-molecular-weight kininogen), one is a cofactor/receptor (tissue factor, factor III), one is a transglutaminase (factor XIII), and the last fibrinogen (factor I) is the substrate for fibrin formation, the end point of blood activation (Table 6-1).

To achieve hemostasis via the process of blood coagulation, the circulating blood coagulation factors need to be concentrated at the site of injury. This is accomplished by blood coagulation reactions occurring on exposed collagen, tissue factor, and cell membranes, including platelet–phospholipid membranes. Amplification of the blood coagulation system, which occurs locally, is a powerful mechanism to form thrombin. It is estimated that from one molecule of activated FXII, more than 1 million molecules of thrombin can be generated. The primary thrombin function is to convert fibrinogen to fibrin. Fibrin holds the platelet-aggregates

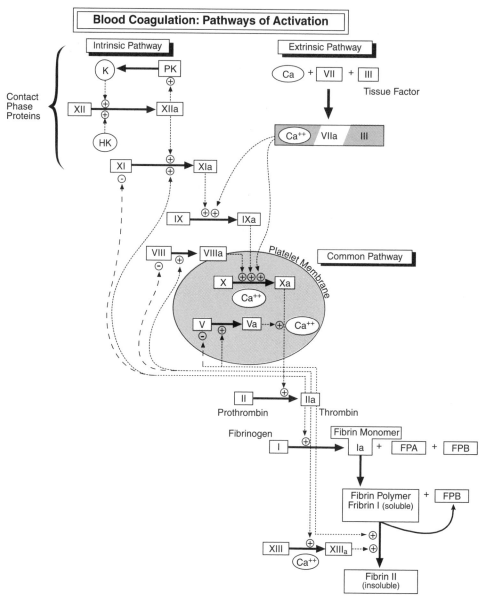

Figure 6-2. The activation of proteins that lead to blood coagulation. A positive-feedback system (amplification) causes magnification of initial pathway reactions. A negative-feedback system (inhibitions) serves as a countervailing force and limits coagulation. Dotted arrows and + signs indicate facilitation of process. Dashed arrows and − signs indicate inhibition of process. See text for abbreviations

at the site of vascular injury and changes the unstable platelet-plug (primary) into a stable, permanent hemostatic plug.

The Pathways of Blood Activation

Traditionally, the mechanisms of blood activation are separated into the extrinsic and the intrinsic pathways. This division is artificial and does not occur *in vivo*, but it facilitates the interpretation of *in vitro* laboratory tests.

TABLE 6-1. *THE BLOOD COAGULATION FACTORS*

FACTORS	NAME	SYNTHESIS	T 1/2	GENE LOCATION	FUNCTION
I	Fibrinogen	Hepatocyte	4–5 days	Chromosome 4	Substrate
II	Prothrombin	Hepatocyte/ **vitamin K**	3 days	Chromosome 11	Enzyme
III	Tissue factor	EC + many other cells	—	—	Receptor/ cofactor
V	Labile factor	Hepatocyte EC/platelets	12–15 hr	Chromosome 1	Cofactor
VII	Proconvertin	Hepatocyte/ **vitamin K**	4–7 hr	Chromosome 13	Enzyme
VIII	Antihemophilic factor	Sinusoids of liver	8–10 hr	Chromosome X	Cofactor
IX	Christmas factor	Hepatocyte/ **vitamin K**	1 day (~24 hr)	Chromosome X	Enzyme
X	Stuart–Prower factor	Hepatocyte/ **vitamin K**	2 days	Chromosome 13	Enzyme
XI	Plasma thromboplastin antecedent factor	Hepatocyte	2–3 days	Chromosome 4	Enzyme
XII	Hageman factor	Hepatocyte	1 day	Chromosome 5	Enzyme
XIII	Fibrin-stabilizing factor	Hepatocyte/ platelets	8 days	Chromosomes 6,1	Transglutaminase
—	Prekallikrein (PK) or Fletcher factor	Hepatocyte	—	Chromosome 4	Enzyme
—	High-molecular-weight kininogen (HK) or Williams or Flaujeac or Fitzgerald factor	Hepatocyte	—	Chromosome 3	Cofactor

The Extrinsic Pathway. The major pathway of blood activation *in vivo* is considered to be the extrinsic pathway (Fig. 6-3). The components of this pathway include tissue factor (TF, FIII), its inhibitor (tissue factor pathway inhibitor, TFPI; Fig. 6-12), and plasma factor VII (FVII). TF is an intrinsic membrane glycoprotein, present in many cells that are in contact with blood; it is not accessible to blood unless proteases are formed or cell injury occurs *in vivo*. TF functions as a cofactor/receptor, which in the presence of calcium activates factor VII. FVII is a single-chain glycoprotein (M_r 50,000), produced by hepatocytes, that circulates in blood as a zymogen. It contains 10 γ-carboxyglutamic acid residues (Gla domain), which require vitamin K for their biosynthesis.

Activation of Factor VII leads to exposure of its active serine center. It results primarily from binding of FVII to TF/Ca^{2+}. However, FVII can also be activated by

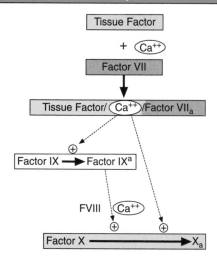

The Extrinsic Pathway of Blood Activation

Figure 6-3. $FVII_a$ helps to activate FIX in the intrinsic pathway and FX in the common pathway. FVIIIa and Ca^{2+} are also needed to help FX activation.

minor proteolytic action of other serine proteases of the blood coagulation (e.g., thrombin, FXIIa, FIXa, and FXa), as well as autoactivation. Autoactivation contributes to only minor FVII activation *in vivo.* The $TF/FVIIa/Ca^{2+}$ complex acts on two substrates—FX and FIX—to generate thrombin.

The Intrinsic Pathway. The intrinsic pathway of blood activation is defined as coagulation initiated by components entirely contained within the vascular system. It exists *in vivo* concomitantly with the extrinsic pathway. The components of the intrinsic system are factors XII (FXII), XI (FXI), IX (FIX), VIII (FVIII), the cofactors high-molecular-weight kininogen (HK) and prekallikrein (PK), and their respective inhibitors (Fig. 6-4).

The initiation of FXII activation begins when negatively charged surfaces (e.g., collagen) are exposed within the vessel wall, where autoactivation of FXII leads to conformational changes with exposure of its active serine center (FXIIa). The availability of small amounts of FXIIa leads to activation of its substrates: PK, HK, and FXI (Fig. 6-4). PK and FXI bind to the activating surfaces through HK; in the absence of HK, activation of both these zymogens does not occur. Bound HK may be cleaved by kallikrein (K) or surface-bound FXIIa to initiate the reciprocal activation of the PK–FXII systems. Since plasma PK and FXI both exist in bimolecular complexes with HK, this facilitates direct delivery of more PK and FXI to attach to the surface, where FXII is being activated. Surface-bound FXIIa then cleaves FXI to FXIa and prekallikrein to kallikrein. The mechanism of reciprocal activation of FXII and prekallikrein is much faster than autoactivation of FXII and accounts for amplification of FXII activation system. Once formed, kallikrein converts HK to HKa and bradykinin. The net result of these initial contact reactions is to position HKa/K and Hka/FXIa complexes in the vicinity of FXIIa, where activation of blood coagulation, fibrinolysis, and complement activation are initiated (Fig. 6-4).

The kallikrein complexed with HKa is not tightly bound to the surface, and it is released into the fluid phase to act on a variety of substrates, including FXII, plasminogen, prorenin, and complement C1 (Fig. 6-4).

Kallikrein also acts on FXIIa to form FXII fragment (FXIIf), which retains the active serine site but loses the binding domain. This negative-feedback regulation by kallikrein switches off surface-bound coagulation. The FXIIf in the fluid phase can act as a potent activator of prekallikrein, and it converts FVII to FVIIa and C1 to activated C1. In contrast, FXIa bound to HKa remains tightly bound to the surface, where it positions the zymogens in close proximity to FXIIa. FXIa also cleaves HK, destroying its cofactor activity, which allows FXIa to separate from the site of surface activation. FXIa converts FIX to FIXa, both in the fluid phase and on membrane-bound platelet-phospholipid (Fig. 6-4).

Vitamin K is necessary for postribosomal carboxylation of the terminal glutamic acid residues of all **vitamin K–dependent blood coagulation factors, FX, FIX, FVII, FII** (the mnemonic is "1972"), and two coagulation factor inhibitors (C and S). This carboxylation allows the binding of calcium, which is needed for the expression of the phospholipid binding site and activation of all the vitamin K–dependent proteins.

Although activation of FIX is initiated by either FXIa or FVIIa/TF(III) (see Fig. 6-2), the latter is considered the most important pathway of blood activation *in vivo*. Activated FIX requires the presence of calcium and a cofactor, FVIII, to attach to platelet-membrane phospholipid and to convert FX to FXa. FVIII acts as a powerful accelerator of the latter enzymatic reaction.

Factor VIII, also called *antihemophilic factor*, is a single polypeptide synthesized by various tissues, including the endothelial cells of hepatic sinusoids. It is coded by a large gene (186 kb) located in the tip of chromosome X. Analysis of FVIII cDNA has identified two internal repeats in the protein organized with the following do-

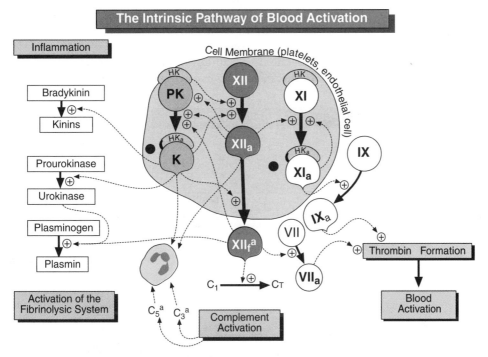

Figure 6-4. Autoactivation of FXII and reciprocal activation of FXII and PK result in powerful activation of the intrinsic coagulation pathway with many positive feedback/facilitated reactions. Conversion of FXII$_a$ to FXII$_f$ by K results in surface-bound coagulation being switched off. See text for further details of this complex story.

mains: A1–A2–B–A3–C1–C2 (Fig. 6-5). Activation of FVIII by thrombin results in heavy- and light-chain FVIII fragments. The A domains are located in both the heavy- and light-chain fragments, whereas the C domains are restricted to the light chain. The coagulant activity of FVIII is associated with both the A and C domains, but not with the B domain (connecting region), which is devoid of procoagulant properties. Molecular analysis of FVIII and another cofactor of blood coagulation, FV, shows similarities between the two molecules. Both FVIII and FV share a common structure (A1–A2–B–A3–C1–C2), with homology between both the A and C domains, where the coagulant activity of both cofactors resides; the B region differs between FVIII and FV but is not associated with the function of either cofactor (Fig. 6-5).

FVIII circulates in blood bound to vWf, a large glycoprotein produced by ECs and megakaryocytes. The vWf serves as the intravascular carrier protein for FVIII (Fig. 6-21). The binding of vWf to FVIII (via FVIII amino acid residues 1649 to 1689) stabilizes the FVIII molecule, prolongs its intravascular half-life, and transports it to the site of injury. Activated FVIII, however, must dissociate from vWf to express its cofactor activity. Exposure of the FVIII/vWf complex to thrombin causes separation of FVIII from its carrier protein and generates the heavy- and light-chain fragments, which are essential to FVIII coagulant activity. One of the other physiologic roles of FVIII/vWf association is the capacity of vWf to increase FVIII concentration at sites of vascular injury. Because circulating vWf binds to both exposed subendothelial tissues and stimulated platelets, it positions FVIII in the area of injury, where it is needed to accelerate FIXa conversion of FX to activated FXa.

FVIII can also be activated by FXa and FIXa in presence of anionic phospholipid and calcium. This reaction occurs at a much slower rate than that of thrombin *in vitro*. Thus it is presumed that thrombin is the major activator of FVIII *in vivo*.

The Common Pathway. The final pathway of blood activation is called the common pathway (Fig. 6-6). In this stage, FXa in association with FVa on phospho-

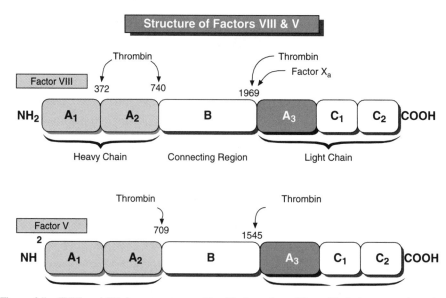

Figure 6-5. FVIII and FV demonstrate considerable homology. Thrombin is important in activating both factors by cleaving them at the indicated regions.

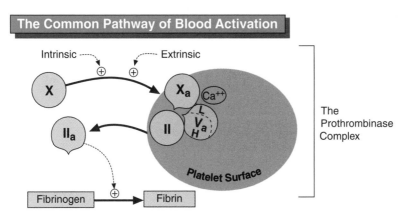

Figure 6-6. FX$_a$, FV$_a$ phospholipid and calcium (the prothrombinase complex) convert FII (prothrombin) to FII$_a$ (thrombin). See Figs. 6-2 and 6-5. (L = FV$_a$ light chain. H = FV$_a$ heavy chain.)

lipid surface, and in presence of calcium (called prothrombin complex), converts prothrombin (FII) into thrombin (FIIa).

Prothrombin is the most abundant of the vitamin K–dependent blood coagulation factors in plasma. It is synthesized by hepatocytes as a prepropeptide. Post-translational processes modify preprothrombin to the mature molecule by including carboxylation of glutamic acid residues, and incorporation of carbohydrate side chains. The mature prothrombin molecule contains four domains: the first two bind to calcium and phospholipid, the third appears also to be involved with calcium binding, and the fourth contains the active serine protease precursor (Fig. 6-7).

Prothrombin activation to thrombin can occur by various pathways. Physiologically, the most important pathway is by the action of prothrombinase complex (FXa + FVa + phospholipid + calcium). Prothrombinase cleaves prothrombin at two positions (Arg 320 first, and then Arg 271). The predominant, measurable cleavage products are α-thrombin (amino acid residues 272–579) and prothrombin fragment 1.2 (amino acid residues 1–271; Fig. 6-7). FXa in presence of calcium without FVa can also cleave prothrombin at the same points (in reverse order), but at a much slower rate (300,000-fold). Thrombin itself may cleave prothrombin at amino acid locations 155 and 284.

Factor V inactive profactor circulates in plasma as single polypeptide, asymmetric glycoprotein. It is synthesized both in the liver and in the megakaryocytes, with the former contributing the plasma FV and the latter contributing to platelet FV.

The factor V in the prothrombin interaction is supplied by platelet secretion with binding and expression of FV on the platelet cytoskeleton through a site on the plasma membrane that contains all elements of the prothrombin complex (Fig. 6-6). FV serves as a receptor for anchoring FXa to the activated platelet at the site of injury. FVa also binds prothrombin, facilitating the FXa interaction with prothrombin. The cDNA analysis of FV shows a domain structure similar to that of FVIII, as previously described (Fig. 6-5). The FV gene is located on chromosome 1. FV is converted to the active cofactor (FVa) by limited proteolysis by thrombin and by FXa. Thrombin excises the B domain, changing the single-chain FV polypeptide into a two-chain polypeptide, the FVa.

The binding of FVa, to the platelet phospholipid membrane or cell surfaces, occurs via the amino-terminus of the light chain. Once assembled on the cell sur-

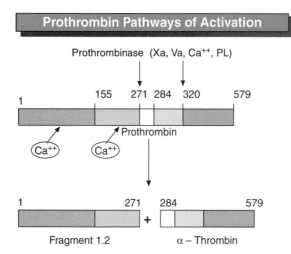

Figure 6-7. The prothrominase complex cleaves prothrombin at the amino acid sites indicated. Fragment 1.2 and α thrombin result from cleavage at amino acids 271–272. Thrombin itself cleaves at amino acid locations 155 and 284.

face, FVa acts as part of FXa receptor. For this binding site to remain functional, FVa must contain intact light and heavy chains. FV forms a binary interaction with each of the components of the prothrombinase complex. The FVa bound to the membrane then modulates the conformation and orientation of both the enzyme and the substrate. Although the phospholipid provides the template for concentration of the enzyme and substrate, FVa markedly accelerates the FXa conversion of prothrombin to thrombin (Fig. 6-6).

Thrombin causes hydrolysis of fibrinogen to fibrin (Fig. 6-8). Fibrinogen (M_r 340,000) is a complex glycoprotein consisting of two sets of three different polypeptide chains, including two α chains, two β chains, and two γ chains. It is a product of three genes, each coding one of the polypeptide chains; the genes are grouped together on the long arm of chromosome 4. Fibrinogen is synthesized primarily by hepatocytes, but it is also present in megakaryocytes and platelets. Its synthesis is markedly induced by tissue damage, inflammation, and stress (acute-phase states). Fibrinogen plays an essential role in normal hemostasis, and it is commonly involved in disorders of hemostasis. Thus bleeding or thrombosis is a common manifestation of either qualitative or quantitative changes in fibrinogen.

Thrombin first cleaves the arginine-glycine bonds of fibrinogen, releasing two peptides (fibrinopeptide A [FPA] and fibrinopeptide B [FPB]) and forming fibrin monomers (Fig. 6-6). The monomers polymerize with each other side by side (fibrin I) and are held together by hydrogen bonds (soluble fibrin complexes). Further hydrolysis by thrombin of these complexes results in further release of FPB. In addition, thrombin activates FXIII, which in the presence of calcium, links the side chains of the polymers (lysine to glutamine residues) by isopeptide bonds. Numerous cross-links are formed between the monomers leading to a highly interconnected network of fibrin fibers (fibrin II), which are mechanically strong, and capable of holding the platelet mass at the site of injury (Figs. 6-8 and 6-15).

Biological Functions of Thrombin. In addition to fibrin formation, thrombin activates platelets, activates coagulation factors and procofactors, and extends its activity beyond the mechanism of blood coagulation (Fig. 6-9). Thrombin activates the fibrinolytic system and stimulates ECs and white blood cells. It also causes migration of white cells and regulates vascular tone. Finally, by stimulating cell growth, thrombin contributes to tissue repair.

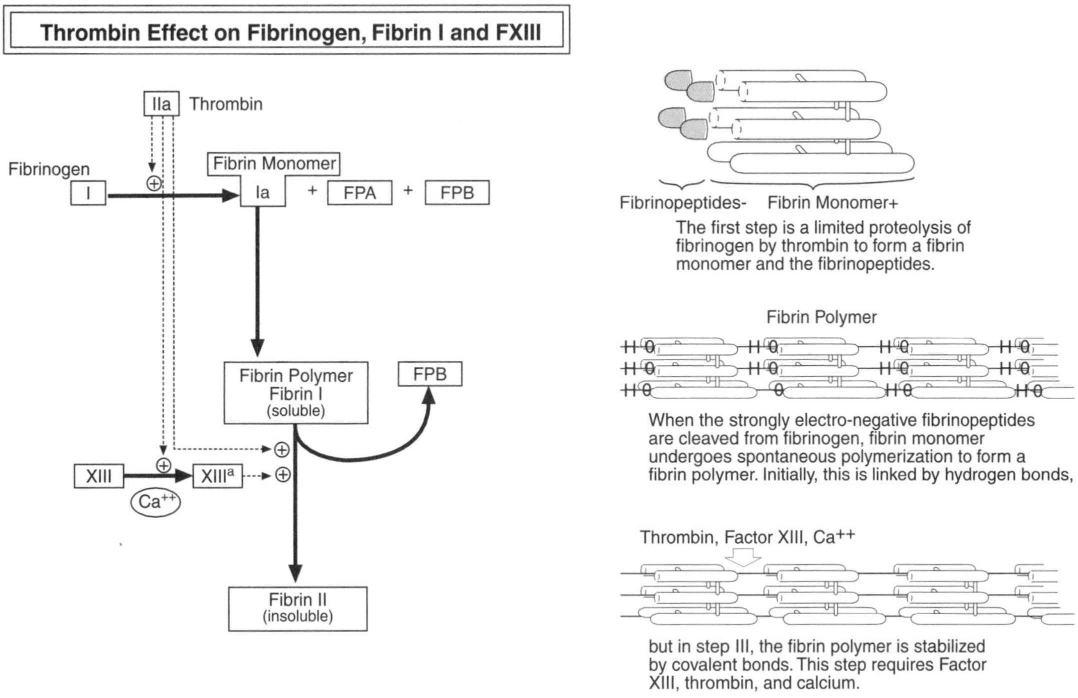

Thrombin Effect on Fibrinogen, Fibrin I and FXIII

IIa Thrombin

Fibrinogen
I ⊕ → Fibrin Monomer Ia + FPA + FPB

Fibrin Polymer
Fibrin I
(soluble) → FPB

XIII ⊕ → XIIIᵃ → ⊕
Ca⁺⁺

Fibrin II
(insoluble)

Fibrinopeptides−   Fibrin Monomer+

The first step is a limited proteolysis of fibrinogen by thrombin to form a fibrin monomer and the fibrinopeptides.

Fibrin Polymer

When the strongly electro-negative fibrinopeptides are cleaved from fibrinogen, fibrin monomer undergoes spontaneous polymerization to form a fibrin polymer. Initially, this is linked by hydrogen bonds,

Thrombin, Factor XIII, Ca⁺⁺

but in step III, the fibrin polymer is stabilized by covalent bonds. This step requires Factor XIII, thrombin, and calcium.

Figure 6-8. Thrombin's multiple actions are shown. The fibrinogen molecule is shown in diagrams on the right as it undergoes transformation to insoluble fibrin. (Right figure redrawn from Hirsh J, Braun E, eds. *Hemostasis and Thrombosis: A Conceptual Approach,* 2nd ed. New York: Churchill Livingston; 1983.)

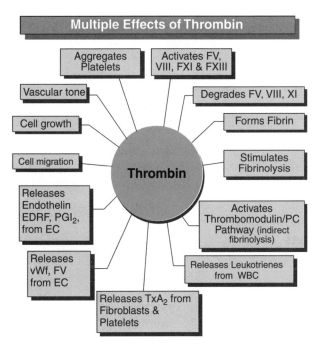

Multiple Effects of Thrombin

- Aggregates Platelets
- Activates FV, VIII, FXI & FXIII
- Vascular tone
- Degrades FV, VIII, XI
- Cell growth
- Forms Fibrin
- Cell migration
- Stimulates Fibrinolysis
- Releases Endothelin EDRF, PGI₂, from EC
- Activates Thrombomodulin/PC Pathway (indirect fibrinolysis)
- Releases vWf, FV from EC
- Releases Leukotrienes from WBC
- Releases TxA₂ from Fibroblasts & Platelets

Thrombin

Figure 6-9. The multiple actions of thrombin are shown. They are not restricted to actions on fibrin and fibrinogen.

Some of the general characteristics of blood coagulation factors are summarized in Table 6-2. The blood coagulation factors (FI–FXIII) are measured in plasma. Plasma is prepared by adding a calcium chelating agent (e.g., sodium citrate) to whole blood. When blood is allowed to clot in a glass tube, in absence of a chelating agent or anticoagulant, serum is obtained. Serum does not contain fibrinogen, FII, FV, and FVIII; these factors are utilized in the process of clot formation. Once FV and FVIII are activated by trace amounts of thrombin in the test tube or *in vivo*, their respective activities decay rapidly. For the latter reason, FV and FVIII are called labile coagulation factors.

Regulation of Blood Activation

Activation of blood coagulation *in vivo* is modulated by several regulatory mechanisms, which limit the reactions to the site of injury and prevent massive intravascular thrombosis. These include blood flow and hemodilution, hepatic and reticuloendothelial clearance, proteolytic action by thrombin (feedback mechanism), inhibitors of serine proteases, and fibrinolysis.

Blood Flow and Hemodilution. Rapid blood flow dilutes active serine proteases and transports them to the liver for clearance. It also disperses and frees bound platelets from the periphery of the platelet aggregates limiting the size of the growing hemostatic plug.

Hepatic and Reticuloendothelial Clearance. The soluble active serine proteases are inactivated and removed from circulation by hepatocytes and reticuloendothelial cells of the liver (Kupffer cells) and other organs.

Proteolytic Effects of Thrombin. Thrombin accelerates fibrin deposition at the site of tissue damage by potentiating activation of factors XI, V, and VIII (Fig. 6-2). However, thrombin also plays many roles in limiting hemostasis. It causes proteolysis and degradation of factors XI, V, and VIII (Fig. 6-2), which facilitates their inactivation by the respective inhibitors and rapid clearance. Thrombin further contributes to hemostatic control by initiating activation of the fibrinolytic system via the protein C pathway, which ultimately causes dissolution of fibrin and by stimulating white cells (cellular fibrinolysis).

TABLE 6-2. *SOME GENERAL CHARACTERISTICS OF BLOOD COAGULATION FACTORS*

CONTACT PHASE FACTORS	VITAMIN K–DEPENDENT FACTORS	OTHER FACTORS
XII, XI, PK, and HK	X, IX, VII and II	V, VIII, XIII, and I
Stable	Stable	Labile (V and VIII)
Ca^{2+} independent	Ca^{2+} dependent	Ca^{2+} independent
Present in serum	All in serum, but II	Only XIII in serum
No bleeding with deficiency, except XI	Bleeding with deficiency	Bleeding with deficiency

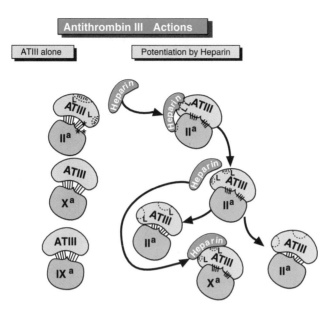

Figure 6-10. Interaction of AT III with Factors, II_a, X_a, and IX_a without and with heparin. Not shown is XII_a which is also inactivated by AT III. (AT III, antithrombin III; L, lysine binding sites; *, arginine reactive center of AT III; serine protease (II_a, X_a, IX_a); **, serine protease center.)

Inhibitors of Active Serine Proteases. The blood coagulation process is tightly controlled by naturally occurring plasma proteins (inhibitors), which limit the extent of the proteolytic reactions and protect against thrombus formation.

The major inhibitors of blood coagulation factors are antithrombin III (AT III), heparin cofactor II (HC II), protein C (PC), protein S (PS), tissue factor pathway inhibitor (TFPI), protease nexin-1 (PN-1), C1 inhibitor (C1-Inh.), α_1-antitrypsin (α_1AT), and α_2-macroglobulin (α_2M). Most of these inhibitors, with the exception of TFPI and α_2M, belong to a superfamily of proteins homologous with α_1-proteinase inhibitor, named serpins. The term *serpin* is a contraction of *serine protease inhibitor*.

The mechanism of inhibition of most protease inhibitors involves the formation of a tight stoichiometric complex with the protease, followed by slow hydrolysis of the inhibitor, and rapid hydrolysis of the loosely bound substrate. The mechanism of inhibition by serpins is different! The inhibition results from interactions between the substrate-binding site of the activated blood coagulation factor and the reactive site of the inhibitor. As a result of this interaction, the enzyme reactive site is blocked, without hydrolysis of the inhibitor reactive site, and the serine protease is not released. The function of the serine protease inhibitors, *in vivo*, is to limit blood activation by rapidly complexing with the serine proteases. This process does not shut down blood activation completely but restricts the systemic amplification of blood activation and confines it to the site of injury.

According to their mechanism of inhibition, the blood coagulation inhibitors are grouped as (1) serpins (AT III, HC II, PN-1, C1-Inh, α_1-AT); (2) kunins (e.g., TFPI), which are proteins with homology to aprotinin (pancreatic trypsin inhibitor), explained in detail later; and (3) α_2-macroglobulin, a scavenger inhibitor (the active site of the serine protease is not involved in the complex formation with α_2M).

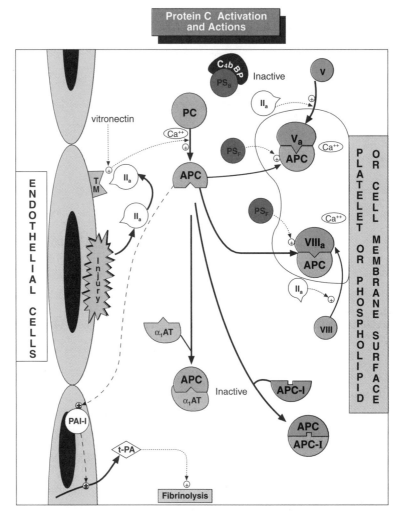

Figure 6-11. Protein C is activated quickly by the TM-II_a complex or II_a alone (slower). APC affinity for cell membrane/phospholipid is enhanced by PS and renders FV_a and $FVIIIa$ more easily accessible to APC-mediated cleavage and inactivation. C_4bBP binds PS and renders it inactive. α_1 AT or APC-I bind APC and render it inactive. Because APC inhibits PAI-1, it stimulates fibrinolysis via increased t-PA activity.

Serpins.

Antithrombin III (AT III) is a serpin and the major inhibitor of thrombin, FXa, and FIXa. It also inactivates FXIa and FXIIa. AT III neutralizes thrombin and the other serine proteases by forming a covalent bond, resulting in an inactive 1:1 stoichiometric complex between the enzyme and the inhibitor, involving the interaction of the arginine reactive site on AT III and the active serine center of thrombin (Fig. 6-10). The rate of neutralization of serine proteases by AT III proceeds slowly in the absence of heparin (anticoagulant), but it is greatly accelerated in its presence (1,000- to 100,000-fold).

AT III is an α_2-glycoprotein (M_r 58,0000) produced by the liver. It is also called *heparin cofactor I*. Heparin has two binding sites to AT III, and thrombin has one. Heparin binds to lysyl residues on AT III and causes conformational changes in the AT III molecule, which allow its arginine-reactive center to be more accessible to the active serine site of thrombin. The binding of heparin to AT III accelerates the rate of thrombin–AT III–heparin complex formation. The covalent bond between the active serine site of thrombin and the arginine site of the AT III–heparin complex produces inactivation of the active serine protease. Once the complex between AT III and thrombin is formed, heparin dissociates from the complex and binds to another AT III molecule, generating multiple rounds of enzyme inactivation. Neutralization by AT III of the activated forms of other blood coagulation factors occurs by a similar mechanism, but at different rates of inactivation. Heparin binding to AT III alone is sufficient to catalyze FXa inhibition; however, heparin must bind to both thrombin (FIIa) and AT III to catalyze thrombin inhibition by AT III (Fig. 6-10).

Approximation between AT III and the active enzymes of blood coagulation may also be mediated by other mucopolysaccharides and heparan sulfate. Since these substances are present in the vessel wall, a role played by them in controlling blood activation is suspected. The importance of AT III, as a major modulator of blood activation, is further emphasized by the development of thrombotic tendency in individuals with congenital or acquired AT III deficiency.

Heparin cofactor II (HC II), a serpin, inhibits thrombin, but not other coagulation proteases, in the presence of heparin or dermatan sulfate. HC II is secreted by the liver into the bloodstream, where it circulates for approximately 2.5 days, but HC II–thrombin complexes are cleared much more rapidly by a serpin–enzyme complex receptor on hepatocytes. Although the inhibitory effect of HC II on thrombin in circulation is secondary to that of AT III, HC II equilibrates with the extravascular compartment, where dermatan sulfate is present, and here it may have a critical role on thrombin inhibition. Thrombin has a variety of activities unrelated to blood coagulation or platelet activation, such as proliferation of fibroblasts and other cells, induction of monocyte chemotaxis, promotion of adhesion of neutrophils to endothelial cells, stimulation of prostacyclin production and other mediators by ECs, and inhibition of neurite outgrowth (see Fig. 6-9). The ability of HC II to block these thrombin activities may contribute to regulation of wound healing, inflammation, or neural development.

Protease Nexin-1 (PN-1), a serpin, is another secondary inhibitor of thrombin, which prevents thrombin binding to cell surfaces.

α_1-*antitrypsin* (α_1-AT) neutralizes FXIa and activated protein C (APC).

C1 inhibitor (C1-Inh) is also a serpin, and the major inhibitor of the contact system serine enzymes. It neutralizes 95% of FXIIa and more than 50% of all kallikrein formed in circulation. Its deficiency results in angioneurotic edema. FXIa is mainly neutralized by α_1-AT and by AT III.

Protein C (PC) is a vitamin K–dependent protein, synthesized by hepatocytes, which circulates in its inactive form in blood. It consists of a light chain (with glutamic acid domain and two epidermal growth factor–like domains) and a heavy chain (serine protease domain). Protein C (glutamic acid residues) binds to EC surfaces via calcium bridges.

PC is activated by trace amounts of thrombin; this reaction is markedly accelerated by *thrombomodulin*, an endothelial cell surface protein that binds thrombin (Fig. 6-11). The interaction between thrombin and thrombomodulin appears to be mediated by another protein, called *vitronectin*. Thrombomodulin is responsible for 60% of thrombin binding sites on endothelial cells. The thrombin bound to thrombomodulin becomes an anticoagulant protein capable of activating the serine protease, PC. The thrombin–thrombomodulin complex is internalized by the EC, where thrombin is degraded, and the thrombomodulin is recycled to the surface.

Protein S (PS). Activated protein C (APC) in the presence of its cofactor protein S cleaves and inactivates FVa and FVIIIa (Fig. 6-11). The activity of PC is potentiated by PS, also a vitamin K–dependent protein, which is synthesized by hepatocytes and by ECs. Protein S binds to both the EC membrane and APC, and forms a cell surface–bound complex. Since FVa binds to EC in the proximity of PS, this process facilitates acceleration of PC activation. APC cleaves FVa at the Arg 506 and FVIIIa at the Arg 562, resulting in loss of their respective coagulant activities. Since factors VIIIa and Va are cofactors for the generation of FXa and thrombin, respectively, PC exerts its anticoagulant effect through two linked assembly systems on the cell membrane. The activated PC inhibits *free* FVa, but *not* FVa *bound* to FXa; however, this protection of FVa that is bound to FXa does not exist in the presence of PS (the cofactor of PC activation) with the result of inhibition of both *free* and *bound* FV, causing augmented anticoagulant effect of APC. APC activity is controlled by its own circulating plasma inhibitor (APC inhibitor) and α_1-AT.

Impairment of PC activation occurs in pathologic conditions associated with production of factors such as hypoxia, endotoxin, IL_1, $TNF\alpha$, and high levels of homocysteine. All these substances are known to accelerate blood coagulation by inducing tissue factor expression by ECs and by suppressing transcription of thrombomodulin.

Activated PC, by a feedback mechanism, suppresses production by ECs of plasminogen activator inhibitor 1 (PAI-1), leaving t-PA unchecked. This indirectly stimulates the fibrinolytic system and augments the anticoagulant activity of APC (Fig. 6-11).

Both PC and PS are important modulators of blood coagulation activation, and their respective congenital deficiencies are associated with severe thrombotic tendency. The clinical significance of the PC system is illustrated by the increased thrombotic tendency (thrombophilia) in individuals born with an abnormal FV. The abnormal FV molecule (called FV Leiden) demonstrates resistance to *in*activation by APC! The mutation in FV results from the single nucleotide substitution of adenine for guanine 1691, which results in the replacement of glutamine for arginine at amino acid position 506. This single-nucleotide and single-amino-acid abnormality in FV eliminates its APC cleavage site, thus preventing FV *in*activation by APC, and causes subsequent unchecked thrombosis.

Kunins

Kunin inhibitors are a superfamily of proteins homologous to aprotinin, also called pancreatic trypsin inhibitor. They contain one or more kunitz domains. A kunitz domain contains 58 amino acid residues (which is much smaller than the serpin domains). Kunins are also recognized by the absolute conservation of cysteine residues. Unlike serpins, whose structure does not depend on disulfide bonds, kunins depend on the correct formation of three disulfide bonds per domain. Of the inhibitors of blood serine proteases, the tissue factor pathway inhibitor (TFPI) is a kunin type of inhibitor. TFPI is the FXa-dependent inhibitor of FVIIa–TF complex (Fig. 6-12).

Tissue factor pathway inhibitor (TFPI) is a glycoprotein (40 kDa) consisting of an acidic amino acid terminal, three kunitz-type domains, and a basic carboxy terminal end. The inhibitory activity of TFPI is associated with the first and second kunitz domains. The first kunitz domain binds to the TF–FVIIa complex, the second binds FXa, and the third binds to lipoproteins and is devoid of inhibitory activity. TFPI is mainly synthesized by endothelial cells, and to a small extent by mononuclear cells and hepatocytes. There are three intravascular pools of TFPI: 50–90% in EC, 10–50% in

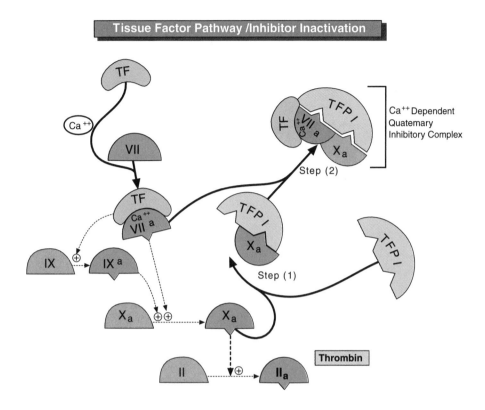

Figure 6-12. The two-step process by which TFPI inactivates FX$_a$ and FVII$_a$. See text for details and abbreviations.

plasma, and 2.5% in platelets. The plasma pool is mainly associated with lipoproteins, with only 5% free TFPI. However the inhibitory activity is confined to the *free* TFPI.

Inactivation by TFPI occurs in two steps. TFPI first binds to and inactivates FXa (1:1 stoichiometric complex), in the absence of calcium; then the TFPI–FXa complex binds to and inactivates the TF–FVIIa complex, forming a calcium-dependent quaternary inhibitory complex (Fig. 6-12). Unfractionated heparin, fractionated heparins such as low-molecular-weight heparins, and pentosan polysulfate stimulate the release of TFPI and potentiate its anticoagulant activity. The acceleration of the inhibitory effect of TFPI by heparin compounds and heparin affinity for TFPI are postulated as the reasons for the anticoagulant properties of the endothelium, which contains heparin family molecules. By inhibiting small amounts of TF, TFPI plays an essential role in maintaining normal hemostasis.

Fibrinolysis. The final stage in the reparative process following damage of a blood vessel is accomplished by activation of the fibrinolytic system (fibrinolysis), which results in dissolution of the fibrin plug and initiation of vessel wall repair (Fig. 6-15). Fibrinolysis is the major endogenous mechanism that protects against thrombus formation. There are two essential components to fibrinolysis: the plasma fibrinolytic activity and cellular fibrinolysis.

The Plasma Fibrinolytic System. The plasma fibrinolytic system consists of plasminogen (the zymogen), plasmin (the enzyme), plasminogen activators, and respective inhibitors. Activation of the fibrinolytic system leads to the generation of *plasmin*, a potent proteolytic enzyme, with multiple actions *in vivo*. The precursor of plasmin, *plasminogen*, is a single-chain glycoprotein (92 kDa), produced by the liver, eosinophils, and the kidney. The native plasminogen molecule consists of an A-chain with five domains (kringles, like Danish pastry), a B-chain (catalytic domain), and an N-terminal containing glutamic acid (Glu-plasminogen). Plasminogen has a half-life of 2.2 days; a slightly degraded form (Lys-plasminogen) has a much shorter half-life of 0.8 days. Plasminogen has a strong affinity for lysyl residues; the kringles confer to the plasminogen the ability to bind to exposed lysyl residues in fibrin, α_2-antiplasmin, histidine-rich glycoprotein, cell surface receptors, extracellular matrix, thrombospondin, and immunoglobulin.

Activation of Plasminogen. Conversion of plasminogen to plasmin is catalyzed by *plasminogen activators* and is closely regulated by various *inhibitors*. The latter inactivate both plasmin and the plasminogen activators (Fig. 6-13).

The plasminogen activators are produced either by the vessel wall (intrinsic activation) or by tissues (extrinsic activation). Activation of the fibrinolytic system via the intrinsic activation pathway involves the activation of the contact phase blood proteins: FXII, FXI, PK, HK, and kallikrein (Fig. 6-4). Although, this is an important pathway of plasminogen activation, the major activation of plasminogen is via tissue or extrinsic activation pathway and results from the action of tissue plasminogen activator (t-PA) released from endothelial cells. t-PA is also produced by other cells: monocytes, megakaryocytes, and mesothelial cells.

t-PA is a serine protease (half-life approximately 4 minutes) that circulates in blood complexed to its PAI and has a high affinity to bind to fibrin. This dependence of t-PA on fibrin localizes plasmin generation by t-PA to the area of fibrin accumulation. At the earliest stages of fibrin formation, t-PA and Glu-plasminogen bind to the fibrin strands. Once small amounts of t-PA and plasminogen are bound to the fibrin, the catalytic action of t-PA on plasminogen is enhanced many-fold. The plasmin formed then degrades fibrin, exposing new lysyl residues to which another plasminogen activator (single-chain urokinase [scu-PA]) binds. Plasmin activates scu-PA to its active two-chain form (u-PA), leading to further conversion of plasminogen to plasmin and dissolution of fibrin (Fig. 6-13).

Urokinase (scu-PA) is found in large amounts in urine. Like t-PA, it is a serine protease. Its major function is exerted in tissues, in the degradation of the extracellular matrix, which enables cells to migrate. Urokinase is produced by fibroblasts, monocytes/macrophages, and endothelial cells. It has a half-life of about 7 minutes and does not circulate bound to PAI, as does t-PA. scu-PA potentiates the effect of t-PA when injected after but not before t-PA. Both t-PA and urokinase have been synthesized by recombinant DNA methods and are available as therapeutic agents.

Other plasminogen activators (nonphysiologic) are streptokinase (produced by hemolytic streptococci), anisoylated plasminogen-streptokinase activator (APSAC), and staphylokinase (produced by *Staphylococcus aureus*). The first two are pharmacologic thrombolytic agents currently used in the treatment of acute thrombosis.

The major function of plasmin is to digest fibrin, to maintain blood vessel patency. Plasmin, however, degrades a wide range of other substrates, including fib-

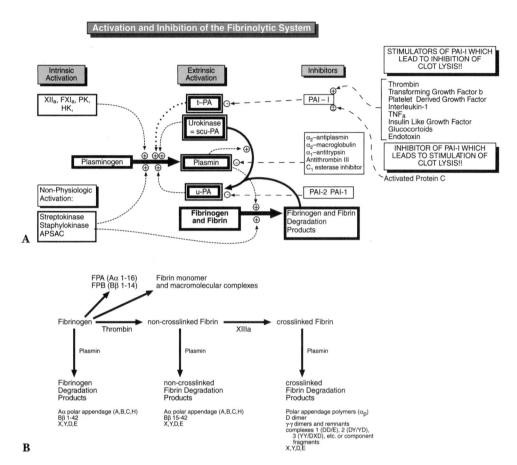

Figure 6-13. Panel A shows the activation and inhibition of the fibrinolytic system. Many complex interactions are seen. See text for details and abbreviations. Panel B shows the transformation of fibrinogen to fibrin as it is cross-linked and degraded. (Redrawn from Butler E, Lichtman MA, Coller BS, Kipps TJ, eds. *Williams Hematology,* 5th ed. New York: McGraw-Hill, 1995.)

rinogen, FV, FVIII, FX, FIX, vWf, and platelet glycoproteins; it also activates components of the complement cascade (C1, C3a, C3d, and C5).

Plasmin cleavage of peptide bonds in fibrin and fibrinogen produces various smaller-molecular-weight derivatives named fibrin(ogen) degradation products (FDP) or fibrin(ogen) split products (FSP). The largest derivative is called fragment X, which still retains arginine-glycine bonds for further action by thrombin. Fragment Y (an antithrombin) is smaller than X and delays fibrin polymerization by acting as a competitive inhibitor of thrombin. Two other, smaller fragments, D and E, inhibit platelet aggregation (Fig. 6-14).

Plasmin in circulation (fluid phase) is rapidly inactivated by naturally occurring inhibitors, but plasmin in the fibrin clot (gel phase) is protected from the action of inhibitors, and it lyses fibrin locally. Thus under physiologic conditions, fibrinolysis is localized to the areas of fibrin formation (gel phase)—that is, to the hemostatic plug. However, under pathologic conditions fibrinolysis can be generalized, affecting both phases of plasmin formation (fluid and gel phases). Pathologic conditions can lead to a lytic state (fibrinolytic state or active fibrinolysis), which is

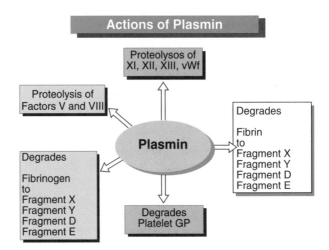

Figure 6-14. Plasmin's many actions on fibrinogen, other coagulation factors, and platelets.

characterized by formation of excessive fibrin(ogen) degradation products in circulation and clinical bleeding.

Like the active serine proteases of the blood coagulation, the activity of plasmin and plasminogen activators is modulated by *inhibitors.*

The **inhibitors of plasmin** are α_2-antiplasmin (α_2AP), α_2-macroglobulin (α_2M), α_1-antitrypsin (α_1AT), antithrombin III (AT III), and C1 esterase inhibitor (C1-inh).

α_2-*Antiplasmin* is a serpin, and the major inhibitor of plasmin in circulation. It has three main properties: it inhibits plasmin rapidly, it interferes with plasminogen adsorption to fibrin, and it undergoes cross-linking with α-chains of fibrin during fibrin formation. It is produced by the liver. When plasmin is formed in excess in circulation, the order of its neutralization is as follows: α_2-antiplasmin, $\alpha_2$macroglobulin, α_1-antitrypsin, AT III, and C_1 inhibitor, respectively. Despite the presence of various inhibitors to neutralize plasmin *in vivo,* the inherited deficiency of α_2-antiplasmin is manifested clinically by a severe bleeding, suggesting that plasmin activity is not well controlled by the other inhibitors.

α_2-*Macroglobulin* is a second-line inhibitor of plasmin and other proteases (e.g., kallikrein and t-PA). It acts as a scavenger protease inhibitor.

Plasminogen Activator Inhibitors 1, 2, 3 (PAI-1, PAI-2, and PAI-3). PAI-1 is the principal inhibitor of t-PA and two-chain u-PA, but it does not inactivate single-chain u-PA (scu-PA). It is produced by endothelial cells, smooth muscle cells, megakaryocytes, and mesothelial cells. PAI-1 is stored in platelets in its inactive form, and it is a serpin. PAI-1 is highly regulated and increased in circulation in many pathologic conditions. Its production (and subsequent inhibition of clot lysis) is stimulated by thrombin, transforming growth factor-β, platelet-derived growth factor, interleukin 1, TNFa, insulin-like growth factor, glucocorticoids, and endotoxin. Activated protein C inhibits PAI release from endothelial cells and thereby stimulates clot lysis (see Figs. 6-11 and 6-12).

The major function of PAI-1 is to limit the fibrinolytic activity at the site of hemostatic plug by inhibiting t-PA. PAI-1 accomplishes that easily, because of its molar excess over t-PA in the vessel wall. Thus at the site of injury, activated platelets release excessive amounts of PAI-1, preventing premature lysis of fibrin.

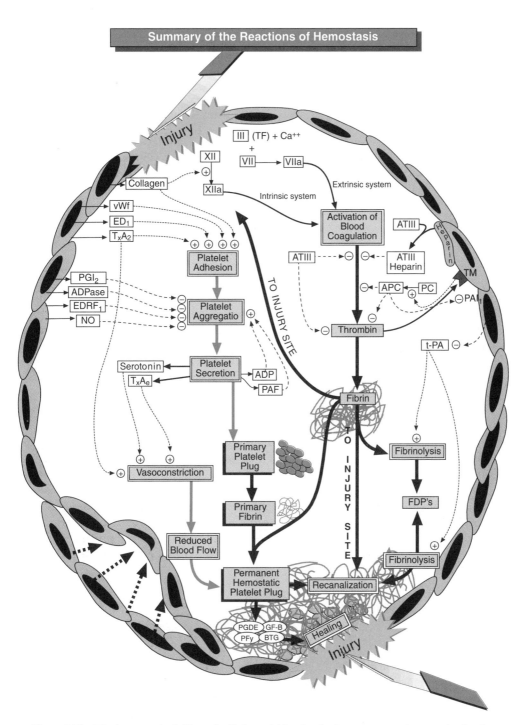

Figure 6-15. The integrated soluble and cellular activities that lead to permanent hemostatic plug formation and vessel wall repair. See text for details and abbreviations.

PAI-2 is the major inhibitor of two-chain u-PA.

C1 esterase inhibitor (C1-Inh) inactivates contact-phase-dependent fibrinolysis, such as the conversion of single-chain u-PA (scu-PA = urokinase) to two-chain u-PA.

Histidine-rich glycoprotein (HRG) is another competitive inhibitor of plasminogen. High plasma levels of PAI-1 and HRG are associated with increased thrombotic tendency.

The Cellular Fibrinolytic System. Cellular fibrinolysis is derived from white cells, macrophages, endothelial cells, and platelets. It contributes to the fibrinolytic activity of both localized and systemic fibrinolysis. White cells are attracted to the area of fibrin deposition by chemostatic substances released by platelets, by kallikrein formation, and by products of fibrin. In addition to the effect of esterase and other proteases on digesting fibrin, white cells and macrophages phagocytose fibrin and cellular debris accumulated at the site of injury.

HEMOSTATIC RESPONSE

In summary, the response to vascular injury depends on multiple linked interactions between the blood vessel wall, the circulating platelets, the blood coagulation factors, their inhibitors, and the fibrinolytic system (Fig. 6-15). The hemostatic process is modified by several positive- and negative-feedback loops, which maintain promoters of vessel wall constriction and platelet–fibrin formation, and those of fibrin dissolution and vessel relaxation, allowing return to the normal state.

DISORDERS OF HEMOSTASIS

Defects in the normal hemostatic mechanism are clinically manifested by either bleeding or thrombosis. Bleeding may occur because of failure of any of the processes involved in the formation of the permanent hemostatic plug formation and stabilization. Thrombosis may result from either excessive activation or defective modulation of the hemostatic mechanism. The steps of blood activation leading to fibrin and platelet aggregates are common to both hemostatic plug formation and thrombus formation. The major difference between these two processes is their location. The permanent hemostatic plug is formed extravascularly, whereas the thrombus is formed intravascularly.

BLEEDING DISORDERS

Pathogenesis

Abnormal bleeding may be caused by defects involving each of the components of normal physiologic hemostatic mechanism described earlier. These defects can be inherited or acquired and are usually classified according to their place of action in the hemostatic mechanism as vascular defects; platelet defects (both quantitative and or qualitative); blood coagulation factor defects; or fibrinolytic defects (excessive fibrinolysis).

Vascular defects of the inherited type consist of structural vessel wall abnormalities (e.g., defective collagen), and the acquired ones result from inflammatory or immune disorders that affect the blood vessels. The acquired defects are also called vascular purpuras and are common in medical practice.

Platelet defects include disorders of the quantity ($<100,000/\mu L$; i.e., thrombocytopenia) or of the quality of platelets (thrombocytopathy). Acquired platelet disorders are much more common than congenital ones (Chapter 5).

Blood coagulation defects such as vascular and platelet defects are also inherited or acquired. The latter are also much more frequent in medical practice. The defects in blood coagulation may result from (1) absolute failure of synthesis of one of blood coagulation factors; (2) reduced synthesis of blood coagulation factor(s); (3) production of an abnormal blood coagulation factor molecule; (4) excessive destruction of blood coagulation during pathologic conditions of blood activation (e.g., disseminated intravascular coagulation [DIC]), followed by rapid clearance; and (5) destruction of blood coagulation factor(s) activity due to acquired circulating inhibitors (antibodies).

Fibrinolytic defects are characterized by excessive production of fibrinolytic activity leading to severe bleeding diathesis. These include (1) inherited deficiency of α_2-antiplasmin, manifested by a lifelong severe bleeding disorder, secondary to unchecked plasmin in circulation; (2) excessive production of the activators of plasminogen (e.g., t-PA and urokinase); (3) failure of inactivation of plasminogen activators secondary to lack of inhibitors or impairment of their mechanisms of clearance (e.g., liver disease). Acquired disorders of fibrinolysis are also much more common than congenital disorders.

Clinical Consequences of Bleeding

Mortality and morbidity are consequences of abnormal bleeding. Although mortality is rare, morbidity is very common, and it is manifested by different clinical forms. Acute blood loss alone leads to acute anemia, which results in anoxia and hypovolemic circulatory failure. Chronic bleeding causes anemia due to iron deficiency. Excessive bleeding may produce pressure on vital structures such as the pharynx, causing asphyxia, or in the brain, resulting in severe neurologic deficit. Bleeding into joints and muscles also has dangerous consequences, leading to joint deformities and muscle contractures, respectively.

Clinical Presentation

The History. In the evaluation of patients with a bleeding disorder, the history, physical examination, and laboratory testing (screening and specific tests) evolve from an understanding of the basic mechanisms of normal hemostasis. The *history* (see Chapter 2) should address the type of bleeding (e.g., local versus generalized), severity and frequency of bleeding, and site of bleeding manifestations (e.g., skin and mucouscutaneous areas versus bleeding into joints or muscles). It is also important to determine whether the bleeding occurred spontaneously or followed drug intake, trauma, dental extractions, or other types of surgery. The *family history* establishes whether the bleeding disorder is inherited, and the mode of inheritance (e.g., X-linked, autosomal dominant or recessive). A positive family history is of great value in establishing the diagnostic etiology of bleeding, but a negative history does not exclude the possibility of an inherited bleeding diathesis. Patients with inherited disorders have bleeding manifestations that usually began in childhood; often they have a positive family history of bleeding and a history of bleeding after trauma or surgery. In the *social history*, alcohol and drug use are important, including the use of over-the-counter drugs, especially aspirin and related compounds that may be contained in combination medications. The *past medical history* provides information about illnesses that may have caused or worsened the bleeding.

The Physical Examination. The physical examination (Chapter 2) should focus on the type and location of the bleeding manifestations (e.g., skin, oropharynx, eyes, joints). Common bleeding manifestations include the following:

Petechiae. These are pinhead-sized red spots that occur in crops over the skin and mucous membranes of various parts of the body. These red spots represent extravasated red blood cells (cells that have escaped from blood vessels as a consequence of either increased permeability of the wall [e.g., vascular purpuras] or a problem with platelets whose physiologic task it is to plug normal gaps between endothelial cells). Platelets may be reduced in number or defective in function. Petechiae do not blanch under pressure because the escaped red blood cells cannot be squeezed back into the blood vessel.

Purpuras. These result from confluent petechiae and are caused by the same factors noted under "petechiae."

Ecchymosis. An ecchymosis, or bruise, is a large multicolored flat area of the skin caused by extravasated blood. It results from trauma to the vessel wall and occurs in patients with either vessel wall or platelet disorders. It is also a clinical manifestation of an inherited or acquired coagulation disorder.

Hematoma. A hematoma is a large collection of extravasated blood that infiltrates the subcutaneous tissues and muscles, and causes elevation and bluish discoloration of the skin above it. Hematomas are the clinical manifestation of an inherited or acquired blood coagulation factor(s) deficiency.

Hemarthrosis. Hemarthrosis, or bleeding into a joint, is caused by a severe blood coagulation factor defect, such as factor VIII deficiency (hemophilia A); factor IX deficiency (hemophilia B); in rare cases, severe factor XI deficiency (hemophilia C); or deficiency of factor V, factor X, or factor II.

Hematuria. Hematuria, or blood in the urine, occurs frequently in hemophilia A and B, von Willebrand disease (vWD), and severe vitamin K deficiency; but it also can be caused by local renal lesions.

Epistaxis. Epistaxis, or nose bleeding, is usually caused by minor trauma (e.g., nose blowing) to dilated blood vessels in the anterior nares, but it can also be secondary to a platelet or blood vessel wall disorder or to vWD.

Telangiectasia and angiomas. Telangiectasia and angiomas are malformations that produce red spots or patches that blanch on pressure.

After taking the history and noting physical findings, a few routine laboratory tests are indicated. These include a search for blood in the stool and urine, examination of a blood film (peripheral blood smear), a complete blood cell count, liver function tests (to consider liver disease), and blood urea nitrogen and creatinine (to consider renal failure). These are followed by the so-called screening blood tests for bleeding, which are needed to characterize the bleeding diathesis.

Laboratory Testing. Laboratory evaluation of bleeding disorders should address each of the components of hemostatic mechanism: vessel wall, platelets, blood coagulation factors, and components of the fibrinolytic system.

The *laboratory screening tests for bleeding* include the following:

1. Platelet number (estimate and measurement);
2. Peripheral blood smear;
3. Bleeding time (BT), if a qualitative platelet disorder or vWD is suspected;
4. Activated partial thromboplastin time (aPTT);
5. Prothrombin time (PT).

In acquired bleeding disorders, such as disseminated intravascular coagulation (DIC), two more screening tests are required:

6. Fibrinogen level;
7. Fibrin split (degradation) products (FDP), or the D-dimer level (see later).

1. Platelet count is the number of platelets that can be estimated by simple inspection of the blood film under the microscope. The number of platelets counted under the high-power field is multiplied by $10,000/\mu L$. A more accurate platelet count is obtained by either automated counting (e.g., the Coulter counter) or manual-phase microscopy methods.

2. Blood smear examination of the blood film provides additional clues to the cause of an abnormal platelet count. Thus the finding of a low number of large platelets together with fragmented red blood cells or schistocyte (see Chapter 3) suggests increased platelet destruction as the cause of the low platelet count with release of young, large platelets of the bone marrow. The presence of myeloblasts and a low number of small platelets in the peripheral blood implies bone marrow invasion by leukemic cells, causing decreased platelet production.

Bleeding in a patient with a platelet problem may result from a either a low number of platelets (*thrombocythopenia*) ($<100,000/\mu L$) or normal platelet number with impaired platelet function, or qualitative platelet disorders.

3. Bleeding Time (BT) measures vascular integrity following platelet–blood vessel wall interactions. It is determined by a modified Ivy template method. After applying a blood pressure cuff to the upper arm and maintaining the pressure at 40 mmHg, an incision (1 mm by 9 mm) is made in the flexor surface forearm skin with the aid of a disposable template. The bleeding time represents the time taken for the bleeding to cease. The range of the normal BT is 3–8.5 minutes. The BT has been standardized for platelet counts above $100,000/\mu L$. Lower platelet counts are associated with progressive prolongations of the bleeding time. The BT is abnormal in primary vessel wall disorders (e.g., vascular purpuras), qualitative platelet disorders, and vWD.

4. Activated partial thromboplastin time on a (aPTT, Fig. 6-16) measures the intrinsic blood coagulation factors (XII, PK, HK, XI, IX, VIII) and the common pathway factors (X, V, II, and I). The test employs an activating agent (e.g., micronized silica or kaolin), a platelet membrane phospholipid substitute, calcium, and patient citrated plasma or normal plasma. When the activating agent is added to the plasma, it exposes the active serine center of factor XII leading to subsequent activation of both the intrinsic and the common pathway blood coagulation factors. The phospholipid (reagent) substitutes for platelet membrane phospholipid, which anchors the activated factors IX, X, V, and II to accelerate clot formation, in the presence of added calcium. The clot end point is recorded in seconds. The normal range for the aPTT is 25–38 seconds.

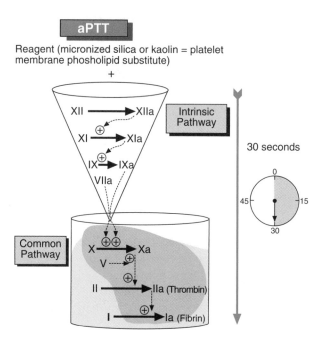

Figure 6-16. What the aPTT does. It measures intrinsic and common pathway integrity. If there is a problem with either one, the aPTT is prolonged.

The aPTT is prolonged in deficiencies of both the intrinsic blood coagulation factors (XII, PK, HK, XI, IX, and VIII) and the common pathway blood coagulation factors (X, V, II, and I).

5. *Prothrombin time* (PT) (Fig. 6-17) measures the extrinsic blood coagulation factor VII and the common pathway factors (X, V, II, and I). The PT assay is performed by adding the reagent tissue factor and calcium to the patient plasma. Tissue factor activates factor VII, which in turn activates the common pathway factors (factor X, factor V, Ca^{2+}, and factor II) leading to thrombin formation. Thrombin transforms fibrinogen into fibrin. The PT bypasses the intrinsic pathway blood coagulation factors. The normal range for the PT is 10–14 seconds.

The PT may be expressed as the international normalized ratio (INR). The INR is calculated as follows: INR = (Patient PT seconds/Normal mean plasma PT)^{ISI}; ISI = International Sensitivity Index, a value derived from calibrating the tissue factor reagent from animal sources against a human tissue factor standard. The INR result is used to monitor the effect of oral anticoagulants. It was recommended by the World Health Organization in an attempt to achieve accurate control of anticoagulant therapy and to improve interlaboratory correlation.

The PT is prolonged in patients with hereditary deficiency of factors VII, X, V, II, or I, or in acquired combined deficiencies of these blood coagulation factors (e.g., vitamin K deficiency or use of oral anticoagulants).

INTERPRETATION OF LABORATORY TESTS.

Prolonged aPTT. As a result of screening or preoperative coagulation testing, it may be discovered that the aPTT is prolonged. Platelet studies, PT, and BT should then be performed after careful history and physical examination are completed. The laboratory evaluation of a patient with a prolonged aPTT, normal platelet count, normal PT, and BT should follow the sequence of laboratory tests and interpretations depicted in Fig. 6-18 (see also Figs. 6-2, 6-16, and 6-17). Critical in this flowchart is the clinical determination of the patients hemorrhagic status. (Is the patient a bleeder or a nonbleeder?)

If the patient first comes to medical attention because of bleeding problems, then performance of platelet evaluation, aPTT, PT, BT must be done, after history and physical examination data are obtained.

A *bleeder* with a *prolonged aPTT* and normal platelet count, PT, and BT, requires that the aPTT be done in a plasma mixture (1 volume of normal plasma + 1 volume of patient plasma). This is called the 1:1 mix aPTT test. If the prolonged aPTT corrects with a 1:1 mix test, a deficiency of either factor VIII, IX, or XI is suspected, since less than 30–50% of normal level is all that is needed for a normal aPTT. In contrast, in the bleeding patient if the prolonged aPTT does not correct with a 1:1 mix test, an inhibitor is suspected. The inhibitors, which neutralize the activity of factors VIII or IX, are the most frequent, but an inhibitor against factor XI activity is also possible.

A *bleeder* with a *prolonged aPTT*, and a normal platelet count and *PT, but* a *prolonged BT* requires consideration of problems which affect the intrinsic pathway as well as qualitative platelet function (Fig. 6-19).

A *nonbleeder* with *prolonged aPTT*, normal platelet count, and correction of the aPTT with the 1:1 mix test has a deficiency in one of the contact phase blood coagulation factors (e.g., FXII, PK, or HK). In contrast, a nonbleeder with prolonged aPTT without correction in the 1:1 mix test most likely has a lupus—like inhibitor, which is associated with thrombosis, not bleeding complications (Fig. 6-18).

In the following clinical situations it will be useful to refer to Figs. 6-2, 6-16, and 6-17 to understand why certain factor deficiencies or factor inhibitors can be predicted by the clinical laboratory data provided.

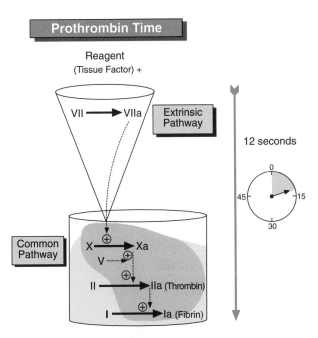

Figure 6-17. What the PT does. It measures extrinsic and common pathway integrity. If there is a problem with either one, the PT is prolonged.

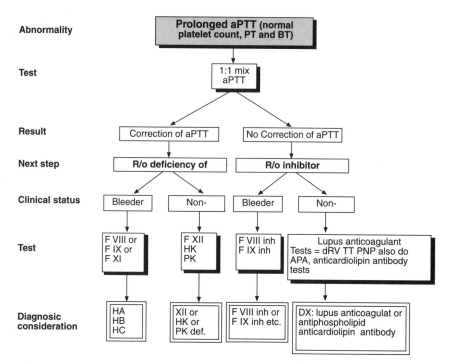

Figure 6-18. The evaluation of a prolonged aPTT is both a laboratory and clinical exercise. Repeating the aPTT and confirming that it is indeed prolonged is a necessary first step. A logical second step is learning if a prolonged aPPT does or does not correct with 1:1 mix. However, the hemorrhagic history and current bleeding status of the patient are of critical importance in guiding the pace and direction of the workup. See text for abbreviations.

Prolonged PT. A *bleeder* with a *prolonged PT* (normal aPTT, platelets, and BT) probably has factor VII deficiency.

Prolonged aPTT and Prolonged PT. A *bleeder* with *prolongation of both aPTT and PT* (normal platelets and BT) and correction with the 1:1 mix test may have one of the following conditions: (1) deficiency of FX, FV, FII, or FI (the common pathway factors); (2) vitamin K deficiency (reduction in all FX, FIX, FVII, and FII); (3) warfarin therapy effect (reduction of vitamin K–dependent factors, as discussed earlier); (4) liver disease (reduced synthesis of coagulation factors); (5) disseminated intravascular coagulation (see later); or (6) active fibrinolysis (secondary to therapy or to a pathologic process).

A *bleeder* with *prolongation of both aPTT* and *PT* (normal platelets and normal BT) but without correction in the 1:1 mix test has an inhibitor in one of the common pathway factors. Factor V inhibitor is the most frequent, but inhibitors to FX or FII are also possible.

A *nonbleeder* with prolongation of both *aPTT* and *PT* (normal platelets and normal BT) without correction in the 1:1 mix test usually has a lupus anticoagulant-like inhibitor.

No Routine Hemostatic Test Abnormalities. Patients with *a mild bleeding history* but *no abnormalities* on the *routine blood screening tests* (normal platelet count, BT, PT and aPTT) may have a FXIII deficiency or α_2-antiplasmin deficiency. Factor XIII de-

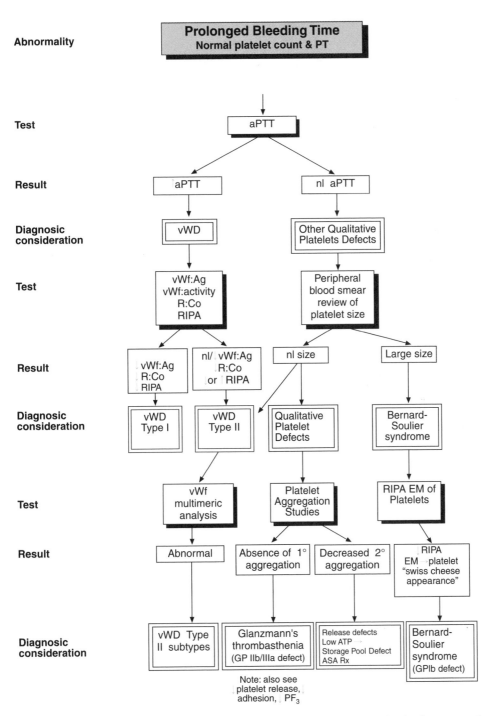

Figure 6-19. The evaluation of a prolonged bleeding time first demands that the platelet count and PT be assessed. If these are normal, then evaluation of aPTT is necessary. If confirmed as prolonged, correction with 1:1 mix may suggest factor deficiency, but the prolonged BT suggests a platelet and/or blood vessel wall abnormality as well. The bleeding status of the patient is important, but it must be emphasized that vWD may occur in those who have had no significant personal or family hemorrhagic problems. In the face of seemingly normal or inconsistently abnormal laboratory values, life-threatening bleeding may be unmasked at the time of trauma or severe hemostatic stress. See text for abbreviations.

ficiency can be demonstrated by a screening test, which measures the solubility of the fibrin clot in 5 M urea. Factor XIII cross-links fibrin clots (by covalent bonds), making the clot insoluble in urea. Absence of FXIII causes fibrin links (hold by hydrogen bonds), to dissolve in 5 M urea.

Special Tests for Blood Coagulation Factors. The special tests required to define the cause of the bleeding disorder after obtaining a detailed and complete history and physical examination include the following:

1. Specific coagulation factor assays;
2. Platelet function tests (platelet adhesion, aggregation, secretion, procoagulant activity);
3. vWf assays (quantity and function);
4. Inhibitor assays (e.g., lupus anticoagulant or specific factor VIII or IX inhibitor assays);
5. DIC screening tests (PT, aPTT, platelet count, fibrinogen level and FDP or D-Dimer assays);
6. Tests for pathologic fibrinolysis;
7. Specific tests of blood coagulation activation.

Specific Blood Coagulation Factor Assays. The *functional activity of blood coagulation factors* is measured in clinical laboratories by assays that employ a modification of the aPTT or PT methods. The modification consists of add to the reaction mixture a congenital plasma deficient in the coagulation factor in question. This plasma is called "substrate", and it contains normal quantities of all blood coagulation factors, except the one to be measured. The corrective effect of the patient plasma on the prolonged time of the deficient substrate plasma is compared with the corrective effect of known concentrations of the factor being tested in the normal plasma (e.g., factor VIII—100%, 75%, 50%, 25%, 10%, 5%, and 1%). The results are expressed in percent of normal pooled plasma activity; 1 mL of pooled normal plasma = 100% activity or 1 U/mL. Other assays to measure activity of blood coagulation factors employ chromogenic (colorimetric) substrates. The latter are susceptible to cleavage by the enzymatic action of the serine proteases of the blood coagulation factors; this allows the development of a titration curve and the measurement of the particular blood coagulation factor.

The *concentration of the blood coagulation proteins* is determined by various immunologic assays, such as enzyme-linked immunoabsorbent assay (ELISA), radioimmunoassay (RIA), or quantitative immunoelectrophoresis (Rocket electrophoresis or Laurell technique, QIE).

Platelet Function Tests. See Chapter 5 for a discussion of platelet function tests.

Tests for von Willebrand Disease. *vWf Activation.* The ristocetin cofactor (R:CO) is measured by a modification of a platelet aggregation testing. The assay employs ristocetin as the aggregating agent and lyophilized platelet membranes from normal individuals. The ristocetin binds to vWf; the latter interacts with GP-1b and GP-IIb/IIIa in the platelet membranes, inducing platelet-to-platelet interaction (platelet aggregation). The effect of the patient (vWf) plasma in the test system is compared to the effect of known concentrations of normal vWf. The results are expressed as percentage of normal plasma vWf activity (Fig. 6-20).

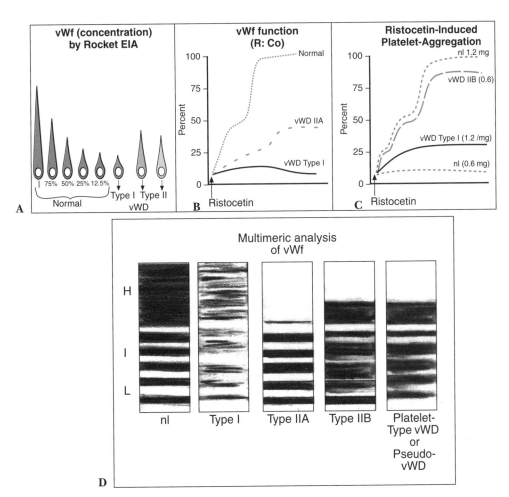

Figure 6-20. Depictions of vWf concentration by Rocket RIA (**A**), vWf function by R:CO assay (**B**), and RIPA (**C**) in normal and selected vWD patients. Multimeric analysis of vWf (**D**) (H = high, I = intermediate, L = low) displayed in normal and selected vWD patients. See text for abbreviations.

Ristocetin-induced platelet aggregation (*RIPA*) is another test to assess platelet response to normal and suboptimal concentrations of ristocetin. RIPA differs from R:CO in that RIPA the patient's *own* platelets are suspended in their *own* plasma as a source of vWf (in R:CO, normal lymphilized platelets are used). RIPA is used to separate variants of vWf disease (e.g., abnormal vWf protein such as type IIb) from classic type I vWD (decreased synthesis of vWf). Patients with vWD-type IIb respond fully to half-normal concentration of ristocetin (0.6 mg/mL), whereas platelets of normal subjects require 1.2 mg/mL of ristocetin to exhibit a similar response. The response of platelets to low concentrations of ristocetin is unique to type IIB-vWD (Fig. 6-20).

vWf concentration (vWf antigenic concentration, *vWf:Ag*) is measured by *QIE, ELISA, or RIA assays.* Figure 6-20 depicts the QIE assay. Briefly, agarose is combined with rabbit anti-vWf antibody and poured onto plastic slides. Wells are punched along one side of the slide to hold 10 mL of diluted plasma standard or patient samples. Electrophoresis is performed overnight. After washing and staining the slides, the height of each rocket formed by the precipitated antigen and antibody is determined. The height of the rockets are directly proportional to the concentration of vWf. The height of the patient sample (rocket) is read off the standard curve. This is an accurate, practical, and inexpensive clinical assay. ELISA and RIA (not illustrated) have the advantage of measuring large numbers of samples simultaneously, and can detect minute vWf concentrations. Multimeric analysis of vWf subunits by SDS-agarose gel electrophoresis is the method used to identify the various subtypes of vWD (type-II A-H), which result from an abnormal structure of the von Willebrand protein (Fig. 6-20).

Tests for Inhibitors. Inhibitors of specific blood coagulation factors (e.g., FVIII, FIX, and FV) are screened by mixing sequential dilutions of the patient's plasma with normal plasma and incubating the mixture at 37°C for 2 hours. At the end of this incubation period, the aPTT is repeated in the plasma mixtures. If no correction is obtained, levels of the specific factor in question (e.g., FVIII) are determined in each sample. The test sample producing a residual factor activity of 50% of normal is considered to have one Bethesda Unit (BU) of inhibitor per milliliter. The inhibitor titer equals the reciprocal of the dilution of test plasma that neutralizes 50% of normal plasma factor activity (e.g., FVIII). One Oxford inhibitor unit (United Kingdom) corresponds to 1.21 BU (United States).

Lupus anticoagulant (LA) prolongs both the aPTT and the PT; low titers only influence the aPTT. To demonstrate LA activity in plasma two clinical tests are used: the diluted Russel viper venom time (d RVVT) and the platelet neutralizing procedure (PNP). In the d RVVT, the RVV reagent activates FX directly. Sequential dilutions of RVV generate small amounts of activated FX, which allow weak levels of the LA inhibitor to express its activity against the prothrombinase complex (FXa + FVa + Ca^{2+} + platelet phospholipid) and prolong the clotting time.

The *platelet neutralizing procedure* (PNP) employs lyophilized normal platelet membranes and patient plasma. The LA inhibitor in plasma binds to the normal platelet-membrane Fc receptors. A repeated aPTT done in the supernatant of this mixture shows normalization of the clotting time. Characterization of the *LA inhibitor* can be assessed by immunologic techniques employing specific phospholipids (e.g., Sphingomyelin [SM], Phosphatidylethanolamine [PE], phosphatidylcholine [PC], phosphatidylinositol [PI], and cardiolipin [CL]); the LA inhibitor reacts with SM, PI, CL, and PE and is identified. The use of altered configuration of phospholipids such as *hexagonal phase PE* is another alternative method to confirm the presence of LA inhibitor in plasma.

Anticardiolipin antibodies (ACA) are measured by ELISA assays employing cardiolipin and anti-human immunoglobulin antibodies (IgG and IgM) directed against cardiolipin. Like the lupus coagulation, they may be associated with hypercoagulability.

DIC Screening Tests. See "Tests of Fibrinolysis" below and Table 6-13.

Tests of Fibrinolysis. Screening tests that measure increased fibrinolytic activity in plasma include the following:

1. Shorter whole-blood clotting time, or shorter plasma euglobulin lysis time, than normal;
2. Increased lysis of fibrin plate assays or radioactive fibrin clot;
3. Low plasminogen levels by immunologic techniques;

4. Elevated fibrin(ogen) degradation products (FDP) measured in serum by a variety of immunologic techniques;
5. Elevated plasma levels of D-dimer, which are also indicative of increased fibrinolysis and blood activation.

The *FDP assay* employs polyclonal antibodies raised against plasmic products of fibrin(ogen) to detect fibrinolysis in serum by a simple latex-bead method. This screening test measures fibrinolysis, but it does not distinguish fibrinogen from fibrin derivatives. In contrast, the D-dimer assay detects plasmic-fibrin digests specifically. (Plasmic fibrinogen digests do not yield D-dimer since cross-linked fibrin is required for D-dimer to be released.)

The *D-dimer assay* employs monoclonal antibodies raised against the smallest degradation product (D-dimer) derived from plasmin-lysis of cross-linked fibrin (but not fibrinogen). The levels of D-dimer are measured in plasma by either a latex-bead assay or ELISA. (The latter is more sensitive.) The advantages of the D-dimer over the FDP assay include the detection of the D-dimer in plasma and the measurement of a specific plasmin-fibrin product. The latter implies that blood activation occurred *in vivo*, generating both thrombin and plasmin, which are, respectively, responsible for the cross-linking of fibrin and its degradation into the D-dimer product.

Specific Tests of Blood Coagulation Activation. Tests to assess blood activation *in vivo* are still considered research tools and are not readily available in most clinical laboratories. These tests include (1) fibrinopeptide A and B by RIA; (2) prothrombin fragment 1.2 by ELISA; (3) complex of AT III with thrombin by immunologic and chromogenic assays; (4) protein C–activated peptide, APC–PC inhibitor complex, APC-α_1-antitrypsin complex, APC–α_2-macroglobulin complex, which are measured by ELISA or other immunologic assays; (5) factor IX activation peptide or IXa–AT III complexes, also assessed by immunologic assays; and (6) factor X activation peptide by either RIA or ELISA.

INHERITED BLOOD COAGULATION DISORDERS

Hereditary deficiencies of each of the blood coagulation factors have been reported. Inherited deficiency of a blood coagulation factor is associated with clinical bleeding, except for deficiency of either factor XII, prekallikrein, or high-molecular-weight kininogen (HK).

The three most common hereditary coagulation disorders are factor VIII deficiency (hemophilia A), factor IX deficiency (hemophilia B), and abnormalities associated with von Willebrand factor (von Willebrand disease [vWD]). The mode of inheritance of the blood coagulation factors is shown in Table 6-3.

Hemophilia A

Hemophilia A (HA) is the most common of the hemophilias (80–85% of all cases). In the United States, the incidence of HA is estimated to be 25 per 100,000 males; however, estimates of HA of $30–100/10^6$ of the world population have been proposed. The defect in hemophilia A is absence or reduction in plasma factor VIII coagulant activity (VIII:C), but usually not absence of the factor VIII molecule.

Factor VIII circulates in plasma bound to vWf, which stabilizes its activity and

TABLE 6-3. *MODE OF INHERITANCE OF THE BLOOD COAGULATION FACTORS*

BLOOD COAGULATION FACTORS	MODE OF INHERITANCE
FVIII and FIX	X-linked
vWf* and dysfibrinogenemias	Autosomal dominant
All other factor deficiencies	Autosomal recessive

* Rare vWD variants appear to be autosomal recessive.

regulates its synthesis (Fig. 6-21). Studies of the factor VIII gene (X chromosome) have shown many deletions and point mutations in the affected kindred.

Inheritance and Carrier State Detection. Hemophilia is inherited as an X-linked defect; sons of a hemophiliac female carrier have a 50% chance of inheriting the gene (Fig. 6-22). It is a bleeding disorder of males. All sons of hemophiliac patients are normal, whereas all daughters are obligatory carriers of the trait. Since the defect is located on the X chromosome, males have no normal allele (X^hY) and manifest the clinical bleeding disorder. In contrast, female carriers (X^hX), who inherit a normal allele from the mother, usually do not exhibit a bleeding tendency. Factor VIII coagulant activity in carriers should be 50% of normal; however, this is not always the case, because of the wide range of factor VIII:C (50–200%) in the population, and the rise of FVIII level after exercise, with pregnancy, stress, and various other clinical conditions. FVIII:C level alone detects carrier state in only 60%. Adding the measurement of factor VIII antigen (VIII:Ag) to the level of FVIII:C and finding a 2:1 ratio (FVIII:Ag to FVIII:C) have improved the detection of the carrier state from 60% to 90%. Carrier state and prenatal diagnosis have become even more accurate by analysis of factor VIII gene. Two methods used are restriction fragment length polymorphism (RFLP) and reverse transcriptase–polymerase chain reaction (RT–PCR). Each method requires small samples of blood or of chorionic villi

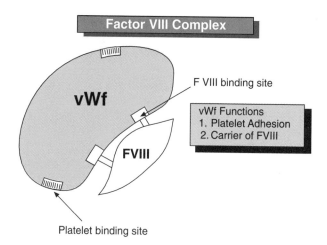

Figure 6-21. Von Willebrand factor acts as a bridge between platelet and blood vessel wall and carries and transports FVIII.

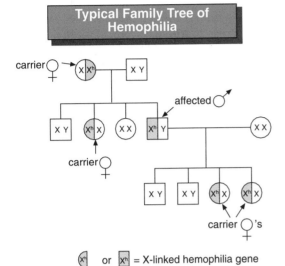

Figure 6-22. The X-linked transmission of the hemophilia gene shown in a typical pedigree.

biopsy, permitting prenatal diagnosis of hemophilia at very early stages of pregnancy (8–12 weeks).

Hemophilia A is rare in a female, but it can occur in the offspring of a hemophiliac male and a hemophiliac carrier. Other, even less frequent possibilities are extreme Lyonization of the normal X chromosome in a heterozygous female (carrier) or a genetic defect for hemophilia in a female with only one X chromosome, as occurs in Turner's syndrome.

Clinical Severity and Bleeding Manifestations. The severity of bleeding in hemophilia (A or B) can be predicted by the plasma levels of FVIII or FIX procoagulant activity (FVIII:C, FIX:C; Table 6-4).

Patients with levels below 1% have spontaneous and severe bleeding complications starting in early childhood (e.g., as a result of circumcision). The bleeding characteristically affects joints (hemarthrosis) and muscles (hematomas) and may lead to handicap unless the patient receives immediate and adequate treatment. Moderately affected patients (FVIII:C or FIX:C levels of 1–5% of normal) bleed after trauma or surgery, and may develop spontaneous bleeding. Patients with mild

TABLE 6-4. *LABORATORY CHARACTERISTICS AND CLINICAL MANIFESTATIONS OF HEMOPHILIAS*

LABORATORY DEFECTS (%)	CLINICAL MANIFESTATIONS	BLEEDING SYMPTOMS
<1	Severe	Early childhood, spontaneous
1–5	Moderate	After minor trauma or surgery May be spontaneous
5–20	Mild	Only after trauma or surgery

hemophilia (FVIII:C or FIX:C levels 5–20%) bleed only after trauma or surgery. Excessive bleeding after dental extractions is common to all hemophiliac patients. Hematuria and gastrointestinal bleeding are also frequent, specifically if the patient has a local lesion (e.g., an ulcer, polyp, or an inflammatory process).

Posttraumatic and surgical bleeding are life-threatening in all types of hemophilia, including the mild forms. Posttraumatic bleeding leads to the formation of large hematomas that can produce pressure on nerves or cause severe vascular occlusion and gangrene. Trivial injury to the mouth or tongue in hemophilia can cause oropharyngeal bleeding, one of the most dangerous types of bleeding, leading to severe respiratory obstruction and death by asphyxia. Minor trauma to the head, in any type of hemophilia, is considered life-threatening and needs to be treated promptly. Spontaneous intracranial bleeding is not common in hemophilia, but when it occurs in patients with severe hemophilia, it is an important cause of death.

Pseudotumors of the long bones, pelvis, and fingers result from recurrent subperiosteal hemorrhages; the latter lead to bone destruction, new bone formation, and tendency to pathologic fractures.

Laboratory Diagnosis. The following laboratory tests should be used for diagnosis:

Prolonged aPTT, normal PT, and normal bleeding time;
aPTT 1:1 mix tests = correction at both zero time and at 37°C after 2 hours incubation (this indicates FVIII deficiency, not FVIII inhibitor);
Factor VIII:C activity: reduced or absent;
Factor VIII:Ag concentration level: normal or reduced.

Therapy. The general principles of therapy include replacement with factor VIII concentrates or administration of desmopressin (DDAVP), and social and psychological support. The majority of patients receive their medical care from groups of specialized health care professionals (hemophilia centers), which provide care to the patient and family members. Parents are advised to bring up children with hemophilia as normally as possible. However, avoidance of injury begins during early childhood (e.g., padding of cribs, elimination of sharp toys). Later, the child is encouraged to participate in noncontact sports. Regular, preventive dentistry is also required. At minimal signs of bleeding the family and/or the patient (self-therapy) are trained to provide supportive therapy.

Such therapy includes local measures, as well as immediate infusion of FVIII concentrate, which is kept in the patient's refrigerator. Implementation of these measures has diminished the occurrence of crippling hemarthrosis and reduced the rate of hospital admissions. Patients with mild hemophilia can use nasal or infused desmopressin (1-desamino-8D-arginine vasopressin [DDAVP]) immediately after trauma or hemorrhage.

Therapy for spontaneous bleeding requires infusion of factor VIII concentrates to raise the factor VIII:C level in plasma to 30% of normal. Although the factor VIII:C level should be raised to 100% in preparation for major surgery, to stop posttraumatic bleeding, or to arrest hemorrhage in a dangerous site. This dose of FVIII concentrate, called the *loading dose*, is followed by a maintenance dose (half of the loading dose), every 12 hours until healing has occurred (7–10 days). Adjustments of the maintenance dose require frequent FVIII:C plasma level determinations, at least every other day, to achieve adequate therapy.

The amount of factor to be replaced is calculated as follows:

Loading dose (units of FVIII) = desired FVIII level × weight (kg);

Maintenance dose = half of the loading dose. (The dosage of FIX to be infused is calculated similarly, but the frequency of treatment is once daily, since the biological half-life of FIX [about 24 hours] is longer than that of FVIII [8–12 hours].)

Other therapeutic principles in the hemophilias include the following:

1. To minimize the development of chronic synovitis or progressive arthropathy, treatment of acute hemarthrosis must include replacement immediate and intensive therapy.
2. Treatment of chronic arthropathy should include physical therapy, wedging casts, night splints, or traction in conjunction with regular infusions of factor concentrates;
3. Treatment of chronic synovitis requires intense replacement therapy, physical therapy, and, in severe cases, surgical synovectomy.
4. Treatment of severe arthropathy can include analgesics and surgical joint replacement;
5. In addition to preventive dentistry, FVIII or FIX concentrates must be infused before dental surgery. The use of antifibrinolytic agents, such as epsilon amino caporic acid (EACA) or transexamic acid, reduces the amount of the factor concentrate to be infused as well as the frequency of infusion. Most patients will require only one infusion prior to surgery. Occasionally, in some patients a repeated infusion after surgery is necessary.

A new therapeutic approach to cure the hemophilias, gene therapy, is under investigation. Genes have been transfected into human fibroblasts, and the cells have been transplanted into mice. The mice have produced human blood coagulation factors!

Complications of Therapy. Ten to 20% of patients with hemophilia produce antibodies (inhibitors) directed against the factor VIII infused. This complication is associated with severe bleeding, and it is difficult to manage. In 70% patients with FVIII inhibitor, the titer of the inhibitor rises upon exposure to the factor VIII infused and falls at a variable rate after infusion. These patients are nonresponders to human factor VIII concentrate therapy; they require other therapeutic modalities to control hemorrhage. In the other 30% of patients the FVIII inhibitor level remains in circulation unchanged or rises minimally post FVIII infusion. They are responders to therapy with high doses of human FVIII concentrate.

Patients with low FVIII inhibitor level (<5 BU) are treated with porcine FVIII in enough quantity to raise the factor VIII:C level in plasma to 30–50 U/dL.

Patients with intermediate FVIII inhibitor level (5–30% BU) receive human factor IX infusions containing activated factor X (to bypass the FVIII) as first-choice therapy; this is followed by infusion of either porcine FVIII or a very high dose of human FVIII concentrate. If these therapeutic measures are insufficient to stop the bleeding, then aggressive plasmapheresis or one of the several methods of extracorporeal immunoadsorption is tried.

Patients with high FVIII inhibitor level (more than 30 BU) are first treated with plasmapheresis, followed by porcine or human FVIII infusions. Patients refractory to these therapeutic modalities may respond to infusions of highly purified concentrate containing activated FVII.

Rapid reduction of antibody titers can be achieved by immunoglobulin therapy. This product contains a high concentration of anti-idiotype antibodies, which neutralize the inhibitory activity. Immunosuppressive agents aimed at reducing antibody production, when used in conjunction with infusions of human FVIII concentrate, have also been effective. The use of these agents is discouraged in young patients because of their potential carcinogenic and leukemogenic side effects. Therapy with recombinant FVIII preparations or highly purified FVIII concentrates is also in current use.

In nonhemophiliac patients antibodies to FVIII may be associated with certain illnesses, pregnancy, and some medications. They may also arise spontaneously in the elderly. (See the following discussion and Table 6-10.)

Besides development of inhibitors, patients may suffer from other problems. Complications of multiple transfusions of concentrates of FVIII or FIX, or other blood products in hemophiliacs also include contraction of infections, such as hepatitis B and C, HIV (human immunodeficiency virus), or cytomegalovirus (CMV). Acquired immunodeficiency syndrome (AIDS) is now the leading cause of death in severe hemophilia. To prevent viral contamination, donor testing has been made more accurate, and procedures of viral inactivation of blood products are in routine use. In addition, recombinant human FVIII, free of viral contamination, is also currently available.

Another complication seen in these patients includes drug addiction resulting from the frequent use of pain medication. In addition, many social and psychological problems afflict both the patient and family members, which result from this life-long, expensive therapy ($15,000 to $90,000/year), and crippling illness.

Hemophilia B

Hemophilia B (Christmas disease) is caused by a deficiency in factor IX, the result of a X-linked mutation/deletion in the FIX gene. Hemophilia B causes bleeding manifestations as described earlier for hemophilia A (e.g., hemarthrosis and hematomas), but its incidence is much lower than that of FVIII deficiency (1/5).

Patients with hemophilia B may synthesize a nonfunctional FIX or have a true absence of synthesis of the factor IX molecule.

Laboratory Diagnosis. The following tests are used for diagnosis:

The aPTT is prolonged, but the PT and BT are both normal.
aPTT (1:1 mix) = correction at zero time and at 37°C after 2 hours of incubation. (This indicates FIX deficiency, not FIX inhibitor.)
FIX:C activity: reduced or absent.
FIX:Ag concentration: reduced or absent.

Carrier detection and antenatal diagnosis can be done by measuring plasma levels of both FIX:Ag and FIX:C. Carrier state or antenatal diagnosis of FIX deficiency, however, is more accurate by gene analysis in blood samples, or in antenatal chorionic biopsy samples using DNA probes and RT-PCR techniques.

Therapy. The principles of FIX replacement therapy are similar to those described for hemophilia A. Factor IX concentrates are used to treat severe bleeding episodes. Fresh-frozen plasma is still used to treat minor bleeding.

Complications of factor IX concentrate therapy include thrombosis (e.g., deep vein thrombosis, pulmonary embolism, disseminated intravascular coagulation) and viral infections (all as described for FVIII therapy). Concomitant use of heparin to prevent thrombosis is recommended, especially in patients undergoing major surgery. Ethanol precipitation, immunoaffinity purification of FIX concentrates, and recombinant FIX products, now available, have minimized the infectious risks. Gene therapy, to cure FIX deficiency, is at early stage of investigation.

Von Willebrand Disease

Von Willebrand disease (vWD) is a heterogenous group of inherited (more than 20 subtypes) and acquired disorders of the von Willebrand factor (vWf). Both types of vWD are manifested clinically by bleeding into the skin and mucous membranes. vWD results from an abnormality in the quantity or quality of the vWf.

vWf Biosynthesis. vWD is produced by endothelial cells and megakaryocytes, where it is stored in organelles. In ECs the vWf is stored within the Weibel-Palade bodies, and in platelets, in the α-granules. Most of our understanding of vWf synthesis is derived from studies of vWf in ECs in culture. In ECs, vWf synthesis is initiated in the endoplasmic reticulum, as a pre–pro-vWf molecule, which is disulfide-bonded at the C-terminus, resulting in a pro-vWf C-terminal-linked dimer. The dimer undergoes glycosylation and processing during transport via the Golgi apparatus. During formation of the Weibel-Palade body secretory granule, the pro-vWf dimer undergoes two important steps: N-terminal disulfide bonding, followed by high-molecular-weight multimerization (of vWf), and cleavage of the propolypeptide (vWf:Ag II). The processing of pro-vWf into the mature vWf form is achieved by the action of a paired amino acid cleavage enzyme (PACE), or furin, which cleaves the vWf:Ag II from the mature vWf form. Both forms, the high-molecular-weight multimerized form (vWf) and the cleaved propolypeptide (vWf:Ag II), are stored in the Weibel-Palade body secretory granule. Upon stimulation, both ECs and platelets release vWf and vWf:Ag II. The function of vWf:Ag II *in vivo* is unknown.

Structure and Function of Normal vWf. The vWf (mature form) has two major functions in plasma: (1) *Platelet adhesion* to the collagen exposed in the vessel wall is bridged by vWf, which binds to glycoprotein Ib and IIb/IIIa (GIb, GPIIb/IIIa) on the platelet membrane and to discrete ligands on the collagen. (2) vWf stabilizes the FVIII molecule by prolonging its half-life and transporting it to the sites of active hemostatic plug formation (see Fig. 6-21).

vWf has a high molecular weight (about 16 million), but its binding functions are localized to discrete domains (Fig. 6-23). The domain for FVIII binding is located at the N-terminus of the mature vWf, at the 272-amino-acid residue; the binding sites for GPIb, heparin, and collagen are located at amino acids 449–728, with an additional collagen binding domain residing at amino acids 911–1114. The binding domain for GPIIb/IIIa in the vWf is located at amino acids 1744–1747.

The vWf Gene. The authentic vWf gene (178 kb) is located on chromosome 12, and a pseudogene (98% homology with vWf gene) is present on chromosome 22. There is conclusive evidence that the pseudogene is not functional in humans. The complete exon/intron structure of the vWf has been established, and it has provided better diagnostic tools to define the molecular defects of some subtypes of

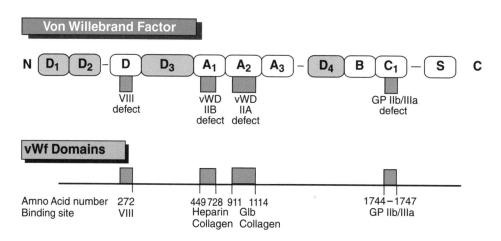

Figure 6-23. Depiction of amino acid numbers and binding sites for a variety of vWf functions and

vWD, but not of type I vWD. Many of the molecular mutations in the subtypes of vWD (e.g., types IIA and IIB) have been located within exon 28. The latter encodes (A1 and A2 repeats) the region of the vWf which interacts with platelet GPIb (domain A2) and the portion of the vWf containing the N-terminal multimerization site(s) (Fig. 6-23).

The genetic alterations of the vWf gene reported include deletions, insertions, point mutations, alternative splice junctions, and premature transcription termination sites.

Mode of Inheritance. vWD is the most common of the inherited bleeding diathesis, with a prevalence in the general population estimated at 1%. Since its first description by Eric von Willebrand (1926) in patients from the Åland Islands, Finland, vWD has been recognized to be inherited as an autosomal dominant trait; thus both males and females have a similar prevalence (Fig. 6-24). Many studies have confirmed the autosomal dominant pattern; however, some variants of vWD (or type III and some cases of type IIC) appear to be inherited as autosomal recessive traits.

Clinical Manifestations. Patients with vWD have symptoms of mucocutaneous bleeding. They present with epistaxis, ecchymosis, menorrhagia, postpartum hemorrhage, gastrointestinal bleeding, hematuria, and history of excessive bleeding after minor trauma or surgery (e.g., tonsillectomy or dental extractions).

Studies of large kindred of vWD have demonstrated that severe bleeding symptoms occur in 65% of the phenotypically abnormal (with laboratory abnormalities) vWD patients and in 25% of the phenotypically normal (without laboratory abnormalities) patients. Thus history alone, or in combination with laboratory tests, is inappropriate to screen family members of patients with vWD. Problems with vWD laboratory detection are compounded by vWf being an acute-phase reactant protein. Its level increases in plasma during stress, exercise, and pregnancy; with use of oral contraceptives; or after surgery. In these situations the laboratory diagnosis of vWf is inaccurate, if not impossible, to make. Genetic markers of allele inheritance are needed in such cases.

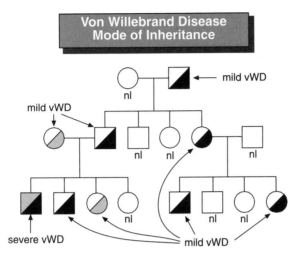

Figure 6-24. The typical autosomal dominant inheritance pattern seen in most forms of vWD.

Laboratory Diagnosis.

Von Willebrand Disease (Type I). Screening tests include the following:
Prolonged BT and aPTT;
Normal platelet count and PT (Fig. 6-19).

Tests for vWf (von Willebrand factor):
vWf:Ag (von Willebrand factor antigen), reduced;
R:CO (ristocetin cofactor), reduced;
RIPA (ristocetin-induced platelet aggregation), reduced.
See Fig. 6-20A and tests for vWd).

von Willebrand Disease (Type II). Screening tests include the following:
Prolonged BT and aPTT;
Normal platelet count and PT.

Tests for vWf:
vWf:Ag is ± reduced, or reduced;
R: CO is either markedly reduced, or ± reduced;
RIPA is markedly reduced, or normal;
RIPA (one-half normal concentration) is increased in vWD-IIB but absent in other type II variants;
Confirmation test: Abnormal multimeric analysis of vWf (Fig. 6-20D).

Classification of vWD. vWD classification is based on the plasma vWf concentration (vWf:Ag), vWf activity (R:CO), and multimeric structure of the vWf. vWf is the carrier protein for FVIII:C. Thus the levels of FVIII are also reduced, explaining the aPTT prolongation. Although this classification has been very useful, there are cases in which the diagnosis of vWD is difficult, because of the wide range of vWf levels in the general population (e.g., lower vWf levels in blood Group O than in A, B, or AB), and the rise in vWf after exercise, during pregnancy, with the use of oral contraceptives, after stress, and after surgery or trauma. During pregnancy, patients with severe vWD normalize the vWf levels, followed by a brisk fall in the postpartum period, which may be associated with severe hemorrhage. Thus the diagnosis of vWD during pregnancy cannot be made by measurements of vWf quantity and function, but only by genetic markers.

The numerous vWD variants can be separated into two major classes: (1) defects of vWf quantity (types I and III), due to reduced synthesis, and (2) defects of vWf quality (types IIA-H, type IIB, type IIM, type IIN), due to abnormal structure of vWf. (Type vWD is also called classic vWD.)

Description of selected subtypes follows (Tables 6-5 and 6-6, and Fig. 6-20).

The platelet-type vWD or pseudo-vWD can be distinguished from vWD type IIB by mixing studies with normal platelets and plasma. The defect is a missense mutation within GPIb on the platelet membrane; this causes an increase binding of vWf high-molecular-weight multimers to the platelet membrane, and loss of multimers from the plasma.

vWD variants types IIC–IIH are now classified under type IIA. vWD type IIC is the only type II variant of vWD that may be inherited as an autosomal recessive trait. The molecular basis of these vWf defects is unclear.

In vWD type IIM, the defect is in the GPIb binding loop of vWf, resulting in decreased affinity of vWf for platelets. Type IIM differs from type IIA by the presence of vWf high-molecular-weight multimers in plasma.

vWD type IIN (vWD Normandy variant) results from a defect in the binding of FVIII to the vWf. Diagnosis is made by the finding of a FVIII:C level disproportionately lower than the vWf level, and assays that measure the ability of FVIII to bind to vWf. The molecular basis is a missense mutation within the N-terminus of the mature vWf, where the vWf binds to FVIII.

Therapy. Treatment is determined by the severity of bleeding and the subtype of vWD. Therapeutic choices include desmopressin (DDAVP), recombinant vWf concentrate, cryoprecipitate, and conjugated estrogens.

DDAVP raises vWf levels in plasma by promoting its release from Weibel-Palade bodies in endothelial cells. This medication can be given as intranasal spray and as intravenous or subcutaneous injection. Individual responses vary, and the response diminishes after several doses as a result of depletion of the storage pools. Thus it is recommended that a trial dose of DDAVP be given prior to surgery to determine its efficacy. DDAVP is most effective in vWD type I, because patients pro-

TABLE 6-5. *von WILLEBRAND DISEASE VARIANTS*

SUBTYPES	vWf:Ag	R:CO	RIPA	RIPA (1/2)	MULTIMERS
Type I	↓ (20–50%)	↓ (20–50%)	↓	Absent	Normal bands
Type IIA	↓ (variable)	↓↓↓	↓	Absent	Absent high and intermediate ↓ satellite
Type IIB	± ↓	± ↓	Normal	Increased	Loss of large bands
Type III	Absent	Absent	Absent	Absent	↓↓↓↓ or undetected bands
Plt-vWD	± ↓	± ↓	Normal	Increased	Loss of large bands

vWf: Ag = von Willebrand's factor antigenic concentration; R: Co = Ristocetin cofactor (vWf function); RIPA = ristocetin-induced platelet aggregation; RIPA (1/2) = one-half normal concentration (0.6 mg/mL); Plt-vWD = "platelet-type vWD" or "pseudo-vWD."

TABLE 6-6. *CLINICAL FEATURES AND THERAPY OF vWD VARIANTS*

SUBTYPES	FREQUENCY (% OF vWD)	MODE OF INHERITANCE	SEVERITY	GENE DEFECT	THERAPY
Type I	70–80	autosomal dominant	Mild to moderate	Unknown	DDAVP, estrogens, vWf concentrate, cryoprecipitate
Type IIA	10–12	autosomal dominant	Mild to moderate	Missence-A2 vWf domain	vWf concentrate, cryoprecipitate
Type IIB	3–5	autosomal dominant	Mild to moderate	Missence-A1 vWf domain	vWf concentrate
Type III	1–3	autosomal recessive	Severe	Deletions; mutations; mRNA expression	vWf concentrate, cryoprecipitate
Plt-vWD (platelet type)	0–1	autosomal dominant	Mild-moderate	Missence mutation GPIb	Platelets

duce a reduced but structurally normal vWf protein. DDAVP therapy is not recommended in vWD type II variants, because these patients synthesize an abnormal vWf, which fails to support platelet adhesion. DDAVP therapy can be dangerous in vWD type II patients, because DDAVP causes the release of abnormal vWf multimers, which aggregate platelets and may lead to thrombocytopenia. vWD type III patients also do not benefit from DDAVP therapy, since they have no effective vWf storage; they require vWf replacement. The side effects of DDAVP are rare and include flushing, headache, hypertension, and fluid retention.

Estrogens are used to control minor bleeding complications in type I vWD. These agents appear to increase the synthesis of vWf.

The major mode of therapy in vWD is replacement with vWf. Two products are available: cryoprecipitate and vWf concentrate. Cryoprecipitate has the disadvantage of transmitting viral infections and is now replaced by vWf concentrate. vWf concentrate has a full spectrum of vWf multimers, and minimal risk of transmitting viral diseases. FVIII concentrates do not contain intact vWF and should not be used in the treatment of vWD patients.

Duration and intensity of vWD therapy are not as well established as they are in hemophilia. In preparation for major surgery, the vWf level should be raised to 80%, maintained at 40% for 3 days postoperatively, and kept at approximately 30% for another 5 days. One unit per killigram of vWf concentrate increases the plasma level by 2 U/dL. Rarely, patients with vWD develop inhibitors. When they do, severe bleeding occurs, and the patient is treated with plasma exchange, extracorporeal absorption columns, or infusions of gamma globulin.

During pregnancy, vWD type I patients have no bleeding complications because the vWf level rises. At delivery vWf level falls rapidly, and the patient needs to be treated with either DDAVP or vWf concentrate. Women with vWD type III and severe vWD types IIA and IIB can have bleeding complications during pregnancy and bleed excessively at partum and postpartum; they require treatment with vWf concentrate.

Acquired von Willebrand Disease. Acquired vWD may result from decreased synthesis of the vWf, a secondary vWf abnormality, or an autoantibody that either interferes with the vWf function or complexes with it, promoting its rapid clearance. The conditions associated with the development of vWD are shown in Table 6-7. Therapy consists of controlling the underlying disease and using vWf concentrate infusions. Removal of the tumor or chemotherapy should be attempted for patients with malignancies. Patients with autoimmune disorders are treated with steroids, immunosuppressive agents, and infusion of gamma globulin, which sometimes are enough to arrest the bleeding. If bleeding persists, then vWf concentrate should be used.

Factor XI Deficiency

Factor XI deficiency is inherited as an autosomal recessive trait and occurs predominantly among Ashkenazi Jews. Bleeding manifestations are usually mild in heterozygous states; homozygous patients for FXI deficiency may have just minor bleeding complications; however, after trauma or surgery they bleed severely (e.g., hemarthrosis and hematomas).

Laboratory Diagnosis. Screening tests include the following:

Prolonged aPTT; normal PT, platelet count and BT;
aPTT 1:1 mix tests = correction to normal; factor deficiency;
FXI:C and FXI:Ag levels: reduced or absent.

Treatment. Replacement of FXI by infusions of fresh-frozen plasma, or recombinant FXI preparation. Prophylaxis prior to dental extractions can be done with ϵ-aminocaproic acid (EACA) or tranexamic acid as described for patients with hemophilia.

Hereditary Deficiencies of Other Coagulation Factors

Hereditary deficiencies of other coagulation factors are all rare, occurring in less than 1 in 1 million members of the population. Most are inherited as autosomal recessive traits. Deficiencies of FXII, PK, and HK are not associated with bleeding, but all other factor deficiencies are. The targeting of specific problem factors is confirmed by demonstrating reductions in their functional activities in plasma as evidenced by aPTT/PT prolongation or reduction in their plasma levels.

TABLE 6-7. *ACQUIRED von WILLEBRAND DISEASE: ASSOCIATED PATHOLOGICAL CONDITIONS*

Hypothyroidism	Mitral valve prolapse
Wilms' tumor	Angiodysplasia
Autoimmune disorders (e.g., systemic lupus erythematosus)	Hereditary telangiectasia
Lymphoproliferative disorders	Adult respiratory distress syndrome
Myeloproliferative disorders	
Multiple myeloma	Pulmonary hypertension
Adenocarcinoma	

Laboratory Diagnosis.

Factor XII, PK, HK Deficiency. Screening tests include the following:

Prolonged aPTT; normal PT and platelet count;
aPTT 1:1 mix tests = Correction of aPTT, factor deficiency;
FXII or PK or HK levels: Reduced or absent.

Factor VII Deficiency. Screening tests include the following:
Prolonged PT; normal aPTT and platelet count;
Factor VII level: Reduced or absent.

Factor V, X, II, I Deficiency. Screening tests include the following:
Prolonged aPTT and PT; normal platelets;
aPTT and PT 1:1 mix tests = Correction of both APTT and PT;
Factors V, X, II & I levels: Reduced or absent.

Fibrinogen Abnormalities. Afibrinogenemia is the most severe quantitative form of fibrinogen abnormality and causes bleeding. Hypofibrinogenemias are usually asymptomatic. Dysfibrinogenemias prolong the aPTT and PT, and show a normal fibrinogen concentration with reduced functional activity. Some of the mutations associated with dysfibrinogenemias lead to bleeding and others to thrombosis or spontaneous abortions. Most defects are autosomal dominant traits.

Factor XIII Deficiency. Factor XIII deficiency (rare, autosomal recessive trait) is manifested by severe bleeding, hemarthrosis, hematomas, poor wound healing, and spontaneous abortions. The screening tests for bleeding (PT, aPTT, platelet count, BT, and fibrinogen) are all normal. Increased solubility of the clot in 5 M urea or 1% monochloroacetic acid is suggestive of XIII deficiency, which is confirmed by FXIII:Ag and FXIII:C levels.

Therapy for all the preceding factor deficiencies associated with bleeding consists in replacement with fresh-frozen plasma (FFP).

ACQUIRED BLOOD COAGULATION FACTOR DISORDERS

The acquired blood coagulation disorders are much more common than the inherited disorders and are usually associated with multiple coagulation factor deficiencies. There are a number of mechanisms by which blood coagulation deficiencies may arise. They are shown in Table 6-8.

Vitamin K Deficiency

Vitamin K is obtained from food (e.g., green vegetables) and from bacterial synthesis in the gut. It is a fat-soluble vitamin that depends on pancreatic lipases, bile, and absorptive ability of the intestine to enter the circulation and be utilized by the hepatocytes. Vitamin K deficiency results from inappropriate diet, pancreatic disorders, biliary obstruction, malabsorption, antibiotic therapy, or use of oral anticoagulants.

Vitamin K is required in the final synthetic steps of factors X, IX, VII, and II; PC; and PS for proper expression of their biologic activities. Vitamin K oxidation to its epoxide form is essential for γ-carboxylation of glutamic acid residues on these vitamin K–dependent proteins. This posttranslational process involves carboxylation of the γ-carbon of several glutamic acid residues in the N-terminus of the proteins. The γ-carboxylated glutamic acid then binds calcium and through it attaches

TABLE 6-8. *ACQUIRED DISORDERS OF BLOOD COAGULATION*
Vitamin K deficiency
Malabsorption of vitamin K (e.g., celiac disease, sprue)
Biliary obstruction
Vitamin K antagonist therapy (e.g., coumarins)
Antibiotic therapy
Hemorrhagic disease of the newborn
Acquired FX deficiency
Liver disease
Massive transfusion syndrome
Acquired inhibitors of blood coagulation
Disseminated intravascular coagulation (DIC)
Fibrinolytic states

to phospholipid receptors on cell membranes (e.g., platelets, ECs); this allows activation of blood coagulation to proceed. During carboxylation, vitamin K is oxidized to epoxide and recycled to its active form by reductases (Fig. 6-25). Oral anticoagulants (e.g., coumarins) inhibit vitamin K epoxide reduction, preventing efficient recycling of the vitamin K to its active enzyme form and limiting the action of the carboxylase. Patients on coumarins produce inactive vitamin K–dependent factors and have hypocoagulable blood.

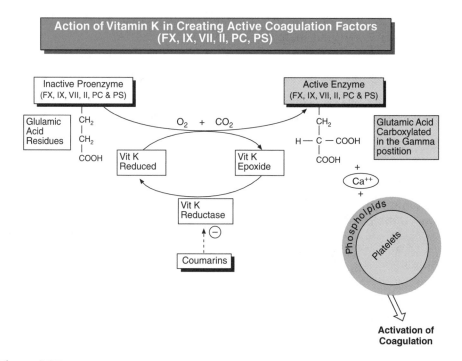

Figure 6-25. How vitamin K influences the activation of FX, IX, VII, II, PC, and PS. See text for abbreviations and details.

Children and adults with vitamin K deficiency are bleeders. The bleeding can be severe and is usually manifested by ecchymosis, hematomas, gastrointestinal and genitourinary bleeding, and hematuria. Vitamin K deficiency is suspected by the patient's mode of presentation (associated diseases) and by blood test abnormalities.

Screening tests include the following:

Prolonged aPTT and PT;
Normal platelet count;
aPTT and PT 1:1 mix tests = correction of both APTT and PT;
FVII, FIX, FX, and FII activities = all reduced;
FVII, FIX, FX, and FII antigenic concentrations = normal.

The finding of nonfunctional vitamin K–dependent factors confirms the vitamin K deficiency.

Clinically, the diagnosis of vitamin K deficiency can be established by treating the patient with vitamin K and demonstrating normalization of both the PT and aPTT.

The principles of therapy include correction of the underlying the disorder, vitamin K administration, and transfusion with FFP for severe bleeding. Correction of the causative disorder is not always possible. For prophylaxis vitamin K is given orally; for treatment of active bleeding or prior surgery, it is given parenterally. The PT improves partially after 7 hours, because of recovery of FVII (half-life, $T_{1/2}$ of 4–7 hours). Vitamin K dose is repeated daily for 3 days, since the other vitamin K–dependent factors have longer half-lives (FIX = about 1 day; FX = about 2 days; and FII = about 3 days). After 3 days both PT and aPTT are completely corrected.

Hemorrhagic Disease of the Newborn

Vitamin K deficiency in the newborn is a different syndrome. Hemorrhagic disease of the newborn occurs on the second to fourth day of life. It results from decreased synthesis of vitamin K–dependent blood coagulation factors. The causes of vitamin K deficiency include reduction of stores of vitamin K and functional immaturity of the liver, lack of bacterial synthesis of vitamin K in the intestine, low quantity of vitamin K in breast milk, and rarely, drug intake by the mother (e.g., such drugs as asprin and phenytoin).

Screening tests include the following:

Prolonged aPTT and PT;
Normal platelet count;
aPTT and PT 1:1 mix tests = correction;
FVII, FIX, FX, and FII activities = all reduced.

Vitamin K_1 (phytomenadione) is given at birth to all infants, except those suspected of having G6PD deficiency (since red blood cell hemolysis can result [see Chapter 3]). For bleeding infants: vitamin K and infusion of FFP are administered.

Acquired Factor X Deficiency

Factor X deficiency is seen in association with amyloidosis. This is the result of FX selective adsorption by the amyloid protein. The patients have a bleeding diathesis, characterized by ecchymosis, hematomas, gastrointestinal, and genitourinary bleeding.

Screening tests include the following:

Prolonged aPTT and PT;

Normal platelets;
aPTT and PT 1:1 mix tests = correction of both PT and aPTT;
FX:C and FX:Ag levels = reduced or absent.

Liver Disease

The coagulopathy of liver disease is associated with bleeding, which sometimes is severe. It results from multiple hemostatic abnormalities summarized in Table 6-9. Defective synthesis of vitamin K–dependent factors in liver disease results from intrahepatic cholestasis, impaired utilization of vitamin K, malabsorption of vitamin K, and poor diet. Reduction in the synthesis of other factors that are not dependent on vitamin K (factors V, XI, XII, and XIII, and fibrinogen) contributes also to the bleeding tendency. In addition, patients with liver disease have chronic activation of both the blood coagulation and of the fibrinolytic systems. The regulatory mechanisms (natural inhibitors) of the latter systems are also markedly impaired.

Platelets in liver disease are decreased in number and impaired in function. The causes of reduced platelets are decreased platelet production by the bone marrow; increased platelet splenic sequestration due to splenomegaly; and increased platelet destruction occurring in the liver and spleen. The mechanism(s) responsible for platelet dysfunction is not clear, but increased fibrinolysis and abnormal fibrinogen are suspected to bind to the platelet membrane and impair their response. Dysfibrinogenemia (decreased content of sialic acid in the fibrinogen) occurs in some patients and also contributes to the hemostatic defect.

Accelerated fibrinolysis is the result of increased levels in plasma of t-PA due to impaired hepatic clearance, lack of appropriate rise in plasminogen activator inhibitors (PAI), and decreased synthesis of α_2-antiplasmin. Hyperfibrinolysis occurs also in response to blood activation.

In *chronic liver disease*, activation of blood coagulation is postulated to result from release of tissue factor by necrotic cells, combined with impaired clearance of activated coagulation factors, and decreased synthesis of the major regulatory proteins (AT III, PC, PS, HC II). In *acute and severe hepatocellular damage*, acute activation is superimposed on the chronic activation of coagulation. The causes postulated to contribute to these acute changes include release tissue function by the necrotic cells of tissue factor, other procoagulants, interleukins (e.g., TNFα, IL-1), endotoxin, and accumulation of activated factors in the expanded low-flow portal system. This leads to thrombin and plasmin formation, via activation of both the blood coagulation and fibrinolytic systems. The presence of thrombin and plasmin *in vivo* re-

TABLE 6-9. *COAGULOPATHY OF LIVER DISEASE*

Reduced synthesis of blood coagulation factors
 ↓ vitamin K–dependent factors (X, IX, VII, II)
 ↓ non-vitamin K–dependent factors (V, XI, XII, XIII, I, PK, HK)
Activation of blood coagulation factors (e.g., disseminated intravascular coagulopathy)
Dysfibrinogenemia
Thrombocytopenia and impaired platelet function
Reduced synthesis and increased consumption of inhibitors
Increased fibrinolysis (↑ t-PA, ↓ α_2-antiplasmin)

sults in both thrombosis of the microcirculation and severe bleeding diathesis, which is called *disseminated intravascular coagulation* (DIC) and is described later.

Laboratory testing shows the following: PT is prolonged; aPTT is slightly prolonged or prolonged; platelet count = 80,000–120,000/μL; fibrinogen is low; FSP, very high specific factor levels: FX, FIX, FVII, FII (vitamin K–dependent) are decreased; FV, FXI, FXII, PK, HK, FXIII, and fibrinogen are also all decreased; FVIII:C is normal; vWf:Ag is increased (acute-phase reactant); plasminogen is reduced; AT III, PC, PS, and α_2-antiplasmin are decreased; α_2-M and PAI are increased.

Therapy consists of correction of vitamin K deficiency. Administer vitamin K (parenterally) and assess corrective effect on the PT in 6–8 hours. Replacement therapy consists of transfusion with large volumes of FFP (6–8 U), which contains all the coagulation factors and inhibitors that help to control bleeding. In severe bleeding, during and after surgery, transfusions with FFP every 6–12 hours are needed to control hemorrhage. In some patients, additional measures are required to achieve hemostasis, such as exchange transfusion, use of prothrombin-complex concentrates (activated FX may cause DIC), platelet transfusions, and AT III concentrates.

Other therapies may include DDAVP, which can be administered to patients with profound qualitative platelet defects. Antifibrinolytic agents (e.g., EACA) are used in preparation for tooth extraction.

Preparation for major surgery may include (1) treatment with vitamin K and FFP; (2) platelet transfusions to maintain platelet count of approximately 100,000/μL. Platelet transfusion in preparation for endoscopy, thoracentesis, paracentesis, and lumbar puncture is generally indicated in patients with platelet counts of less than 50,000/μL.

Massive Transfusion Syndrome

Massive transfusion syndrome, an acquired bleeding disorder, develops after transfusion with large volumes of stored blood. Many factors contribute to the bleeding diathesis following transfusion.

The severity of bleeding depends on the amount and rate of blood transfused, storage time of the blood products, and preexisting/underlying disorders.

1. *Amount and rate of blood transfusion.* Patients transfused with more than 10 U of stored blood, given in less than 24 hours, may develop bleeding. After transfusion with 10 U of blood, the platelet count may fall by 50%. Because platelets in stored blood are reduced in number and qualitatively abnormal, the faster the rate of infusion, the worse the thrombocytopenia and bleeding. Transfusions of packed red blood cells (PRBC) and volume expanders (e.g., dextran) cause dilution of platelets as well as blood coagulation factors. In addition, dextran impairs platelet function by coating the platelet membranes, further contributing to bleeding.
2. *Storage time of blood products.* After 24 hours storage at 4°C, platelets aggregate and lose function. Some coagulation factors also slowly lose their activity. Two labile factors, VIII and V, fall to 80% of their original values. Activation of blood coagulation factors, platelet microaggregates, damaged or activated white cells, bacteria, and viruses when infused into the patients may initiate or accelerate DIC.
3. *Preexisting/underlying clinical disorders.* Excessive blood loss results in a fall of platelets, reduction of blood coagulation factor levels, and reduction of natural inhibitors. The severity of the hemostatic defect due to massive transfusions is much more profound when the production of platelets or blood co-

agulation factors is impaired. This occurs in patients with preexisting blood disorders such as liver disease, idiopathic thrombocytopenia, and DIC.

Laboratory testing shows prolongation of PT and aPTT with correction on a 1:1 mix test. Platelet count is low.

The hemostatic defect can be prevented by administration of 2 U of FFP and 5 U of platelets for each 10 or more U of blood transfused. Calcium preparations may also be necessary because citrate—phosphate dextrose (CPD) used as an anticoagulant for blood products can chelate the patient's calcium and cause hypocalcemia. Treatment of bleeding should include transfusion with FFP and platelets, in addition to treatment of the underlying disease.

Acquired Inhibitors of Blood Coagulation

Acquired inhibitors of blood coagulation, also known as circulating anticoagulants, are antibodies that directly inhibit coagulation factors or their reactions. The inhibitors can occur as the result of transfusion with plasma protein, as in patients with hemophilias, or appear spontaneously in patients with previously normal hemostatic mechanisms. Most acquired inhibitors of blood coagulation cause bleeding, and some are associated with thrombosis (lupus anticoagulant/antiphospholipid antibodies).

Acquired FVIII Inhibitors. Inhibitors to FVIII developed by patients with hemophilia A were described previously. Spontaneously arising FVIII inhibitors have an equal sex incidence, and most are seen in the seventh decade of life. Half of the patients have no associated diseases; the others suffer from immunologic disorders, collagen vascular diseases, malignancies, or drug reactions. A small number of FVIII inhibitors (about 7%) occur in young postpartum women, without evidence of underlying disease. Overall spontaneous remission of FVIII inhibitors is estimated in 38% of the patients, and mortality from bleeding is estimated to occur in approximately 22%. The disorders associated with FVIII inhibitors are listed in Table 6-10. FVIII inhibitor in postpartum women is rare. The inhibitor occurs at birth of the first or second child. Bleeding tendency may become evident immediately or after 2–5 months. The clinical course is variable, but the inhibitor disappears in most patients spontaneously, after 12–18 months. The cause of these postpartum inhibitors is unclear.

Like inhibitors arising in hemophiliac patients, spontaneously acquired FVIII inhibitors are IgG antibodies, which do not fix complement, and are species specific. Both are temperature dependent and require incubation for 1–2 hours at 37°C to

TABLE 6-10. *DISORDERS ASSOCIATED WITH FVIII INHIBITORS*		
IMMUNOLOGIC DISORDERS	**MALIGNANCIES**	**MISCELLANEOUS**
Systemic lupus erythematosus	Monoclonal gammopathies	Postpartum women
Rheumatoid arthritis	Lymphoproliferative disorders	
Dermatitis herpetiformis	Myelofibrosis	
Inflammatory bowel disease	Solid tumor (squamous cell carcinomas)	
Multiple sclerosis		
Penicillin allergy		

demonstrate their inhibitory capacity. However, there is a difference in their reaction kinetics. Laboratory testing shows a prolonged aPTT that does not correct with the 1 :1 mix test. PT is normal. FVIIIC activity is reduced, and FVIII inhibitor levels are present. Although a linear relationship between the inhibitor concentration and the amount of FVIII inactivated is observed with inhibitors of hemophilic patients, it is not seen with spontaneous inhibitors. Although most patients have no measurable FVIII activity in plasma, an occasional patient has some FVIII activity. It has been proposed that vWf may partially shield FVIII epitopes from inhibitor interaction.

Management of bleeding is similar to that described for patients with hemophilia, who develop FVIII inhibitors. Long-term management for patients with underlying diseases also includes immunosuppression of autoantibody production.

Acquired FV Inhibitors. Acquired FV inhibitors may occur in factor V–deficient patients, but this is rare. Most FV inhibitors, however, develop late in life, in patients who have had recent surgery, antibiotic therapy, or infections (e.g., tuberculosis), and in patients without any obvious disease; some of these inhibitors disappear spontaneously. Rarely, FV inhibitors have been reported in patients with myelofibrosis, multiple myeloma, amyloidosis, and carcinoma of the rectum. The inhibitors to FV are an IgG, IgG-IgM, or IgG-IgA.

Prolonged PT and aPTT, and no correction with the 1:1 mix test are characteristic. Absent or decreased FV activity and increased FV inhibitor titer are seen.

The best management of severe bleeding in patients with FV inhibitor is platelet transfusions. Platelets contain FV in the α-granules and Fc receptors on their membranes. The FV inhibitor binds to the Fc receptors, and the platelet-FV inhibitor complex formed is removed from circulation by the reticuloendothelial system. The FV that escapes the inhibitor action and the platelet intracellular FV are then free to provide hemostasis.

Acquired FII inhibitors occur in association with systemic lupus erythematosus (SLE), cirrhosis of the liver, and prosthetic cardiac valves in postsurgical patients. Laboratory testing shows that the PT and aPTT are prolonged without correction on the 1 : 1 mix test; thrombin time (TT) (see Chapter 11) is prolonged due to the inhibitor to FII; FII activity level is reduced or absent; and FII inhibitor titer is high.

Acquired FVII inhibitors are autoantibodies (IgG) associated with severe bleeding, described in patients with monoclonal gammopathy, patients with severe aplastic anemia, and those without underlying disease. Laboratory testing shows that the PT is prolonged without correction on the 1 : 1 mix test; aPTT is normal; FVII activity is absent; and FVII inhibitor is elevated.

Acquired FIX inhibitors are extremely rare; these have occurred in SLE patients and in postpartum women. Most disappear within 1–7 months of the onset.

Acquired FXI and FXII inhibitors have also been demonstrated in SLE and chlorpromazine therapy. Except for hereditary FXI-deficient patients, who developed FXI antibodies after transfusion with plasma, none of the other patients who developed inhibitors to the contact phase factors bled.

Acquired autoantibodies to fibrinogen (I), fibrin stabilization (FXIII), and fibrin polymerization have also been reported in association with SLE, monoclonal gammopathies, and treatment with isoniazid. The latter agent interferes with fibrin stabilization (inhibitor to FXIII). The inhibitors to FXIII are of three types. Type I inhibitors are directed against the FXIII activation but do not interfere with the transamidase activity of FXIII. Type II inhibitors interfere with the transamidase activity.

Type III inhibitors prevent the interaction of activated FXIII with the fibrin substrate. Spontaneous inhibitors to FXIII (fibrin stabilizing factor) can lead to severe bleeding complications, including death. Treatment includes control of the underlying disorder(s), withdrawal of the causative therapeutic agent, and plasma infusions.

Acquired heparin-like anticoagulants, which are spontaneously developed inhibitors of this type, have been reported in patients with plasma cell malignancies, various neoplasms, or adrenocortical or prostate carcinoma undergoing therapy with a drug called suramin. Some patients manifest severe hemorrhagic complications. All inhibitors in plasma exhibit glycosaminoglycan properties and are neutralized by protamine sulfate or heparinase. Treatment with protamine sulfate in patients with severe bleeding has been successful.

Disseminated Intravascular Coagulation

Acute disseminated intravascular coagulation is an acquired thrombohemorrhagic disorder that results from the effects of excessive formation of thrombin and plasmin in circulation. DIC is always secondary to an underlying pathologic process that triggers activation of blood and generation of thrombin. Via its multiple actions, thrombin causes widespread fibrin deposition into the microcirculation with consumption of platelets (platelet aggregation) and of specific coagulation factors. Plasmin, by causing proteolysis of fibrin and coagulation factors, further adds to the bleeding complications of DIC (Fig. 6-26).

Synonyms for DIC include consumption coagulopathy, defibrination syndrome, intravascular coagulation with secondary fibrinolysis, consumptive thrombohemorrhagic disorder. DIC is triggered by diseases that promote release into circulation of procoagulants, cause widespread endothelial injury, or result in platelet/macrophage stimulation. Acute DIC is associated with the conditions listed in Table 6-11. DIC can also be chronic or localized.

Three major pathways of injury lead to DIC (Fig. 6-26):

1. *Tissue injury.* The entry of procoagulants (e.g., tissue factor) into circulation triggers activation of blood coagulation primarily through FVII activation. This type of injury occurs in most obstetrical complications, in malignancies, after trauma, after surgery, in necrosis of the liver, in intravascular hemolysis, in some snake bites, and in some infections (e.g., malaria).

2. *Endothelial injury.* This allows collagen exposure in the subendothelial region, which causes activation of the contact-phase coagulation factors and platelets and leads to excess thrombin formation. In this type of injury the physiologic properties of the endothelium are changed from a predominantly anticoagulant to a powerful procoagulant surface, which activates blood continuously. Bacterial products and agents (e.g., endotoxin; Gram-negative bacteria, including meningococci; and Gram-positive bacteria), certain viral infections (e.g., herpes virus leading to purpura fulminans), severe burns, acute lung injury, and metabolic disorders are all conditions that cause widespread endothelial injury.

3. *Platelet/macrophage injury.* Direct platelet stimulation leading to intravascular platelet microaggregates can also be the trigger for DIC. Viruses, some bacteria, endotoxin, and immune complexes can directly, or via stimulation of macrophages (e.g., platelet activating factor [PAF]), affect platelets.

TABLE 6-11. *CONDITIONS ASSOCIATED WITH ACUTE DISSEMINATED INTRAVASCULAR COAGULATION*

Infections
  Gram-negative septicemia
  Gram-positive septicemia
  Rocky Mountain spotted fever
  Severe falciparum malaria
  Typhoid fever
  Viral infections (purpura fulminans)

Obstetric complications
  Abruptio placenta
  Amniotic fluid embolism
  Eclampsia
  Retained placenta

Malignancies
  Acute promyelocytic leukemia
  Other acute leukemias (AML, AMML)
  Mucin-secreting adenocarcinomas
  Tumor lysis syndrome, lymphomas

Hypersensitivity reactions
  Transfusion reactions
  Intravascular hemolysis
  Anaphylactic shock

Metabolic disorders
  Hyper/hypothermia
  Acute hypoxia
  Hypotension

Tissue injury
  Surgical trauma
  Extracorporeal circulation
  Crush injury
  Head injury

Miscellaneous
  Acute hepatic necrosis
  Snake venoms
  Severe burns
  Adult respiratory distress syndrome

AML = Acute myelogenous leukemia; AMML = acute myelomonocytic leukemia.

Activation of blood coagulation via any of these pathways leads to excessive thrombin and plasmin formation, whose actions cause the manifestations of DIC shown in Table 6-12.

Thrombin generation during early stages of DIC causes large, soluble fibrin–fibrinogen complexes and fibrin microthrombi to develop, which obstruct the microcirculation and lead to multiple organ failure. At this stage the patients show signs of organ injury manifested by obtundation, decreased urinary output, difficulty in oxygenating blood, progressive abnormalities in liver function tests, and manifestations of altered hemostasis.

In later phases of DIC, bleeding results from thrombin-induced platelet consumption and depletion of blood coagulation factors (I, II, V, VIII, XIII), as well as

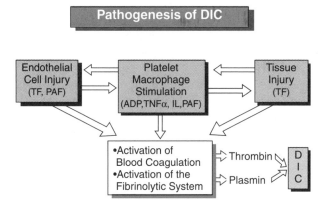

Figure 6-26. A simplified presentation of DIC pathogenesis. See text for abbreviations and details.

TABLE 6-12. *ACTIONS OF THROMBIN AND PLASMIN*

THROMBIN	PLASMIN
Fibrin formation (causing decreased FI and decreased FII)	Digestion of fibrin (causing FSP marked increase)
Platelet aggregation (causing decrease in platelet number)	Digestion of fibrinogen (causing decrease in levels of FI)
Activation of FV and FVIII (causing decrease in levels of FV, FVIII)	Proteolysis of FV and FVIII (causing decrease in levels of FV and FVIII)
Activation of FXIII (causing decrease in levels of FXIII)	Proteolysis of vWf, FXII, FXI (causing decrease in levels of vWf, FXII, FXI)
Activation of PC/PS system (causing decrease in levels of PC and PS)	Proteolysis of FXIII (causing decrease in levels of FXIII)
Activation of fibrinolytic system	Changes in platelet membrane GP

the effects of fibrinolysis. With continuous activation of blood, consumption of natural inhibitors of active serine proteases (AT III, PC, PS, and TFPI) follows. Consumption of such inhibitors leads to thrombus formation. Thrombin also promotes expression of thrombomodulin by EC, a prerequisite for activation of the PC/PS system (Fig. 6-11). Until it is depleted, activated PC inhibits activated factors V and VIII (contributing to hemorrhage); in addition, APC suppresses PAI release by a negative feedback mechanism on the EC, allowing t-PA release to be unchecked (Fig. 6-11). Damage or stimulation of ECs by endotoxin and other mediators of inflammation results in more t-PA release, thereby causing stimulation of conversion of plasminogen to plasmin (Fig. 6-13). Therefore simultaneous and sequential thrombosis and bleeding tendencies develop.

Plasmin formation in DIC worsens the effects of thrombin, leading to further reductions in factors (V, FVIII, fibrinogen, and XIII) and induction of a lytic state, indicated by high levels of fibrin split products (FSP). Proteolysis of vWf and modification of platelet membrane glycoprotein receptors by plasmin prevent platelet–vessel interaction and impair primary hemostasis. At this latter stage of DIC, patients develop hemorrhagic necrosis of tissues and manifest variable signs of bleeding.

Clinical Evaluation of Patients with Acute DIC. The patient with acute DIC shows signs of both microvascular thrombosis and severe bleeding diathesis. Fever occurs in 58%; hypotension in 50%; microangiophatic hemolytic anemia in 15%.

Signs of thrombi in the microcirculation are manifested by the following:
Skin: acrocyanosis; blue toes, ischemia, superficial gangrene;
Neurologic: multifocal signs as well as obtundation, delirium, or coma;
Pulmonary: respiratory failure, acute respiratory distress syndrome;
Gastrointestinal: stress ulcers;
Hematologic: intravascular hemolysis (fragmented red blood cells), which leads to hyperbilirubinemia, causing a pale-yellow skin and sclerae color to develop;
Renal: oliguria, azotemia, cortical necrosis.

Signs of bleeding in acute DIC are manifested by the following:

Skin: petechiae, purpuras, ecchymoses, hematomas, and bleeding from venipuncture sites;

Neurologic: intracerebral bleeding;

Gastrointestinal: massive bleeding;

Mucous membrane: epistaxis, gingival bleeding, vaginal bleeding;

Renal: hematuria.

Laboratory diagnosis of acute DIC depends upon tests that measure platelet depletion, consumption of blood coagulation factors, and secondary fibrinolysis. Table 6-13 shows tests commonly ordered to assist with the diagnosis of DIC.

Factor V and VIII levels are reduced in DIC. These tests are not needed to establish the diagnosis of DIC unless the patient has liver disease. In the uncomplicated coagulopathy of liver disease FV (a non-vitamin K–dependent clotting factor) is reduced because damaged parenchymal cells do not produce it. FVIII is within the normal range. FVIII (another non-vitamin K–dependent clotting factor) is not manufactured by parenchymal cells and is an acute-phase reactant protein; therefore it rises nonspecifically with inflammation and may be normal or elevated in liver disease. If DIC is superimposed upon liver disease, both FV and FVIII are markedly reduced or absent. AT III, PC/PS, α_2-anti-plasmin are all depleted in DIC.

Other research tools to demonstrate intravascular coagulation (e.g., prothrombin fragment 1.2, fibrinopeptide A/B ratio, activated PC peptide, thrombin/AT III complexes and others) may be helpful in considering DIC; however, these tests are not routinely necessary to establish the diagnosis of DIC.

Examination of the peripheral blood smear may show fragmented red blood cells (schistocytes); their presence is consistent with DIC, but their absence does not rule out DIC.

Management principles for Patients with Acute DIC:

1. Treatment of the underlying disease (e.g., infection or malignancy);
2. Supportive measures such as aggressive correction of hypoxemia and hypovolemia;
3. Heparin therapy to arrest blood activation (controversial, see later);
4. Replacement therapy with AT III concentrates, PC concentrate, FFP, cryoprecipitate, and platelets.

TABLE 6-13. *SCREENING TESTS FOR ACUTE DISSEMINATED INTRAVASCULAR COAGULATION (DIC)*

BLOOD TESTS	DIC	NORMAL RANGE
Platelet count	<150,000/μL	150,000–400,000/μL
PT	>15 sec	12–14 sec
aPTT	>37 sec	25–38 sec
Fibrinogen	<150 mg %	150–350 mg %
FDP	>20 μg/mL	2–10 μg/mL
D-dimer	Positive	Negative

The use of heparin therapy in DIC patients, with a severe bleeding diathesis, has been controversial, partly because of lack of general understanding of the cause of bleeding in DIC (e.g., thrombin induced). Some studies have shown a reduction in mortality from 90% to 18% with the use of heparin therapy in DIC. Some patients with depletion of AT III require simultaneous infusion of either AT III concentrate or FFP for heparin cofactor replacement.

Many believe that the use of FFP without simultaneous heparin therapy provides more substrate for the reactions to continue and DIC to progress (fuel-to-the-fire theory).

New therapies with recombinant hirudin, antibodies to TNF await clinical trials.

The clinical and laboratory criteria to monitor response to heparin therapy in DIC patients are shown in Table 6-14.

Chronic DIC

This condition occurs in association with the following:

1. *Retained dead fetus.* Tissue injury with release of TF leads to DIC;
2. *Malignancy.* This accounts for the majority of chronic DIC cases (70%). Tumors that secrete mucinous material also produce and release procoagulants into circulation. Three types of procoagulants have been identified: tissue factor, an enzyme that converts FX to FXa, and microvesicles (phospholipids) shed from the tumor cell membranes, which act as platelet membrane procoagulant substitutes in hemostasis;
3. *Liver disease.* Cirrhosis of the liver and hepatic necrosis (previously described under coagulopathy of liver disease) are forms of chronic DIC.

TABLE 6-14. *CRITERIA TO MONITOR HEPARIN THERAPY RESPONSE IN ACUTE DIC*

CLINICAL	LABORATORY TESTS
IMPROVED Bleeding stops No new purpura Acrocyanosis disappears	IMPROVED Fibrinogen increases by 40 mg% in 24 hr FDP decreases (by 2 dilutions in 24 hr) PT returns to normal in 24 hr Platelet count ↑ in 4–5 days
PARTIAL Major bleeding stops No new purpura Acrocyanosis disappears	PARTIAL Only two tests improve
UNCHANGED Bleeding continuous No resolution of acrocyanosis	UNCHANGED No improvement in blood results
WORSE Bleeding increases Patient unstable	WORSE All blood tests deteriorate

Localized intravascular coagulation

This condition occurs in certain disease states that are associated with consumption of platelets and blood coagulation factors in strictly defined, localized anatomic sites. These are (1) *aortic aneurysm*; (2) *hemangiomas*—Kasabach-Merritt syndrome (benign tumors with convoluted mass of vascular channels that sequester and consume platelets and coagulation factors); (3) *renal diseases* (e.g., SLE, hemolytic uremic syndrome); (4) *ARDS* (acute respiratory distress syndrome), especially if secondary to trauma.

Laboratory tests show (1) reduced platelet count in all; (2) increased FSP or positive D-dimer; (3) normal or prolonged PT and aPTT; (4) fibrinogen and FVIII levels that are increased with malignancies but reduced in most other conditions. Clinical presentation and recognition of the associated clinical disorders are important in establishing the diagnosis of chronic or localized intravascular coagulation, because there is considerable overlap between laboratory findings of acute and chronic DIC. Patients with malignancies, aortic aneurysm without rupture, and hemangiomas respond to heparin therapy with clinical and laboratory improvement. In retention of dead fetus, removal of the fetus is followed by normalization of hemostasis.

Acquired Fibrinolytic States

Acquired defects of fibrinolysis are classified into two types: hyperfibrinolytic states caused by excessive activation or defective inhibition; and hypofibrinolytic states secondary to defective activation or excessive inhibition. These pathologic disturbances of fibrinolysis can result in bleeding or thrombosis.

Hyperfibrinolytic states associated with bleeding result from either *excessive activation* or *defective inhibition* of fibrinolysis.

Excessive activation of fibrinolysis is caused by the following:

1. Increased release in circulation of plasminogen activators (e.g., t-PA, urokinase), as in patients with benign or malignant prostatic disease (primary fibrinolysis);
2. Defective clearance of the activators (e.g., liver disease);
3. Localized excessive release of activator (e.g., menorrhagia, prostatectomy);
4. Iatrogenic, secondary to thrombolytic therapy.

Defective inhibition of fibrinolysis is seen in DIC and liver disease. It may be secondary to decreased plasmin synthesis, complex formation between plasmin–antiplasmin, and/or PAI.

Laboratory tests show that platelet count is normal; D-dimer level is not elevated in primary fibrinolysis because this is primarily lysis of fibrinogen or non-cross-linked fibrin, but it is elevated in secondary fibrinolysis (as in DIC), which causes plasmic digests of cross-linked fibrin. Cross-linking of fibrin that is induced by thrombin and FXIII is required for the D-dimer to be released by plasmic digests. FSP levels are elevated, and levels of fibrinogen, plasminogen, t-PA, PAI, α_2-anti-plasmin, FV, and FVIII are decreased.

Patients with bleeding diathesis should be managed with the following: (1) correction of underlying disorder; (2) antifibrinolytic therapy; (3) FFP to replace plasminogen, fibrinogen, and inhibitors (PAI, antiplasmins).

Hypofibrinolytic states associated with thrombosis result from (1) defective activation of fibrinolysis due to inadequate release of t-PA (congenital or acquired), as in ARDS; or (2) excessive inhibition of fibrinolysis—congenital due to excessive production of plasminogen activator inhibitors (PAI) or secondary to therapy with antifibrinolytic agents (epsilon amino caproic acid [EACA]). Management of patients with thrombosis involves the use of thrombolytic agents or anticoagulants (heparin and warfarin).

DISORDERS OF THROMBOSIS

Definition and Thrombus Composition. A thrombus is formed by an intravascular mass of fibrin and blood cells; the relative proportion of cells to fibrin depends on hemodynamic factors. Arterial thrombi formed under high flow rates are composed primarily of platelet aggregates held together by fibrin strands (white thrombi). In contrast, venous thrombi, originating in areas of stasis, are composed of large numbers of red blood cells, fibrin, but relatively few platelets (red thrombi). Thrombi occurring in areas of slow to moderate blood flow are a mixture of red blood cells, fibrin, and platelets (mixed platelet–fibrin thrombi).

Localization. Thrombi may form in veins, in arteries, in the heart, or in the microcirculation of any organ.

Fate of Thrombi. A thrombus undergoes continuous structural changes with age. Leukocytes are attracted to the thrombus by chemotactic factors, produced by blood (e.g., kallikrein) and platelet activation, and accumulate around the platelet aggregates in the thrombus. The platelets in the thrombus begin to swell and lyse, and in 24 hours are replaced by fibrin. The subsequent fate of the thrombus depends on forces that promote either accumulation or dissolution of the thrombotic material. The thrombus is dissolved by fibrinolytic enzymes (e.g., plasmin), formed as a consequence of t-PA and urinary kallikrein released from endothelial cells and by elastases produced by leukocytes. The thrombus may organize, adhere to the vessel wall, lyse, propagate, or undergo phagocytosis by leukocytes. When the thrombogenic factors override the mechanisms of dissolution, the thrombus may continue to grow.

Clinical Consequences of Thrombus Formation. A thrombus formed in any part of the vascular system leads to the development of ischemia (lack of blood supply) by either vascular obstruction or embolization and obstruction of a distal part of the circulation.

Occlusive Versus Nonocclusive Thrombus. An *arterial thrombus* remains at the vessel wall, as a *mural* thrombus (nonocclusive), because it usually forms in regions of disturbed and rapid blood flow. In contrast, a *venous thrombus* usually forms at areas of slow blood flow and tends to obstruct the circulation (occlusive).

The *mural thrombus* acts as a site for continued platelet interaction. The fresh platelet thrombus may embolize or continue to grow and form platelet thrombus layers of varying ages. This platelet thrombus, eventually becomes incorporated into the vessel wall, releasing platelet-derived growth factor, which promotes rapid acceleration of fibroblast proliferation and atherosclerotic plaque formation. If the mural thrombus embolizes, it may cause serious distal ischemia and organ damage. Both arterial and venous thrombosis are very common in clinical practice and are among the leading causes of morbidity and mortality in Western countries.

Pathogenesis of Thrombosis. More than 150 years ago Rudolph Virchow proposed that the pathophysiology of thrombosis involved three interrelated factors (*Virchow's triad*): changes in the vessel wall, changes in blood flow, and changes in the coagulability of blood. The first two factors have been proven repeatedly, but the third is only now beginning to be explained at a molecular level. The changes in blood coagulability are now called the *hypercoagulable states*. Hypercoagulability of blood, also known as *prethrombotic state*, is defined as the tendency to thrombose under circumstances that would not cause thrombosis in normal individuals. Several inherited and acquired risk factors for thrombosis have been identified as hypercoagulable states and are associated with arterial (Table 6-15) or venous thromboem-

---

TABLE 6-15. *RISK FACTORS IN ARTERIAL THROMBOGENESIS (ACQUIRED HYPERCOAGULABLE STATES)*

Hereditary*,†
Homocystinuria*,†
Males†

Hypertension†
Sex (males)†
Diabetes mellitus†
Hyperlipidemia†
Smoking†
Gout†
Obesity†

Oral contraceptives
Malignancy
Cardiac disease
Elevated fibrinogen
Elevated FVII
Surgery
Trauma
Myeloproliferative disorders (e.g., polycythemia vera and essential thrombocythemia)
Inflammatory vasculopathies
Inflammatory bowel disease
Paroxysmal nocturnal hemoglobinuria
Heparin-associated thrombocytopenia and thrombosis
Antiphospholipid syndrome/lupus anticoagulant
Systemic lupus erythematosus
Hyperviscosity syndromes
Nephrotic syndrome
Stroke
Pregnancy/puerperium

* = Inherited risk factor; † = atherosclerosis risk.

TABLE 6-16. *HEREDITARY CAUSES OF THROMBOPHILIA: (PRIMARY HYPERCOAGULABLE STATES)*

COMMON CAUSES	FREQUENCY IN VENOUS THROMBOSIS (%)	RARE CAUSES	FREQUENCY IN VENOUS THROMBOSIS (%)
ATIII deficiency	1–5	Dysfibrinogenemia	?
PC deficiency	1–9	Hypo- or dysplasminogenemia	?
PS deficiency	1–8	Heparin cofactor deficiency	?
APC resistance (FV mutation)	20–60	High plasminogen activator Inhibitor (PAI-1)	?
Hyperhomocysteinemia	19	Histidine-rich glycoprotein (↑)	?
		Abnormal thrombomodulin	?

bolism (Tables 6-16 and 6-17). The term *thrombophilia* is used to describe the inherited tendency to develop thrombosis. What causes thrombus formation? A thrombus forms when there is an imbalance between thrombogenic factors and protective mechanisms of hemostasis.

The known *thrombogenic factors* include stimulation or damage to the vessel wall, activation of platelets, activation of blood coagulation factors, inhibition of fibrinolysis, and stagnation of blood (stasis). The *protective mechanisms* against thrombosis include intact anticoagulant activities of the endothelium, normal quantity and function of the natural inhibitors of serine proteases, clearance of active proteases by hepatocytes and by the reticuloendothelial system, and intact fibrinolytic system.

TABLE 6-17. *RISK FACTORS IN VENOUS THROMBOSIS (ACQUIRED AND INHERITED)*

Secondary to stasis (acquired)
Immobilization (postsurgery)
Obesity
Cardiac failure
Stroke
Dehydration
Hyperviscosity (polycythemia vera)
Pregnancy
Postmyocardial infarction
Varicose veins

Secondary to hereditary hemostatic disorders (inherited)
ATIII, or PC or PS deficiency
APC resistance (FV mutation)
High PAI
Heparin Cofactor II deficiency
Abnormal fibrinogen and plasminogen
Abnormal thrombomodulin
High histidine-rich glycoprotein
Hyperhomocysteinemia

Secondary to blood activation (acquired)
Major surgery
Major trauma
Malignancy
Pregnancy and puerperium
APA/LA syndrome
Oral contraceptives
Estrogen therapy
Nephrotic syndrome
Tx with FIX concentrates

Secondary to platelet disorders (acquired)
Hyperreactive platelets (as in myeloproliferative disorders)
Thrombocytosis
Paroxysmal nocturnal hemoglobinuria

Secondary to multiple factors (acquired)
Age
Sepsis
High fibrinogen
High factor FVII

The thrombogenic and anticoagulant forces of hemostasis have been described earlier in this chapter. A thrombus evolves from the same exact steps, except for its location in the intravascular space. Excessive amount of thrombogenic factors or failure of the protective mechanisms are the major causes of thrombus formation. Although the pathogenesis of a thrombus is broadly similar in the various parts of the circulation, there are some key differences between arterial and venous thrombus formation that warrant a separate discussion.

Arterial Thrombogenesis

Platelet activation is an essential factor in arterial thrombus formation, as well as acceleration of atherosclerosis. The arterial thrombus is formed mainly by platelets and fibrin. It usually occurs in a diseased vessel wall (e.g., atheromatous or ulcerated plaque), where blood is exposed to perturbed or damaged endothelial cells, and to subendothelial structures. These endothelial changes abolish the thromboresistant properties of the normal endothelium, also known as *anticoagulant properties.* The latter consist of the ability of the endothelium to neutralize active serine proteases, inhibit platelet adhesion and aggregation, and provide a surface for activation of fibrinolysis. Under pathologic conditions, the injured endothelium allows platelets to adhere, aggregate, release their contents, and provide a surface for blood coagulation activation.

Both the collagen and tissue factor at the damaged vessel wall activate the blood coagulation system, resulting in *thrombin* formation, which aggregates platelets and forms fibrin. Stenosis of the diseased blood vessels, and turbulence of flow, are also important factors causing further platelet aggregation at the site of thrombi. Both TxA_2 released from activated platelets and endothelin-1 produced by injured ECs cause vasoconstriction; the latter reduces blood flow and contributes to further growth of the thrombi (Fig. 6-15). Activation by thrombin of the thrombomodulin PC/PS pathway limits the extent of the thrombus by indirect stimulation of fibrinolysis (Fig. 6-11).

Platelet fibrin small emboli may dislodge from the primary thrombus and obstruct the circulation. This occurs frequently from clot in heart chambers (mural thrombi), or from cartoid arteries leading to obstruction of the cerebral circulation. The cerebral ischemia may be transient (transient ischemic attack [TIA]) or permanent (stroke). Platelets in the mural thrombus also release platelet-derived growth factor (PDGF), a promoter of fibroblast growth and atherosclerosis.

Intracardiac thrombosis occurs in relation to damaged valves or endothelium. Valvular damage is seen in association with rheumatic vasculitis, mitral valve prolapse, subacute endocarditis, SLE, and marantic endocarditis of malignancy. Prosthetic heart valves are also associated with a very high incidence of thromboembolism. Mural thrombi may form at any area of endocardial damage.

Some of the acquired risk factors for arterial thrombogenesis are also involved in atherosclerosis and are shown in Table 6-15.

Venous Thrombogenesis

Venous thrombi usually form in regions of slow or disturbed blood flow. The thrombus begins as small deposits occurring most frequently in the large venous sinuses in the calf, in valve cusp pockets in the deep veins of the calf and thigh, or in other veins exposed to direct trauma. At the site of formation the thrombus consists of platelets and fibrin, but with extension of the thrombus, it changes its composition to red blood cells and fibrin, and it occludes the vein.

Venous thrombogenesis differs from arterial thrombogenesis in the type of disturbances affecting the balance between thrombogenic and protective mechanisms. In venous thrombosis increased systemic *hypercoagulability* (blood activation with impaired mechanism of inhibition) and *stasis* are major risk factors. Damage to the vessel wall is not required, but when it is present it is a contributing factor. Platelet activation, however, plays a secondary role (Table 6-17). Occasionally, defective fibrinolysis is the major predisposing factor in the development of venous thrombi. Recurrent venous thrombosis occurs in association with several inherited or acquired disorders, which are characterized by hypercoagulability of blood (Tables 6-15 and 6-16).

The inflammatory response by the vessel wall to a thrombus is variable. Some patients develop a minimal inflammatory reaction and remain asymptomatic; others have a marked vessel wall response manifested by edema, leukocyte infiltration, and massive loss of the endothelium. The inflammatory process and proximal venous obstruction, together with the resultant high venous pressure, explain the tenderness, pain, and swelling experienced by the symptomatic patients with acute deep vein thrombosis (DVT).

The fate of the venous thrombus varies (Fig. 6-27). It may extend, undergo ly-

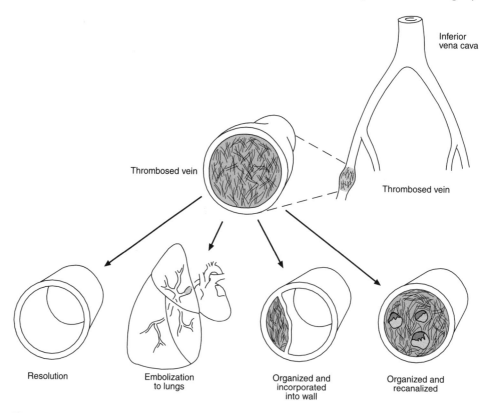

Figure 6-27. The potential outcomes following venous thrombosis. (Redrawn from Cotran RS, Kumar V, Robbins SL, eds., *Robbins Pathologic Basis of Disease,* 5th ed. Philadelphia: WB Saunders, 1996;108.)

sis, become organized, or embolize. Extension of the thrombus is likely if the thrombogenic stimuli persist. Lysis of the thrombus depends on plasmic fibrinolysis and leukocyte elastase, which lead to organization and/or embolization. Most clinical significant pulmonary embolisms arise from thrombi occurring in a proximal large vein of the legs (popliteal, femoral, or iliac veins), and only occasionally from large calf vein thrombi. Fatal pulmonary embolism, however, may occur in association with both proximal and distal vein thrombi.

Complete spontaneous lysis of the thrombus is rare. Thrombus that does not embolize or undergo dissolution slowly will organize and recanalize, causing an abnormal inner-vein surface, which leads to predisposition to recurrent DVTs or to postphlebitic syndrome.

Complications of venous thrombosis include (1) pulmonary embolism (PE), which occurs in 20 of every 1,000 inpatients and causes death in 142,000 Americans each year; and (2) postphlebitic syndrome, whose incidence is difficult to know precisely but is estimated to occur in approximately 500,000 Americans. The latter results from venous hypertension, secondary to valve destruction, venous reflex, or persistent outflow obstruction. The postphlebitic syndrome is manifested by swelling of the ankle and leg, and pain in the calf and ankle on standing or walking; these symptoms are relieved by rest and leg elevation. Because of high intracapillary pressure, red blood cells leak from the blood vessels, and iron is deposited in the skin, causing hyperpigmentation. Edema with prominent collateral circulation develops around the ankle and lower leg. Skin ulcers at the medial malleolus aspect may also be seen.

INHERITED THROMBOPHILIA

AT III deficiency was the first recognized (1965) cause of inherited thrombophilia (also called the hypercoagulable state). In the early 1980s, protein C (PC) and protein S (PS) deficiencies were discovered. Together, these three inherited risk factors accounted for less than 15% of unexplained spontaneous and recurrent DVTs in young individuals (Table 6-16). In 1993, resistance to activated PC, due to a point mutation in the FV gene, emerged as the most frequent cause of inherited thrombophilia (20–60%). In 1994, inherited hyperhomocysteinemia was found to be another risk factor for venous thromboembolism, present in 19% of cases. Although AT III, PC, PS deficiencies, and resistance to APC all result from a single gene defect, hyperhomocysteinemia is caused by multiple gene defects, because different genes control the various enzymes involved in the homocysteine metabolism.

Other rare inherited causes of venous thromboembolism include dysfibrinogenemia, abnormal plasminogen, high levels of plasminogen activator inhibitor 1, high histidine-rich glycoprotein, defective heparin cofactor II, and abnormal thrombomodulin.

Types of Inherited Thrombophilia

Antithrombin III Deficiency. AT III is a single-chain glycoprotein, synthesized by the liver, with a $T_{1/2}$ of 65 hours. The AT III gene is located in chromosome 1. AT III is a serpin inhibitor, which inactivates thrombin as well as other serine proteases (activated factors X, IX, XI, and XII; Fig. 6-10).

AT III deficiency is inherited as an autosomal dominant disorder estimated to occur in 0.2–0.4% of the general population. In patients with venous thrombosis, its frequency is estimated to be as high as 5%. Most affected individuals are heterozygous for the disorder and have plasma levels ranging from 40% to 70% of normal; homozygous patients are very rare. There is a wide range of prevalence of clinical thrombotic complications among AT III–deficient kindred, ranging from 15% to 100% in different families. Two types of inherited AT III deficiency have been recognized. Type I is characterized by both decreased quantity and function of AT III (decreased synthesis). The molecular defect in type I is from gene deletions, short insertions or deletions (frame shift mutations), and single nucleotide changes (nonsense or missense mutations). Type II is expressed by reduced function but normal quantity of the AT III (abnormal synthesis). Type II is subdivided into three subtypes characterized by defective reactive AT III site (inhibition site), defective heparin-binding sites, and defects in both heparin- and protease-inhibition sites. The molecular defect in type II is from missense mutations causing amino acid substitutions.

Protein C and Protein S Deficiencies. Both PC and PS are vitamin K–dependent proteins produced by the liver. Activated PC (APC) inhibits activated factors V and VIII. PC has a $T_{1/2}$ of 7 hours, whereas the $T_{1/2}$ of PS is much longer, at 42 hours. Thrombin activates PC slowly, but thrombin bound to thrombomodulin (EC-thrombin receptor) enhances PC activation by a factor of 20,000. Activated PC inhibition of Va and VIIIa is enhanced by the cofactor PS. Protein S forms a membrane-bound complex with APC, which facilitates APC inactivation of activated factors V and VIII (Fig. 6-11).

Protein C and PS deficiencies are inherited as autosomal dominant traits. Homozygous PC deficiency causes neonatal thrombosis in the form of purpura fulminans, as defined under DIC. The prevalence of heterozygous PC deficiency is 0.3–0.5% in the general population and 1–9% in patients with venous thrombosis. Thus the vast majority of heterozygotes are asymptomatic. However, 50% of heterozygotes from families with a history of symptomatic thrombosis can be expected to develop thrombotic complications.

The frequency of PS deficiency is similar to that of PC in patients with thrombosis. The incidence of PS deficiency in the general population is not known, but extrapolation from cohorts of thrombotic patients has led to estimates of an incidence of 1 in 33,000. Both PC and PS deficiencies have two phenotypes, type I (decreased synthesis) and type II (abnormal synthesis). In type I protein C and S deficiencies, both the antigenic quantity and function are reduced to the same extent, whereas in type II protein C and S deficiencies, the function is disproportionately reduced and the antigen level is normal.

Synthesis of PC is controlled by one gene located on chromosome 2, whereas that of PS is directed by two homologous genes (α and β) located on chromosome 3.

In type I PC deficiency, mutations in the gene (missense type) lead to premature termination of synthesis or disruption of protein folding with loss of stability. Gene deletions and insertions occur rarely (<10%). Type II PC deficiency is secondary to missense mutations, which occur at specific points, such as the protease domain and the thrombin cleavage site, and result in PC dysfunctional inhibitory activity.

Few mutations of the PS gene have been identified, perhaps because of the large size of the gene and the presence of the pseudogene (β). Large deletions of α gene have been found, but the majority of PS defects are point mutations, which lead to premature termination of protein synthesis or incorrect protein folding.

Resistance to Protein C Activation. Resistance to PC activation is the most common cause of inherited hypercoagulability of blood. It occurs in 20–65% of patients with unexplained venous thromboembolism. The resistance to APC is due to a defect in the FV gene, which is located on chromosome 1. Search for the genetic defects to explain resistance to APC involved screening for FV gene mutations affecting the cleavage site (Arg 506–Gly 507) or the APC-binding region to FV (Arg 1865–Ile 1874). A single-point mutation in the FV gene leading substitution of Arg 506 by Gln was found to be the cause for resistance to APC inactivation of FVa. It was present in 80–100% of the patients studied with familial history of venous thrombosis.

Hereditary Hyperhomocysteinemia. Homocysteine is an amino acid derived from methionine. The intracellular metabolism of homocysteine (Fig. 6-28) occurs via remethylation to methionine and transulfuration to cysteine. Three enzymes are involved in the remethylation: methionine synthase (cobalamin is the cofactor), 5,10-methylenetetrahydrofolate reductase, and betaine-methionine methyltransferase. In the transfurylation pathway, homocysteine is transformed to cystathionine by cystathionine—synthase (pyridoxine is the cofactor). In plasma, homocysteine is oxidized to disulfides and mixed disulfides, and exists in both a free and protein-bound form (total homocysteine); normal plasma concentration is 5–16 mmol/L.

The following are some of the inherited enzyme deficiencies associated with hereditary hyperhomocysteinemia: (1) Homozygous cystathionine—synthase deficiency is the most frequent cause of severe hyperhomocysteinemia. Its frequency in the general population is from 1 in 200,000 to 1 in 335,000. Affected individuals have high levels of homocysteine in plasma (>100 mmol/L) and clinically manifest premature arterial vascular disease, and both arterial and venous thrombosis. (2) Heterozygous cystathionine—synthase deficiency causes mild (16–24 mmol/L) or moderate (25–100 mmol/L) hyperhomocysteinemia and has a high frequency of 0.3–1.4% in the general population. (3) A smaller number of patients with homozygous deficiency have inherited defects of the remethylation pathway, such as methyltransferase deficiency. (4) A common defect of the remethylation pathway is a mutant form of methylenetetrahydrofolate reductase, present in 5% of the general population.

Acquired hyperhomocysteinemia is also common and is associated with nutritional deficiencies of cobalamin, folate, or pyridoxine, the cofactors for homocysteine metabolism. Drugs that interfere with the metabolism of any of these cofactors are also associated with high plasma homocysteine levels.

Hyperhomocysteinemia contributes to both arterial and venous thrombogenesis by changing the balance between anticoagulant and thrombogenic properties of the endothelium and, indirectly, by affecting platelets. *In vivo* studies have shown that homocysteine causes endothelial cell desquamation, smooth muscle proliferation, and thickening of the intima (vascular disease). *In vitro* studies have shown that homocysteine can cause several changes in EC behavior. It decreases EC expression of thrombomodulin, interferes with PC activation, inhibits t-PA, impairs nitrous

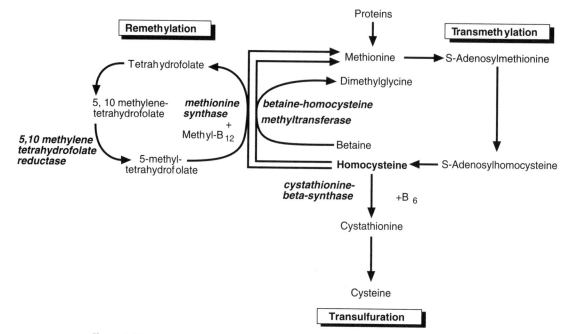

Figure 6-28. The intracellular metabolic pathways of homocysteine. Redrawn after DeStefano V, Finazzi G, Mannucci PM. Inherited thrombophilia: pathogenesis, clinical syndromes, and management. *Blood* 1996; 87:3531–3544.

oxide and PGI_2 production, and suppresses expression of heparan sulfates. Together, these changes markedly reduce the anticoagulant properties of the endothelium. Homocysteine also causes activation of FV and expression of tissue factor by EC, two important thrombogenic effects. In addition, homocysteine-thiolactone, which is increased in plasma of patients with hyperhomocysteinemia, has been shown to cause *in vitro* platelet aggregation and to release TxA_2. This platelet effect, together with endothelial injury by homocysteine, may explain arterial thrombogenesis, a common finding in hyperhomocysteinemia.

Mild to moderate hyperhomocysteinemia is an established independent risk factor for stroke, myocardial infarction, peripheral vascular disease, and extracranial artery stenosis. In young individuals with venous thromboembolism, hyperhomocysteinemia occurs in 19% and is now considered a risk factor for both venous and arterial thrombosis. The clinical manifestations of venous thrombosis do not differ from those of other thrombophilic states. DVT and PE occur in 64%; superficial phlebitis occurs in 24%; and thrombosis of the cerebral or mesenteric veins is found in 12%.

Inherited Defects of Fibrinolysis. Several fibrinolytic defects have been implicated in the pathogenesis of thrombosis. These include hypoplasminogenemia, dysplasminogenemia (abnormal plasminogen), decreased release of tissue plasminogen activator (t-PA), and increased levels of plasminogen activator inhibitor (PAI). These alterations all lead to abnormal or reduced plasmin formation, and impaired (inappropriate) fibrinolytic response to fibrin generation (Fig. 6-13).

Inherited high levels of histidine-rich glycoprotein, which binds plasminogen and prevents plasmin formation, has been found in a family symptomatic for thrombosis. Rare patients with dysfibrinogenemias have increased thrombosis. The latter is secondary to fibrinogen abnormalities, which render the fibrinogen resistant to lysis by plasmin or cause it to bind avidly to thrombin, or to polymerize abnormally. The genetic defects of fibrinolysis in primary hypercoagulable states have not been as well characterized as the inhibitors described earlier.

Clinical Manifestations of Inherited Thrombophilia

The clinical manifestations of patients with AT III, PC, PS, and resistance to APC are similar. Venous thromboembolism occurs in more than 90%. Thrombotic complications may occur at any age; however, the initial thrombotic episode usually manifested in early adulthood. The most common site of thrombosis is in the lower limbs, with embolization to the lungs, but thrombosis in unusual sites such as mesenteric or cerebral veins, and superficial phlebitis can also occur (in approximately 5%). For unknown reasons, superficial thrombophlebitis is more frequent in patients with deficiency of PC and PS, and with resistance to APC than it is in AT III deficiency.

Venous thromboembolism develops in 60–80% of individuals with either AT III, PC, or PS deficiency, usually before age 40 years. AT III–deficient individuals have a higher incidence of thrombosis than those with PC or PS deficiency. Individuals with resistance to APC have a lower tendency to thrombosis than those deficient for AT III, PC, or PS. Although resistance to APC has a higher prevalence in the population, most patients are asymptomatic until late in life. However, resistance to APC in combination with any of the other defects (AT III, PC, or PS) increases the risk to develop thrombosis.

Acquired risk factors for thrombosis (e.g., surgery, pregnancy, puerperium, immobilization) are known to increase the incidence of thrombosis in individuals with a primary hypercoagulable state. Thus women heterozygous for AT III deficiency during pregnancy or puerperium have a frequency of thrombosis of 31–44%; PC- or PS-deficient patients have 10–19%; and those with resistance to APC have 28%. Some studies also show an increased incidence of thrombosis in patients with AT III, PC, or PS deficiencies, and underwent abdominal, orthopedic, or cancer surgery. These clinical observations support the hypothesis that two or more gene interactions involving prothrombotic mutations create an inherited predisposition to thrombosis (hypercoagulable state) but that the thrombotic event is triggered by an acquired prothrombotic stimulus.

Diagnosis of Inherited Thrombophilia

The first step in diagnosing inherited thrombophilia involves taking a complete patient history to consider any acquired risk factors of thrombosis (e.g., SLE, malignancy, antipholized antibody/lupus anticoagulant [APA/LA]). Careful questioning about postoperative problems or sudden death in the patient or family should be done. The second step is to determine familial tendency to thrombosis by creating a pedigree or family tree diagram from information collected. A negative family history does not exclude thrombophilia, especially resistance to APC and hyperhomocysteinemia, because of their low penetrance in the population. The last step involves laboratory testing.

When should laboratory tests for thrombophilia be done and who should be tested? Laboratory diagnosis should be done after resolution of the acute thrombotic event, in stable patients who are not receiving anticoagulants. Laboratory tests to define a hypercoagulable state are costly. Functional assays for blood coagulation inhibitors done during an acute thrombotic event (even if obtained before treatment begins) are misleading, because of consumption of the inhibitory activity of these proteins during thrombus formation. Oral anticoagulants (e.g., warfarin) suppress the vitamin K–dependent PC and PS inhibitors and stimulate ATIII synthesis. Thus measurements of their activities during anticoagulant therapy are unreliable. Heparin therapy also affects the level of functional AT III. Therefore the best time to perform laboratory diagnosis is 1–2 weeks after completing the maintenance anticoagulation therapy (duration is usually 3–6 months).

Laboratory tests to assess AT III, PC, and PS deficiencies are indicated especially in individuals less than 45 years of age who have a positive family history for thrombosis or an unexplained etiology for venous thrombosis. The measurements should include both the concentration and function of each inhibitor. In PS deficiency free and bound PS levels should be determined. Resistance to APC and homocysteine levels should be done in any individual with thrombosis independent of age, because of their high frequency in the general population. Resistance to APC is screened by a functional assay based on the ability of patient plasma to resist the prolongation of the aPTT caused by addition of activated protein C. The sensitivity of the assay is 85%, and the specificity is above 90%. Its accuracy has been improved by addition of FV-deficient plasma to the test system. Only 5–10% patients with borderline results require DNA analysis of the FV gene. The latter assay can be done during the period of therapeutic anticoagulation, but not the former.

Homocysteine plasma levels are done before and 4 hours after an oral methionine load (0.1 g/kg body weight). This improves the separation between normal and heterozygous for cystathionine–β-synthase deficiency. To improve detection of heterozygous states molecular probes are now available to identify gene mutations.

Management of Inherited Thrombophilia

Primary, or Short-Term, Prophylaxis. Patients with thrombophilia (<40 years of years of age) before, during, and after surgery; during pregnancy; and puerperium (4 weeks) should receive prophylaxis with subcutaneous (s.c.) unfractionated or fractionated heparin. ATIII–deficient patients during pregnancy, because of the high risk for thrombosis, must receive either low molecular weight s.c. heparin or adjusted s.c. heparin (aPTT ratio 1.5—2.0). ATIII concentrates can be used during delivery (every other day), followed by heparin s.c. for a total of 4 weeks. ATIII concentrates during pregnancy do not offer any advantage over heparin and are not cost efficient. Low-molecular-weight heparin (fractionated heparin) is another alternative, but it is more expensive than regular unfractionated heparin.

Secondary, or Long-Term, Prophylaxis. All patients, except pregnant women, with thrombophilia who develop a first episode of thrombosis are treated with oral anticoagulant therapy (OAT), warfarin for 6 months (INR 2–3). Patients with multiple defects should be on life-long OAT. Thrombophilic patients with recurrence of thrombosis are also placed on life-long OAT.

Treatment of Acute Thrombosis. Treatment is the same for patients with or without inherited hypercoagulable states. The patient is started on unfractionated heparin intravenously to maintain aPTT ratio between 1.5 and 2.5 for 7 days. Alternatively, after one day of unfractionated heparin, the patient may be started on low molecular weight heparin. Oral anticoagulants are started at 24—48 hours after starting heparin therapy and overlapped with heparin, until therapeutic level (INR = 2–3) is achieved, which usually takes 3–5 days.

Patients with hyperhomocysteinemia are treated for thrombosis as outlined earlier. Prophylaxis with pyridoxine, folic acid, and B_{12} reduces the level of homocysteine, but it is unclear if it prevents further arterial or venous thrombosis.

ACQUIRED THROMBOPHILIA

Postoperative Venous Thrombosis

Postoperative venous thrombosis occurs frequently in the elderly, the obese, those with a medical or family history of venous thrombosis, and those undergoing major abdominal, chest, brain, or orthopedic surgery. Blood activation during surgery, immobilization after surgery, and stasis are the major factors for thrombosis. Similar mechanisms have been suggested in patients with congestive heart failure, myocardial infarction, or varicose veins.

Malignancy

Three types of procoagulants released by malignant cells activate or accelerate blood coagulation and are the triggers of thrombosis. These include tissue factor, enzymes that convert FX to FXa, and microvesicles (phospholipids), which are shed and serve as a template for binding activated coagulation factors (platelet membrane substitutes). These procoagulants are produced by mucin-type adenocarcinomas, such as those of breast, lung, prostate, pancreas, and bowel, which are all associated with a high incidence of venous thrombosis. In addition, in some tumors ineffective fibrinolysis is present.

Blood Disorders

Myeloproliferative disorders (MPD) and myelodysplastic syndromes (MDS), paroxysmal nocturial hemoglobinuria (PNH), sickle cell anemia, and hemolytic anemias are all associated with thromboembolism. In MPD, hyperviscosity of the blood, platelet activation, and endothelial injury lead to blood activation and thrombosis. The leading cause of death in patients with polycythemia vera and essential thrombocythemia is either arterial or venous thrombosis. PNH patients often present with thrombosis of hepatic veins or inferior vena cava (Budd-Chiari syndrome) or portal and mesenteric veins, before the diagnosis of PNH has been established. Platelet and blood activation are the triggers of thrombosis in PNH. The platelets have increased susceptibility to complement activation and to aggregating stimuli. In hemolysis ADP from hemolyzed red blood cells is the inducer of platelet aggregation. Arterial thrombosis is also common in these patients. Sickling of red cells causes obstruction of the microcirculation, and ADP from hemolyzed red cells activates platelets. (These are two important factors for development of either venous or arterial thrombosis in sickle cell anemia.)

Estrogen Therapy

With high-dose estrogen therapy there is a high incidence of thromboembolism. The thrombotic tendency appears to be secondary to increased synthesis of blood coagulation factors (FII, FVII, FVIII, FIX, FX, fibrinogen), decrease in fibrinolysis, decrease in t-PA, reduction of AT III functional activity, and endothelial injury. In low-dose estrogen therapy the risk of thromboembolism is much lower. However, the use of oral contraceptives (low-dose estrogens) in women with primary hypercoagulable states is contraindicated because of increased incidence of thrombosis.

Other Acquired Diseases

Other acquired diseases predisposing to venous thromboembolism are nephrotic syndrome, inflammatory bowel disease (IBD), and bone marrow transplantation. In nephrotic syndrome the patients lose AT III in the urine, platelets are hyperreactive, and injury to the vessel wall is common. In IBD, endothelial injury leading to blood and platelet activation, and reductions in PS, AT III, and PC have been proposed as important factors of thrombosis. Following allogeneic bone marrow transplantation, veno-occlusive disease of the liver develops in 21% of patients, with 45% succumbing from progressive liver disease. Veno-occlusive disease results from endothelial damage of hepatic venules and sinusoids, caused by a combination of radiation and chemotherapy effects. (See Chapter 8.)

Antiphospholipid Syndrome/Lupus Anticoagulant

Definition. Antiphospholipid antibodies (APA) are immunoglobulins (IgG, IgM, IgA, or mixtures) that interact with one or more negatively charged phospholipids in various laboratory assays. They prolong the aPTT and, to a lesser extent, the PT. Lupus anticoagulant (LA) is an antiphospholipid inhibitor with heparin-like activity. However, the clinical significance of APA and LA is the tendency to develop both venous and arterial thrombosis, and not hemorrhage!

APA relation to LA. APAs were first recognized in the detection of syphilis (1906). With the wide use of reagents consisting of a mixture of lipids (cardiolipin, lecithin, and cholesterol), such as the VDRL for syphilis, false-positive results were noted in patients with autoimmune disorders (e.g., SLE, Rheumatoid arthritis [RA], and Sjogren's syndrome). In 1952, two patients with SLE were described to have a circulating anticoagulant (heparin-like activity) that was not associated with bleeding. The anticoagulant was termed *lupus anticoagulant* (LA), a misnomer because the majority of patients with LA do not have SLE.

In 1983, a radioimmunoassay was developed to detect anticardiolipin antibodies (ACA) and suggested that ACA and LA were the same antibodies. Subsequent studies, however, showed that in 60% of patients, these antibodies were concordant, but in the other patients only one antibody was detected. Since then, marked heterogeneity among antibodies has been recognized, both within and between patients. Individual patients may have several antibodies, which react with negatively charged phospholipids. These antibodies may be of different isotypes, and avidity may vary greatly.

Antiphospholipid antibodies are frequently associated with a variety of conditions, such as viral and bacterial infections (e.g., AIDS), autoimmune connective tissue disorders (SLE, RA), malignancy, and medications like procainamide, chlorpromazine, and quinidine. APAs may also be detected in the absence of an underlying disease. The first clinical connection between LA and thrombosis (venous, arterial, livedo reticularis) was made in 1963 in patients with SLE. Many studies have since confirmed the high incidence of both arterial and venous thrombosis in association with APA/LA.

Antiphospholipid syndrome (APS) is defined as the association of antiphospholipid antibodies (LA or moderate to high levels of IgG or IgM anticardiolipin antibody) with venous or arterial thrombosis, recurrent fetal loss, and thrombocytopenia. Where there is no underlying disease, patients are categorized as having primary antiphospholipid syndrome (PAPS). Their symptoms are similar to those with APS associated with autoimmune connective tissue disorders. In APS there is a female-to-male ratio of 9:1; in PAPS this ratio is 2:1. In PAPS thrombocytopenia and antinuclear antibodies occur in 50% of patients, and the antiphospholipid antibody detected is a high-IgG anticardiolipin antibody titer.

Deep vein thrombosis and pulmonary embolism are the most common venous events in APS, but thrombosis in unusual places, such as renal and hepatic veins, may also occur. Arterial thrombosis can affect any artery, especially coronary, cerebral, and peripheral arteries. APS and PAPS are both associated with transient ischemic attacks (TIAs), visual disturbances such as amaurosis fugax, and single or recurrent cerebral infarcts. Patients less than 50 years of age who develop TIAs or strokes should be tested for LA and anticardiolipin antibodies. Vasculitis, rashes, and arthralgia are present in 50% of the patients with APS. Other manifestations include migraine headaches, livedo reticularis, and cardiac abnormalities (e.g., verrucous endocardial lesions affecting the mitral valve).

Characterization of LA and APA. The LA antigen is a hexagonal phospholipid, which requires a plasma cofactor (perhaps prothrombin). LA is detected in plasma by a coagulation assay employing Russel viper venom as reagent (d RVVT), and a platelet-neutralizing procedure (PNP). Results are reported as positive or negative. The anticardiolipin antibody antigen is a lamellar or micellar phospholipid, which requires β_2-glycoprotein 1 (β_2-GP1) as a cofactor. Antiphospholipid antibodies are measured by an ELISA. The results are expressed as mild, moderate, or high IgG or IgM antiphospholipid antibody units (each unit = 1 mg of antibody).

Laboratory diagnosis of APS requires moderate to high positive ACA IgG or IgM or positive LA (done on two occasions 12 weeks apart).

Pathogenesis of thrombosis in APS. A number of mechanisms have been proposed to explain the antiphospholipid antibody-induced thrombosis. Endothelial cells upon exposure to APA change their anticoagulant activities to cause powerful thrombogenic properties such as decreased synthesis of PGI_2, decreased expression of thrombomodulin and heparin sulfate activity, increased tissue factor expression, impairment of fibrinolysis (from a decreased t-PA and increased PAI), and increased platelet activating factor. In addition, patients with APS have been shown to have decreased plasma functional activities of AT III, PC, free PS, antibodies to β_2-GP1, and platelet activation. All these alterations were thought to be induced by APA directed against the specific phospholipids. Recently, however, APAs have been shown not to be directed against the phospholipid but to be directed at the protein bound to the phospholipid. Thus in 1996 Arnout proposed a double-hit mechanism to explain thrombosis in APS. After initial damage, anionic phospholipids are exposed on blood cells (e.g., platelets, neutrophils), on endothelial cells, or on trophoblasts. These reactive phospholipids are covered by phospholipid-binding proteins such as β_2-GP1 or prothrombin. If antibodies to these surface-bound proteins are present in blood, the immunoglobulins concentrate on the cell surface, bind to the Fc receptors, and induce all the thrombogenic changes described earlier. This hypothesis is partly supported by experimental data and by similar mechanisms that are involved in heparin-induced thrombocytopenia with thrombosis.

Management. APS patients are considered at high risk for thrombosis. For prophylaxis prior to and after surgery they are treated with heparin subcutaneously. During pregnancy women are treated with an adjusted dose of heparin, fixed-dose low-molecular-weight heparin, or aspirin together with low-dose steroids. Treatment of patients with acute thrombosis and associated APA is similar to that employed with the other hypercoagulable states with comparable thromboembolic events. Heparin is given IV to maintain the aPTT 2–2.5 times the baseline, and warfarin is started at 24–48 hours, and overlapped with heparin for 5 days. The INR is maintained at approximately 3.0. Patients with APS and recurrent thrombosis are anticoagulated with warfarin for life. Some patients with arterial and venous thrombosis history are placed on both warfarin and aspirin.

ANTITHROMBOTIC THERAPY

Anticoagulants are medications used in the prophylaxis and treatment of both arterial and venous thrombosis. Heparin (administerd parenterally) and coumarins (administerd orally) are the two most widely used anticoagulants in clinical practice.

Parenteral Anticoagulants

Heparin (unfractionated) is an anticoagulant consisting of a mixture of glycosaminoglycans ranging widely in molecular weight (5,000–30,000). Heparin exerts its anticoagulant effect by binding to AT III and potentiating AT III complex formation with active serine proteases of the blood coagulation cascade (thrombin, Xa, IXa, XIa, and XIIa). This complex formation leads to irreversible inactivation of the blood coagulation factors (see Fig. 6-10). Only a small fraction of heparin has AT III binding activity; however, heparin bound to AT III potentiates greatly the AT III inhibitory capacity (by approximately a factor of 1,000). Heparin activates platelets and binds to many others cells (e.g., EC, macrophages, fat cells), and activates lipases and the complement system. Heparin prevents thrombus formation and stops the growth of thrombi.

Heparin is metabolized by the liver and excreted by the kidneys. It is not absorbed by the gastrointestinal tract; thus it has to be administered intravenously or subcutaneously. At a dose of 100 U/kg, the biological half-life of heparin is 1 hour; at lower doses it decreases nonlinearly. Heparin binds to endothelial cells and macrophages, avidly (reason for bolus); the residual heparin is cleared more slowly by the kidneys. In addition, heparin can bind and be neutralized by proteins such as histidine-rich glycoprotein, platelet factor 4, and vitronectin; high levels of these proteins in circulation can cause relative resistance to heparin.

Heparins that are fractionated have a low molecular weight (4,000–8,000) and are designated *low-molecular-weight heparins (LMWHs)*. These act as anticoagulants by binding to AT III and inhibit specifically FXa rather than thrombin. It is unclear whether LMWHs have a lesser effect on platelets than unfractionated heparin.

Administration and Laboratory Monitoring of Heparin Therapy

Intravenous heparin is given continuously or intermittently; for patients with acute thrombosis (e.g., DVT, PE, mural thrombi, and others) continuous IV infusion is the best mode of administration.

Acute venous thrombosis (e.g., DVT) is treated with a heparin bolus followed by IV administered continuously. The dose of heparin is adjusted every 6 hours, to maintain the aPTT 1.5–2.5 × baseline (therapeutic range). In the first 24 hours the aPTT must be maintained within therapeutic range to prevent recurrence of thrombosis.

Oral anticoagulants (e.g., warfarin) should be started at 24 hours or 48 hours and overlapped with heparin for 3–5 days, until the antithrombotic effect of warfarin is achieved. One reason for starting coumadin at 24 hours, and not before, is to delay suppression of PC. (Recall that PC is a vitamin K–dependent clotting factor whose interruption in synthesis by warfarin will cause hypercoagulability and possible thrombus extension or propagation.)

In acute pulmonary embolism (PE) the heparin bolus should be increased in amount, because the heparin mean half-life in the setting of PE is shorter than normal by 20 minutes. The remainder of anticoagulation therapy for PE is similar to that described earlier for DVT and other venous thrombi.

Subcutaneous heparin injections are given intermittently for prophylaxis against thromboembolism. This short-term mode of heparin therapy does not require laboratory monitoring. Long-term subcutaneous heparin treatment for patients with contraindications to oral anticoagulants is useful but can lead to a serious complication, osteopenia and osteoporosis. Adjusted s.c. heparin dosage is recommended for high-risk patients, such as in AT III–deficient women during pregnancy; the dose is monitored by maintaining the aPTT, at 1.5–2.0 ratio (patient aPTT/mean average normal aPTT).

Low-molecular-weight heparins (LMWHs) are now available in the United States for parenteral use. These are administered s.c. once daily, or twice daily in a fixed dose, because of their long biological half-lives (3–18 hours). LMWH therapy is effective, does not require laboratory monitoring, but is much more expensive than unfractionated heparin therapy. It is now recommended for treatment of thromboembolism in cancer patients, pregnant women or others with contraindications to warfarin, and patients undergoing orthopedic surgery. It is now recommended as first-line therapy for DVT and PE. However, low molecular weight heparin preferably inhibits FXa rather than thrombin thus extension of thrombus may occur in acute thrombosis.

Complications of Heparin Therapy

Bleeding can be secondary to excessive anticoagulation, or impairment of platelet function by heparin, or due to heparin-induced thrombocytopenia. In addition, bleeding may result from potentiation of an underlying bleeding defect by heparin or by concomitant administration of antiplatelet agents or thrombolytic agents. Because intravenous heparin has a short half-life (1 hour), interruption of treatment is usually sufficient to correct bleeding caused by excessive anticoagulation. In severe cases of bleeding heparin can be neutralized by protamine sulfate, but protamine in excess can also cause bleeding. LMWHs also cause similar bleeding complications.

Heparin-induced thrombocytopenia (HIT) occurs in about 2% of patients treated with porcine heparin, but its incidence is much lower with heparin from other sources. HIT is an immune-mediated side effect of heparin. Antibodies are developed against a complex between heparin and platelet factor 4 (PF4), a heparin-binding glycoprotein stored in the platelet α-granules, but also having a receptor on the platelet membrane. Heparin-induced IgG binds to these membrane complexes, and then activates platelets via binding to the Fc receptor. Heparin-induced IgG also activates ECs with expression of tissue factor leading to activation of the blood coagulation and thrombus formation. Treatment consists of withdrawing heparin. Some patients may require corticosteroids or immunoglobulin therapy to recover the platelet count to normal. Platelet transfusion is contraindicated.

Heparin-induced thrombocytopenia and thrombosis (HITT) occur in fewer than 1% of the patients who develop thrombocytopenia. Patients at risk of developing HITT are usually post surgery, and the thrombosis can be arterial or venous. The therapy of HITT involves stopping heparin immediately and using alternative anticoagulants (e.g., ancrod, hirulog, LMW heparinoid). Platelet transfusion is contraindicated.

Heparin-induced osteoporosis occurs in patients treated with long-term heparin (>3 months) at doses of 20,000 U or greater daily. This is a problem for bedridden patients, the elderly, or pregnant women. Calcium heparin or calcium treatment must be considered.

New Anticoagulants. Hirudin, which is given parenterally, is a specific inhibitor of thrombin (7k protein), originally found in the salivary glands of leeches (*Hirudo medicinalis*). It binds to the active site of thrombin as well as to the site where thrombin binds to fibrinogen; thus hirudin can inhibit thrombin bound to fibrinogen but heparin cannot. Hirudin also does not require a cofactor to inhibit thrombin, nor does it inhibit any other serine proteases. Both hirudin and its synthetic analog, hirulog, are effective anticoagulants that do not affect the aPTT or cause bleeding complications but are devoid of antiplatelet effect.

Ancrod is an enzyme derived from the Malayan pit viper that cleaves fibrinopeptide A from fibrinogen without activating FXIII, thus preventing formation of cross-linking of fibrin. Soluble fibrin is then easily digested by plasmin. Ancrod therapy causes defibrinogenemia and increased FDPs, without excessive bleeding. Ancrod is effective in the treatment of HITT and has been used for several years in various countries. In the United States is only available for compassionate use and is still an investigational drug.

Oral Anticoagulants

Oral anticoagulants are derivatives of coumarin or indanedione that exert their actions as vitamin K antagonists. Warfarin sodium (coumadin) is the most frequently used in the United States.

Warfarin is almost always given orally, but an injectable preparation is available. Warfarin is a racemic mixture of equal amounts of the two active isomers, the S and the R forms. The isomeric composition of warfarin is important clinically, because the S-warfarin is five times more potent as an antagonist of vitamin K than the R form. Drugs that inhibit the metabolite clearance of the S form potentiate the anticoagulant activity of warfarin much more than those that inhibit the clearance of the R form.

Warfarin is rapidly absorbed by the gastrointestinal tract and reaches peak blood levels within 90 minutes. It circulates in blood mostly bound to albumin, with only 3% in free form in plasma. However, it is this free warfarin that is biologically active. Warfarin has a mean half-life of 36–42 hours. It is metabolized by the liver to an inactive metabolite, which is conjugated with glucuronic acid and ultimately excreted in the urine and stool.

Drugs that interfere with either the binding to albumin or excretion, or that decrease absorption of vitamin K alter the response to both warfarin and diet. Thus the dose-response to warfarin depends on pharmacokinetic factors (e.g., differences in absorption or metabolic clearance of warfarin), pharmacodynamic factors (e.g., differences in the hemostatic response to given doses of warfarin), technical factors (e.g., laboratory errors, poor compliance, poor communication between care givers and patients), and unexplained factors.

Warfarin and other coumarins induce their anticoagulant effect by interfering with the cyclic interconversion of vitamin K and its oxidized form, vitamin K epoxide (Fig. 6-25). Reduced vitamin K is a cofactor for the postribosomal γ-carboxylation of the glutamic acid residues of FII, FVII, FX, FIX, PC, and PS. γ-Carboxylation of these proteins permits conformational change that in the presence of calcium allows binding to phospholipid surfaces, and therefore biological activity. Warfarin therapy reduces the functional activity of these vitamin K–dependent proteins and changes the blood to a hypocoagulable state. The warfarin effect is first observed on the FVII and PC levels, because of the short mean half-life (6 hours) of these proteins; next on FIX, FX, and PS (24–48 hours); and finally on prothrombin (72 hours). Since the goal is to reduce prothrombin to minimize thrombin formation, anticoagulation with warfarin cannot be achieved in less than 3 days.

Warfarin loading dose for elderly patients, women, and patients with hemostatic defects should be low. Other individuals can be started on higher doses. This dose should be repeated for 3 consecutive days and then adjusted according to the prothrombin time or INR. Large loading doses of 20 mg affect the INR rapidly, because of marked suppression of FVII, but the *in vivo* anticoagulant effect on prothrombin takes 3 days. Also, large loading doses can cause dramatic falls in PC levels and predispose to warfarin-induced skin necrosis. (See later.)

Monitoring Oral Anticoagulant Therapy

The prothrombin time (PT) is the test to monitor oral anticoagulant therapy. It has been standardized, as described under laboratory tests, and reported as PT/INR. The recommended therapeutic range for oral anticoagulant therapy is shown in Table 6-18.

Duration of Treatment

The length of treatment for the short term is 1 month in preparation for cardioversion. Short- to medium-term treatment last for 3–6 months for DVT and PE. Long-term treatment exceeds 12 months for recurrent thromboembolism. Life-long or chronic anticoagulation treatment is necessary for patients with atrial fibrillation, prosthetic valve replacement, rheumatic heart disease, arterial grafts, and thrombophilia, or APS.

TABLE 6-18. *THERAPEUTIC RANGE FOR ORAL ANTICOAGULANT THERAPY*

INDICATION	INR
Venous thrombosis Prophylaxis (↑ risk surgery) Treatment DVT and PE	2.0–3.0
Arterial thrombosis Atrial fibrillation, TIAs Cardiomyopathy Hypo- and dyskinesis Acute myocardial infarction Mural thrombi Tissue heart valves Peripheral vascular disease	2.0–3.0
Mechanical prosthetic valves	2.5–3.5
Acute myocardial infarction (to prevent reinfarction)	2.5–3.5
Recurrent systemic embolism	2.5–3.5

Complications of Warfarin Therapy

Bleeding is the main adverse effect of warfarin. The risk of bleeding is influenced by the intensity of treatment. INRs in excess of 4.0 are associated with higher incidence of bleeding than ratios of 2.0–3.0. Minor bleeding (e.g., nosebleeds) is treated with local measures and reduction or temporary withdrawal of the warfarin. Major bleeding (e.g., large hematomas, intracranial or retroperitoneal bleeding) requires aggressive reversal of anticoagulation with fresh-frozen plasma and/or vitamin K (parenterally). Bleeding from the gastrointestinal tract or genitourinary tract suggests an underlying pathology and requires appropriate diagnostic testing.

Purple toe syndrome, which involves *skin necrosis*, is an uncommon complication of warfarin therapy. It occurs between 1 and 6 weeks of therapy and is the result of thrombosis of the venules and capillaries within the subcutaneous fat. (Abdominal and breast fat can be affected too.) In the purple toe syndrome, patients develop pain and blue discoloration of the plantar aspects of the big toe and of the first, second, and third toes. An association between skin necrosis and PC and PS deficiencies has been made. This complication, however, can occur in individuals without PC or PS deficiency and may be associated with large loading doses of warfarin. Patients with underlying disorders (e.g., vasculitis, mural thrombi, large abdominal aneurysms) in whom blood activation exists may develop purple toe syndrome if started on warfarin without previous heparin therapy. Skin necrosis therapy involves stopping the warfarin and starting heparin IV. If patients require long-term anticoagulation and warfarin is contraindicated, they can be treated with heparin or LMWH subcutaneously.

Drugs or other factors interfering with warfarin therapy are shown in Table 6-19.

TABLE 6-19. *FACTORS INFLUENCING WARFARIN THERAPY*

POTENTIATION OF WARFARIN THERAPY	INHIBITION OF WARFARIN THERAPY
Drugs that decrease binding to albumin: phenylbutazone, statins, sulfonamide, clofibrate	Drugs that decrease warfarin action: barbiturates, rifampin, penicillin, alcohol, carbamazepin, griseofulvin
Drugs that inhibit metabolic, clearance: disulfiram, trimethopansulfamthoxozole, phenylbutazone, sulfinpyrazone, cimetidine, omeprazole, statins, amiodarone, allopurinol, tricyclic antidepressants, antifungal agents;	Increased synthesis of blood coagulation factors: oral contraceptives
Drugs that interfere with vitamin K: cephalosporins (1st and 2nd generation), High-dose salicylates	Inherited resistance to warfarin
Drugs that alter the hepatic receptor: thyroxine and quinidine	Pregnancy
Potentiation of anticoagulant action: erythromycin, clofibrate, anabolic steroids, liver disease, increased absorption of vitamin K	

TABLE 6-20. *THROMBOLYTIC AGENTS*	
AGENTS	**HALF-LIFE (min)**
Streptokinase	18–25
Urokinase	13–20
Tissue plasminogen activator (t-PA or rt-PA)	2–6
Single-chain urokinase plasminogen activator (rscu-PA)	5–8
Acylated plasminogen streptokinase activator complex (APSAC)	70–90

Thrombolytic agents act by causing dissolution of thrombi. Several agents are available clinically (Table 6-20). This therapeutic modality is standard for the treatment of acute myocardial infarction and appears to be beneficial for initial treatment of acute peripheral arterial occlusion, massive pulmonary embolism, and selected cases of DVT.

The clinical efficacy of thrombolytic therapy is based on the ability of these agents to generate plasmin from plasminogen in circulation or within the thrombus (Fig. 6-13). Plasmin formed in circulation is rapidly neutralized by antiplasmins under physiologic conditions. However, during thrombolytic therapy, the inhibitors are consumed rapidly, permitting the free plasmin to dissolve fibrin. This creates a lytic state in which the excess plasmin also digests fibrinogen, coagulation factors (e.g., V, VIII, XII, vWf), thrombospondin, and platelet membrane glycoproteins (GPIb, GPIIb/IIIa). The thrombus-bound plasmin is not effectively inactivated by antiplasmins and initiates lysis of the thrombus rapidly.

Laboratory monitoring is unnecessary for single-dose streptokinase, recombinant t-PA, or APSAC. In the treatment of PE with streptokinase or urokinase thrombin time (5–7 times baseline), fibrinogen and FDPs are followed at least twice daily to ensure achievement of the lytic state.

Complications of thrombolytic therapy include bleeding and allergic reactions. Bleeding occurs in 3–40% of patients. The incidence of bleeding is greatly increased in patients who are receiving concomitant antiplatelet agents, calcium channel blockers, or anticoagulants. Bleeding occurs at sites of vascular invasion for diagnostic, therapeutic procedures or monitoring. Avoidance of invasive procedures reduces major bleeding complications to less than 5%. Intracerebral bleeding occurs in up to 2% patients, especially in the elderly, women, low-body-weight patients, patients with previous cerebral vascular disease, and those taking antiplatelet agents or anticoagulants concomitantly.

Allergic reactions occur in association with streptokinase or APSAC therapy as a result of previous streptococcus infections. Contraindications to thrombolytic therapy are shown in Table 6-21.

TABLE 6-21. *CONTRAINDICATIONS TO THROMBOLYTIC THERAPY*	
ABSOLUTE CONTRAINDICATIONS	**RELATIVE CONTRAINDICATIONS**
Recent or active internal bleeding	Major surgery or trauma <10 days
Head injury, surgery, hemorrhage, or stroke <2 months	Bleeding diathesis, congenital or acquired
	PMHx of GI bleeding
Aortic dissection	Traumatic CPR
Intracranial aneurysm or cancer	Thrombocytopenia
Intraspinal neoplasm	Prior organ biopsy; prior arterial puncture (<10 days)
	Subacute endocarditis or left ventricular mural thrombus
	Uncontrolled hypertension
	Pregnancy or delivery (<10 days)

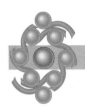

CASE PRESENTATION

A 22-year-old woman comes to see you because of easy bruising. She noticed a month ago that there were many bruises on her thighs and arms that did not develop in association with even the mildest form of traumatic stress. She is also concerned because menstrual periods that always seemed "worse than my friends'" have become heavier and longer. She bruised easily as a child and suffered from occasional nosebleeds but never underwent a surgical procedure, including a tooth extraction. She has never been pregnant. Family history is notable for a mother "who bruises and bleeds easily" and a father who is completely normal. There is a younger sister who has a history similar to that of the patient. The patient takes no medication and is training to be a nurse anesthetist. No alcohol or illict drug history was noted. There were no HIV risk factors. Physical examination shows a well-appearing patient with normal vital signs. Skin examination shows many ecchymoses in various stages of resolution 2–3 cm in diameter over the outside of thighs and upper arms. Mucous membranes are free of petechiae or purpuras. There are no head, ears, eye, nose, or throat (HEENT), neck, lung, or cardiac abnormalities. Abdomen is benign. Extremities show the ecchymoses described earlier, and the neurologic examination is intact. Breast, rectal, and genital examinations are normal as well.

Question 1. What should you be thinking about?

Answer. Von Willebrand disease is the most common inherited bleeding disorder and occurs in approximately one in 1,000 individuals. Hemophilia A has an incidence of one in 10,000 males who inherit one X chromosome to which it is linked. Females would need to inherit two X chromosomes that are abnormal in order for a symptomatic coagulopathy to develop. Especially with a normal father but a symptomatic mother and sister, it is more likely that this woman is suffering from a genetically linked coagulation defect, probably von Willebrand disease. Other hereditary defects would be less likely. An acquired coagulation problem is a possibility, especially since there has been a recent exacerbation of symptoms, but there is a somewhat compelling family history that must be considered.

Question 2. How should you proceed now?

Answer. Laboratory testing should commence with prothrombin time (PT) and activated partial thromboplastin time (aPTT), which assess the soluble coagulation system. Platelets should be assayed first numerically with a CBC and peripheral smear review and then perhaps with platelet function studies. Bleeding time should be the first platelet function assessment. Coagulation factor abnormalities usually lead to the development of ecchymoses and other hemorrhagic problems. Platelet disorders (quantitative or qualitative) cause petechiae and purpuras and other hemorrhagic problems. However, one can see bruising (ecchymosis) with platelet-associated problems as well.

Question 3. PT = 11 sec; aPTT = 34 sec (both normal). Platelet count is 345,000/μL with normal peripheral smear review. Bleeding time is 8 minutes (normal). What do you do next? Can you tell the patient she is normal?

Answer. Although the laboratory values are not abnormal, the aPTT and bleeding time values are at the upper limit of the normal range. Von Willebrand disease is notorious for being manifested by normal or slightly abnormal screening test values at different time points. Hormonal or other factors may be involved in control of the coagulation system that lead to exaceration of clinical or laboratory abnormalities (but the time to check a woman is during the first week or two, the *preluteal phase,* of her menstrual cycle). You ask for this patient's values to be repeated next month.

Question 4. This is done. The aPTT is now 39 seconds and the bleeding time is 9.5 minutes. What is the next step?

Answer. The elevated aPTT is addressed by performing a 1:1 mix (patient's plasma and normal plasma). This will correct a factor deficiency (it did in this patient, with the aPTT falling to 27 seconds) but will not change the value if an inhibitor is present. Given the elevated bleeding time as well as aPTT, one would be justified in making the diagnostic leap that this is von Willebrand disease (a coagulation system defect plus a platelet defect) and doing a von Willebrand disease screen.

The von Willebrand screen was done with the following results; factor VIII: C = 50% (normal = 50–180%). Ristocetin cofactor = 50% (normal = 50–150%). Von Willebrand's antigen = 50% (normal = 50–180%).

Question 5. Have you made a firm diagnosis? Is there more to do?

Answer. The data are fully consistent with von Willebrand disease, but the subtype may need to be better defined because treatment with desmopressin (DDAVP) may cause patients with type IIB von Willebrand disease to consume platelets and thereby exacerbate their coagulation problem. Patients with the most common type (I) have no such complications from DDAVP.

Question 6. How can you define the subtypes?

Answer. Western blot analysis of von Willebrand multimers will provide the answer. This patient turns out to have qualitatively normal multimers, but they are reduced in number. This fits with a type I diagnosis. Now you can give full information to the patient.

Follow-up:
Wisdom tooth extraction was successfully performed with DDAVP coverage 1 year after diagnosis. The patient continues to do well.

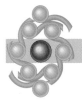

CASE PRESENTATION

A 23-year-old woman has come to the emergency room because of left calf swelling and pain. She has been well most of her adult life and has had no serious illnesses requiring hospitalization. She takes birth control pills daily. Three days prior to admission she noted left calf discomfort; over the last day it has been painful, red, and swollen. Her thigh has begun to ache as well. The patient has never been pregnant. She does not smoke cigarettes, drink alcohol, or take illicit drugs. There are no HIV risk factors. She works as a clerk in a convenience store. There has been no recent travel or immobilization. An uncle died unexpectedly at age 37 following a surgical procedure. Physical examination is significant for left calf swelling, erythema, heat, and tenderness. No cords are noted, but swelling has begun. There is no adenopathy in the groin. Screening laboratory data are normal. She undergoes 2-D Doppler ultrasound, which shows deep venous thrombosis in the calf and thigh. She is begun on heparin, and warfarin is started 24 hours later.

Question 1 . Should this patient be evaluated for the hypercoagulable state?

Answer. Yes. The patient's family history and seemingly unprovoked deep venous thrombosis raise concerns about a hereditary hypercoagulable state perhaps provoked by acquired risk factors such as birth control pills.

Question 2. What studies should be done?

Answer. Although it is certainly not cost effective to screen everyone, many laboratories can now inexpensively do a panel of tests that will assess the more common abnormalities contributing to hypercoagulability. These include tests for antithrombin III deficiency, protein C and S deficiencies, lupus anticoagulant and other associated antiphospholipid antibodies, activated protein C resistance, and homocystine elevation.

Question 3. When is the ideal time to obtain these?

Answer. Blood could have been drawn for these studies prior to beginning heparin or warfarin therapy, because heparin will affect antithrombin III levels and warfarin will affect protein C and S levels. Also, in the face of active clot deposition some of the tests may give misleading results. Therefore waiting for the course of therapy to be completed, allowing another 2 weeks to pass, and then doing these studies would be ideal.

Using a functional assay, the screening test for activated protein C showed a low value for this protein. An Factor V Leiden mutation was subsequently demonstrated.

Question 4. How should you advise her?

Answer. The patient has a common but real predisposition to hypercoagulability because of this disorder. She should probably be advised against taking estrogen-containing birth control pills because estrogen is an inducer of the hypercoagulable state. In addition, if she is immobilized, such as for a surgical operation, prophylactic anticoagulant therapy should be advised. At this point it is unclear whether this patient should be on lifelong anticoagulation if she is free of other risk factors. Anticoagulation during a high-estrogen state such as pregnancy may be needed. It may of value to do screening tests on her relatives so that they can be advised about their risk of hypercoagulability.

Follow–up. The patient informed her relatives of her diagnosis and encouraged them to undergo testing. After much discussion, she decided to discontinue birth control pills, but she decided against taking anticoagulant medication. She agreed to return for consideration of anticoagulation therapy if she became pregnant.

SELECTED READING

NORMAL HEMOSTASIS

Colman WR, Marder VJ, Salzman EW, Hirsh J. Overview of hemostasis. In: Colman RW, Hirsh J, Marder VJ, Salzman EW, eds. *Hemostasis and Thrombosis: Basic Principles and Clinical Practice*, 3rd ed. Philadelphia: JB Lippincott; 1994: 3–18.
This chapter is the most comprehensive general review of hemostasis available in the literature.

Esmon CT. The roles of protein C and thrombomodulin in the regulation of blood coagulation. *J Biol Chem* 1989;264: 4743–4749.
This article was the first to describe the role of protein C and thrombomodulin in blood coagulation.

Furie WA, Furie BC. Molecular basis of vitamin K–dependent gamma carboxylation. *N Engl J Med* 1990;75: 1753–1762.
This article describes in detail the biochemistry of vitamin K–dependent factors.

Hawiger J. Adhesive interactions of platelets and their blockade. *Ann NY Acad Sci* 1991;614: 270–278.
This article describes the mechanisms of platelet adhesion in physiologic hemostasis and in thrombosis. It also discusses the implications of platelet-adhesive inhibition in clinical medicine.

Ruggeri ZM, Ware J. The structure and function of vWf. *Thromb Haemost* 1992;67: 594.
This is an excellent and classic article on the biochemistry, function, and laboratory evaluation of vWf.

Salvesen G, Pizzo SV. Proteinase inhibitors: α-macroglobulins, serpins, and kunins. In: Colman RW, Hirsh J, Marder VJ, Salzman EW, eds. *Hemostasis and Thrombosis: Basic Principles and Clinical Practice*, 3rd ed. Philadelphia: JB Lippincott; 1994: 241–258.
The best review in the subject.

Shen L, Dahlback B. Factor V and protein S as synergistic cofactors to activated protein C in degradation of factor VIIIa. *J Biol Chem* 1994;269: 18735–18738.
An original article; well written and very informative.

DISORDERS OF HEMOSTASIS AND THOMBOSIS

Arnout J. The pathogenesis of the antiphospholipid syndrome: a hypothesis based on the parallelisms with heparin-induced thrombocytopenia. *Thromb Haemost* 1996; 75: 536–541.

Provocative review article.

Asherson RA, Khamashta MA, Gil A, et al. The primary antiphospholipid syndrome: major clinical and serological features. *Medicine* 1989;68:366–374.
Good review article.

Dahlback B. Resistance to activated protein, the Arg 506 to Gln mutation in the factor V gene, and venous thrombosis. *Thromb Haemost* 1995;73:739–742.
Excellent article relating the factor V defect to thrombosis.

Dahlback B, Hildebrand B. Inherited resistance to activated protein C is corrected by anticoagulant cofactor activity found to be a property of factor V. *Proc Natl Acad Sci USA* 1994;91:1396–1400.
Original article identifying the mechanism of resistance to protein C.

De Stefano V, Finazzi G, Mannucci PM. Inherited thrombophilia: pathogenesis, clinical syndromes, and management. *Blood* 1996;87:3531–3544.
This is a very-well-referenced and informative review article.

Feinstein DI. Acquired disorders of hemostasis. In: Colman RW, Hirsh J, Marder VJ, Salzman EW, eds. *Hemostasis and Thrombosis: Basic Principles and Clinical Practice*, 3rd ed. Philadelphia: JB Lippincott; 1994:881–905.
This chapter is an overview of all acquired disorders of hemostasis and their respective management.

Fourth ACCP Consensus Conference on Antithrombotic Therapy. Dalen JE, Hirsh J, eds. *Chest* (supplement) 1995;108:225–521.
State-of-art review of the guidelines for practice of antithrombotic therapy.

Geerts WH, Jay RM, Darmon J-K, et al. A comparison of low dose heparin with low molecular weight heparin as prophylaxis against venous thromboembolism after major trauma. *N Engl J Med* 1996;335:701–707.
State-of-art review article.

Greengard JS, Sun X, Xu X, Fernandez JA, Griffin JH, Evatt B. Activated protein C resistance caused by Arg 506 Gln mutation in Fva. *Lancet* 1994;343:1361–1362.
Excellent article demonstrating elegantly the cause of PC resistance.

Harker LA, Slichter SJ, Scott CR, Ross R. Homocysteinemia: vascular injury and arterial thrombosis. *N Engl J Med* 1974;291:537–543.

Hoyer LW. Hemophilia A. *N Engl J Med* 1994;330:38–47.
Superb FVIII review, and diagnosis and treatment of FVIII deficiency, by one of the greatest authors on FVIII biochemistry and its relation to the vWF protein.

Joist HJ. Hemostatic abnormalities in liver disease. In: Colman RW, Hirsh J, Marder VJ, Salzman EW, eds. *Hemostasis and Thrombosis: Basic Principles and Clinical Practice*, 3rd ed. Philadelphia: JB Lippincott; 1994:906–920.
Comprehensive review on hemostatic alterations in liver disease.

Marder VJ, Feinstein DI, Francis CW, Colman RW. Consumptive thrombohemorrhagic disorders. In: Colman RW, Hirsh J, Marder VJ, Salzman EW, eds. *Hemostasis and Thrombosis: Basic Principles and Clinical Practice*, 3rd ed. Philadelphia; JB Lippincott; 1994:1023–1063.
This is the most comprehensive review in the literature in this subject.

Schaffer AI. Hypercoagulable states: molecular genetics to clinical practice. *Lancet* 1994;344:1739–1742.

This article is stimulating, concise, and very informative.

Scott JP, Montgomery RR. Therapy of von Willebrand disease. *Semin Thromb Hemost* 1993;19:37–47.
Excellent review of vWD diagnosis and therapy.

Triplett DA. Laboratory diagnosis of lupus anticoagulant. *Semin Thromb Hemost* 1990; 16:182–191.
Comprehensive review of the LA laboratory diagnosis.

Triplett DA. Antiphospholipid antibodies and thrombosis: a consequence, coincidence or cause? *Arch Pathol Lab Med* 1993;117:78–88.
This is a comprehensive and stimulating review, with many contributions made by the author.

Weitz JI. Low molecular weight heparin. *N Eng J Med* 1997; 337: 688.
A recent review of mechanisms of action and recommendations for treatment of acute thrombosis with low molecular weight heparin.

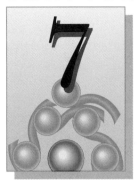

Bone Marrow Failure, Aplastic Anemia

Daniel E. Dunn

Peripheral blood cytopenias (anemia, leukopenia, or thrombocytopenia) can be due to increased loss, sequestration, consumption, or destruction of mature circulating blood elements, or to impaired production of mature cells resulting from a process that affects the origin of these cells, the bone marrow. This chapter will describe only conditions in the latter category, termed *bone marrow failure syndromes*. The mechanism of this impaired production can be either intrinsic to the bone marrow (as with congenital or inherited syndromes), secondary to agents extrinsic to the bone marrow (as with autoimmune, drug-, or virus-related syndromes), or, most commonly, of unknown etiology. This chapter attempts to organize these syndromes on the basis of clinical presentation and/or etiology (when known).

ACQUIRED APLASTIC ANEMIA

Acquired aplastic anemia (AA) is characterized by peripheral blood pancytopenia and bone marrow aplasia (hypocellularity). The absent hematopoietic tissue is replaced by fatty tissue. AA is typically idiopathic; it may be associated with other conditions, but causal relationships have not been established. The presence of clonal disorders (such as malignancy or myelodysplastic syndrome [MDS]) that impair hematopoiesis, however, rules out AA as the diagnosis.

EPIDEMIOLOGY AND ETIOLOGY

Incidence.

1. 2 per 10^6 in Western Europe (and presumably, the United States)
2. Two to three times *higher* in the Far East

Epidemiology. A bimodal age distribution has peak incidences during early adulthood and in the elderly. No predilection with regard to race or gender has been noted.

Etiology.

1. Chemicals: Patients with unrecognized AA are often prescribed antibiotics and nonsteroidal anti-inflammatory drugs (NSAIDs) prior to performance of any blood counts. Thus a cause-and-effect relationship between these drugs and the subsequently identified AA is difficult to establish on an individual-case basis. Certain medications and chemicals, however, have been found to be associated with significantly higher risks of AA; a feature common to many of the implicated agents is the benzene ring.
   a. Benzene: a causative relationship is likely. Related aromatic hydrocarbons (e.g. trinitrotoluene—TNT) and insecticides have also been implicated
   b. Chloramphenicol, NSAIDs (especially indomethacin and phenylbutazone), gold, sulfonamides, certain neuroleptics, antithyroid drugs, anti-convulsants (e.g., diphenylhydantoin and carbamazepine)
   c. Cytotoxic chemotherapeutic agents and ionizing radiation also produce both pancytopenia and a hypocellular bone marrow.
2. Certain viral infections can rarely be accompanied by hypoplastic cytopenias:
   a. Infectious mononucleosis with Epstein-Barr virus (EBV)
   b. Hepatitis (non-A, non-B, non-C)
   c. HIV
   d. Parvovirus B19 causes an isolated erythroid suppression, transient aplastic crisis or pure red cell aplasia (see section on pure red cell aplasia)
3. Immune disorders
   a. Graft-versus-host disease (GVHD): hematopoietic progenitors are targets for alloreactive donor lymphocytes in, for example, transfusion-associated GVHD
   b. Eosinophilic fasciitis
   c. Hypoimmunoglobulinemia
   d. Thymoma and thymic carcinoma
4. Paroxysmal nocturnal hemoglobinuria (PNH)
5. Pregnancy
6. Idiopathic: Most cases of AA are *not* associated with any identifiable etiologic factors

NATURAL HISTORY

Untreated aplastic anemia in the pretransfusion era was typically fatal within 6 months. With improved transfusion practices, patients unresponsive to treatment can now be supported for several years but can become refractory to platelets due to the development of alloantibodies. Persistently neutropenic patients may eventually succumb to bacterial or, increasingly, fungal infections. Spontaneous remission is probably rare.

PATHOPHYSIOLOGY

Multiple lines of laboratory and clinical evidence point to a consistent quantitative deficiency in the most primitive hematopoietic stem cells of AA patients. In most cases, both drug-induced as well as idiopathic, bone marrow suppression is mediated by immune mechanisms. Activated cytotoxic T-lymphocytes (i.e., $CD8^+DR^+$) are often found in the bone marrow and peripheral blood of patients with AA. These cells can produce both interferon ($IFN\gamma$) and tumor necrosis factor ($TNF\alpha$), two antiproliferative cytokines with proven hematosuppressive activity which induce apoptosis in hematopoietic target cells. Hence the early clinical observation that a bone marrow transplant from a *syngeneic* donor (i.e., identical twin, without AA) is often ineffective comes, in retrospect, as no surprise. The immunosuppressive preparative regimen that is routinely administered prior to transplantation of normal marrow, if it does not include radiation, has in several instances been found to induce remissions in the absence of marrow infusions.

DIAGNOSIS

Symptoms and Signs. These are as expected from pancytopenia—bleeding, bruising, infections, lethargy, shortness of breath, etc. Unexplained symptoms (weight loss, pruritus) and signs (lymphadenopathy, hepatosplenomegaly) should trigger a search for another cause of the cytopenia(s).

Severity. *Severe* aplastic anemia (SAA) is defined by a hypocellular bone marrow biopsy and two of the following three criteria:

1. Absolute reticulocyte count $< 40,000/\mu L$
2. Absolute neutrophil count $< 500/\mu L$
3. Platelet count $< 20,000/\mu L$

Very severe aplastic anemia is defined by a neutrophil count $< 200 \, \mu L$, and has a significantly worse prognosis.

Moderate aplastic anemia (MAA) is hypoplastic pancytopenia that does not fulfill these stringent criteria.

Laboratory Studies.

1. In addition to standard chemistry panels (markedly elevated liver function tests, for example, are suggestive of the hepatitis/aplasia syndrome), folate and B_{12} levels, all patients should be tested for HIV and have a Ham's test performed to detect paroxysmal nocturnal hemoglobinuria (PNH)
2. Cytogenetics
3. Depending on the clinical scenario, tests for one or more of the following may be appropriate:
   a. B19 parvovirus: if only the erythroid lineage is affected
   b. Fanconi anemia (FA): occasionally positive in young adults (< 50 years old) despite the absence of characteristic skeletal abnormalities

Bone Marrow Examination.

1. *Biopsy* of the bone marrow *must* be performed because cellularity cannot be quantitated from an aspirate smear. The standard criterion for AA is

TABLE 7-1. *BONE MARROW MORPHOLOGY IN MYELODYSPLASIA VERSUS APLASTIC ANEMIA*

CHARACTERISTICS	MYELODYSPLASIA	APLASTIC ANEMIA
Cellularity	Usually normal, increased	Decreased
Erythropoiesis		
Megaloblastic	Very common	Common
Dyserythropoietic	Very common	Unusual
Maturation defects	Frequent	Not found
Ringed sideroblasts	Often	Not found
Myelopoiesis		
Monocyte prominence	Very common	Unusual
Mid-myeloid predominance	Very common	Unusual
Increased blasts	Yes	Not found
Megakaryocytes		
Atypical morphology	Very common	Not found

By definition ringed sideroblasts and myeloblasts are observed in some of the myelodysplastic syndromes. Dys-erythropoietic red cell precursors show bizarre forms with multiple or irregular nuclei. Megakaryocytes can show defective nuclear polyploidization and increased internuclear spaces, or they may be small, with only a few nuclei and peculiar granulation.

less than 25% cellularity on the biopsy, but cellularity may be patchy. Fat generally comprises the nonhematopoietic balance of the marrow space. Lymphocytes, plasma cells, and macrophages may also be present; if lymphocytes are organized in para-trabecular follicles, the diagnosis of lymphoma should be considered. Reticulin is not increased.

2. *Aspirates* of the bone marrow show little or no hematopoietic tissue. Dysplasia of the erythroid lineage is common; dysplasia of the granulocytic or megakaryocytic lineages is suggestive of MDS.

Differential Diagnosis (Of Pancytopenia With Low Cellularity).

1. Inherited AA: Fanconi's and others
2. Myelodysplastic syndrome (MDS)—hypocellular variant (see Table 7-1)
3. Aleukemic leukemia (AML)
4. Acute lymphocytic leukemia
5. Lymphoma
6. Hairy cell leukemia
7. Infectious causes (mycobacteria, legionella, Q fever)
8. Miscellaneous (anorexia nervosa, starvation, hypothyroidism)

MANAGEMENT

Temporizing measures serve no purpose in the management of patients with AA and serve only to increase the patient's exposure to infectious agents and blood products. A decision regarding immunosuppression versus bone marrow transplantation should be made quickly and then rapidly instituted. Ongoing active medical problems related to the patient's aplasia (e.g., a systemic infection or hepatitis) should not, in general, delay therapy.

Bone Marrow Transplantation. (Chapter 8). An HLA-matched sibling bone marrow transplant (BMT) corrects the two principal pathologies of AA: autoimmunity and the defect in hematopoietic stem cells. This is accomplished at the risk of a new pathology—graft versus host disease (GVHD). An important consideration in BMT that is specific to AA is the increased incidence of graft rejection. This is thought to be due to the underlying autoimmune state in the recipient against the very organ being transplanted—marrow. Attempts to minimize one morbidity often lead to an increase in a second morbidity. Thus if purified hematopoietic stem cells, free of donor lymphocytes, are used for the BMT, GVHD decreases in incidence and severity, but the risk of graft rejection/failure rises. An important prognostic factor in graft rejection is the number of blood products transfused prior to the transplant: more than 40 units of platelets correlates with a significantly increased risk of graft rejection. Thus the decision to transplant should be made as quickly as possible after diagnosis of AA, and implemented promptly. The most important prognostic factor for GVHD is patient age: younger AA patients (< 20 years old) have about a 1 in 4 chance of acute or chronic GVHD; the risk in older AA patients is higher. The standard regimen used to prepare the patient for BMT consists of high-dose cyclophosphamide on four consecutive days. Total body irradiation (TBI) decreases the risk of graft rejection but increases the risk of GVHD and possibly also late complications such as malignant tumors. The long-term survival in AA patients less than 40 years old treated with HLA-matched sibling BMT ranges at various institutions from 60% to 90% but drops significantly with advancing age.

Immunosuppression. BMT from an HLA-matched sibling is available to only a minority of patients. Over the past 20 years, striking progress in immunosuppressive therapy has been made, such that the current standard regimen of antithymocyte globulin (ATG) (or antilymphocyte globulin [ALG] in Europe) plus cyclosporine A (CsA) can be expected to produce remissions in about 70% of patients, regardless of age. Survival at 3 years for all patients who undergo immunosuppression is about equivalent to that for BMT. Figures for longer survival await follow-up of the cohort of AA patients treated with this latest generation of immunosuppressive therapy. Both components of the ATG + CsA regimen produce significant but manageable toxicities. Low-dose methylprednisolone is given for the first 2 weeks as prophylaxis against severe serum sickness, a sequela of ATG/ALG. If severe arthralgia or other complications develop, steroid therapy may be extended but should be tapered as soon as possible. Cyclosporine may cause renal insufficiency, hypertension, gingival hypertrophy, hypertrichosis, myalgia, and arthralgia, and dose adjustments to below the target level of 200–400 ng/mL may be necessary. *Pneumocystis carinii* pneumonia must be prophylaxed against during the period of CsA administration; pentamidine by inhalation is often used to avoid the potential marrow-suppressing activities of trimethoprim/sulfamethoxazole or dapsone. Long-term morbidity from ATG/ALG or CsA is rare.

BMT v. Immunosuppression. Younger patients suffer fewer complications with BMT. Hence if an *HLA-matched* sibling donor is available, this treatment should be pursued. For patients more than 20 years old, both treatment approaches offer distinct advantages and disadvantages. Mortality with BMT is largely secondary to GVHD and is concentrated in the 2 years following transplant. Attrition of patients treated with immunosuppression is more gradual: late sequelae include relapse (which can respond to a second round of immunosuppression) and evolution to clonal disorders such as PNH, MDS, and overt leukemia. Recovery from AA after immunosuppression is, in contrast to BMT, often incomplete, with asymptomatic cytopenias being common. Of note, a small study of 14 patients found no apparent detriment to delaying transplant until after immunosuppression had proven ineffective, despite the increased transfusion exposure of these patients at the time of transplant.

Supportive Measures.

1. *Transfusion.* Because many AA patients require extensive transfusional support, it is important to minimize the potential for allosensitization with each transfusion. This likewise should decrease the chance of graft rejection should the patient proceed to BMT (related or unrelated). This is generally accomplished by filtering blood products through leukocyte-depleting devices. Any candidate for a sibling BMT should *not* receive transfusions from a relative to avoid sensitization. CMV-negative AA patients in whom BMT is being considered should receive CMV-negative (or failing that, leukocyte-depleted) blood products, if feasible. Transfusions given in the course of a BMT should also be irradiated to prevent transfusion-associated GVHD.

   a. *Red cell transfusions.* Standard indications for red cell transfusion apply in AA: transfusions should be given until a hemoglobin level is reached at which the patient suffers no symptoms of anemia. Older patients, in particular those with known or suspected cardiopulmonary disease, should be kept at a higher target hemoglobin, usually 9–10 g/dL. There is *no* evidence that anemia accelerates the erythropoietic drive.

   b. *Platelet transfusions.* The primary concern in severely thrombocytopenic patients is cerebral hemorrhage. Because no reliable harbinger of this catastrophic complication exists, AA patients generally receive prophylactic platelet transfusions when the platelet count falls below a preset threshold. Our current threshold is $10,000/\mu L$. Rapidly spreading purpura, buccal mucosal hemorrhages, or extensive retinal hemorrhages are also used as indications for platelet transfusion. In actively bleeding patients, platelet transfusions should be administered with a goal of keeping the count greater than $50,000/\mu L$. The hemoglobin level should also be aggressively supported (i.e., at greater than 10 g/dL) in bleeding patients in order to achieve optimal hemostasis (Chapter 5). The use of apheresis platelet products (i.e., single-donor) will decrease allosensitization.

2. *Infection management.* Neutropenic fevers should be treated promptly with broad-spectrum antibiotics until a source is identified or the neutropenia resolves. Sustained fevers should prompt a search for fungi, especially in immunosuppressed patients. The role of nonabsorbable antibiotics in the management of AA patients is controversial. The severely neutropenic AA patient differs significantly from the more commonly encountered patient

with neutropenia secondary to chemotherapy in that the latter situation is generally complicated by breakdown of the gut mucosal barrier as a direct result of the chemotherapy.

3. *Growth factors.* AA is not a disease of growth factor deficiency; thus growth factors, primarily G- and GM-CSF, are used primarily in management of life-threatening infections, not for the simple purpose of boosting the neutrophil count in *asymptomatic* patients. Only a subset of AA patients shows a response to these factors. The effects of thrombopoietin on patients with AA needs to be determined in clinical trials.

4. *Iron chelation.* The risk of damage from excessive iron to viscera, especially to the heart, is increased in patients who have received approximately 100 U of red cells. Chelation therapy can be initiated after the patient has received about 50 U of red cells. The current approved therapy is deferoxamine by subcutaneous infusion.

Options for Refractory AA.

1. *Androgens.* There are sufficient examples of red cell transfusion independence following androgen therapy to warrant a therapeutic trial in some refractory patients. A 3-month trial is recommended before deeming androgens a failure. The most common androgens used are danazol, or decadurabolin. The most serious toxicity is hepatic, ranging from abnormal liver function tests (LFTs), which are generally reversible with discontinuation, to peliosis (blood–filled cysts) and hepatic tumors.

2. *Growth factors.* As discussed earlier, there is little evidence that growth factors, alone or in combination, are remittive agents in AA. Thus definitive therapy (i.e., immunosuppression or BMT) should not be delayed pending a trial of growth factors.

3. *Matched, unrelated-donor (MUD) BMT.* The principal drawback to sibling transplants, GVHD, is multiplied several-fold in MUD transplants, such that the long-term survival is on the order of 50% in children, with older patients faring worse.

The constitutive hypoplastic *pan*cytopenic syndromes will be discussed later in this chapter. The remaining bone marrow failure syndromes must therefore, by definition, consist of isolated cytopenias and can be categorized according to the classification scheme presented in Table 7-2.

ACQUIRED PURE RED CELL APLASIA

Pure red cell aplasia (PRCA) is defined by anemia, reticulocytopenia, and absent marrow precursors. PRCA shares many clinical associations and pathophysiologic mechanisms with aplastic anemia.

EPIDEMIOLOGY AND ETIOLOGY

Incidence. Rare—only a few hundred cases have been reported.

Epidemiology. Female predilection—2:1. The mean age of onset is about 60 years.

ACQUIRED CYTOPENIAS	**INHERITED CYTOPENIAS**
TABLE 7-2. *A CLASSIFICATION OF THE SINGLE CYTOPENIAS*	

ACQUIRED CYTOPENIAS	**INHERITED CYTOPENIAS**
Pure red cell aplasia (PRCA)	
Idiopathic	Diamond Blackfan anemia (DBA)
Drugs, toxins	
Immune	
Thymoma	
Transient erythroblastopenia of childhood (TEC)	
Neutropenia	
Idiopathic	Kostmann's syndrome (KS)
Drugs, toxins	Shwachman–Diamond–Oski syndrome (SD)
	Reticular dysgenesis
Thrombocytopenia	
Idiopathic amegakaryocytic	
Drugs, toxins	Thrombocytopenia with absent radii (TAR)

Etiology. Many provocative associations have been noted; the most widely cited is thymoma. Despite the propensity to report such associations, the true proportion of PRCA cases accompanied by thymoma is probably low. Other associated conditions include lymphoid malignancies, chronic myelogenous leukemia (CML), myelodysplastic syndrome (MDS), myelofibrosis, collagen vascular diseases, pregnancy, paraneoplastic syndromes, viruses, and drugs. The list of drugs associated with PRCA is similar to but more restricted than that for AA (see earlier). A causal relationship for diphenylhydantoin has been established by recurrence of the PRCA after readministration to the patient. As with AA, however, most PRCA cases are idiopathic.

PATHOPHYSIOLOGY

The best-understood mechanism of selective red cell aplasia is in the case of persistent parvovirus B19 infection. Patients with chronically immunosuppressed states, either congenital (Nezeloff syndrome), iatrogenic (chemotherapy), or acquired (AIDS), are unable to eradicate the cytotoxic B19 virus. Because of the virus tropism for erythroid progenitors, red cell production is selectively affected. The mechanisms of bone marrow failure in non-B19-related cases of PRCA have been elucidated in many cases and involve both humoral and cellular immune elimination of hematopoietic cells at various stages in the erythroid lineage.

DIAGNOSIS

Anemia, reticulocytopenia, and a bone marrow notable for isolated deficiency of erythroblasts are the hallmarks of PRCA. Proerythroblasts may occasionally be present in small numbers, and the abnormal giant forms (pronormoblasts with a diameter twice that of typical pronormoblasts, with or without nuclear inclusions or cytoplasmic blebbing) suggest parvovirus B19. Megakaryocytic and granulocytic lineages are preserved in number and morphology. Lymphocytes may be present diffusely or in small aggregates. Overall cellularity is normal, in contrast to AA.

Additional Studies. Additional studies should include tests for B19 *virus* (note that the presence of IgG antibody to B19 is *not* evidence of an active viral process) or recent seroconversion (i.e., IgM antibody), and a computed tomographic scan of the mediastinum to address the possibility of a thymoma.

Differential Diagnosis.
1. Hereditary PRCA: Diamond-Blackfan syndrome (DBA) (see later)
2. Nonimmune hydrops fetalis: *in utero* B19 parvovirus infection
3. Self-limited syndromes
   a. Transient erythroblastopenia of childhood (TEC) (see later)
   b. Transient aplastic crisis of hemolysis. Patients with hemolytic anemias may become reticulocytopenic during an acute B19 infection while awaiting sufficient production by their immune system of neutralizing antibodies. Infection of healthy individuals with parvovirus B19, while producing transient reticulocytopenia, generally does not come to medical attention because of the long lifespan of red cells, compared with the time required to mount an adequate immunoglobulin response.

MANAGEMENT

Any suspicious medications should be stopped. In the cases of malignancies, therapy should be directed at this presumed etiology. If PRCA persists after all candidate etiologies have been remedied, treat as autoimmune PRCA.

B19 Parvovirus. IV immunoglobulin is effective because it contains neutralizing antibodies.

Thymoma. Thymic surgery is used. If PRCA does not resolve with surgery, the patient should be treated as having autoimmune PRCA.

Autoimmune PRCA. A stepwise approach of immunosuppressive regimens should be employed until a remission is obtained or all therapeutic modalities have been exhausted. Less toxic regimens should be tried first.

1. Prednisone
2. Azathioprine or cyclophosphamide (oral) ± prednisone; increase azathioprine or cyclophosphamide until either
   a. Reticulocyte count increases (i.e., remission)
   b. WBC falls below 2,000/μL
   c. Platelets fall below 80,000/μL
3. Antithymocyte globulin (ATG) + prednisone; if no response, a second course of ATG may be attempted.
4. Cyclosporine A (CsA) ± prednisone

A standard course of therapy lasts 4–8 weeks. The earliest indicator of response will be the reticulocyte count. Patients must be closely monitored for the known toxicities of these agents. After a remission is achieved, the therapeutic agents should be tapered slowly and discontinued. If patients remain refractory, a trial of androgens, plasmapheresis, IV IgG, lymphocytopheresis and, ultimately, splenectomy may be attempted. Patients dependent on chronic red cell transfusions will eventually require chelation therapy with desferoxamine. This should be initiated after about 50 U have been transfused.

PROGNOSIS

Ultimately, the majority of patients will become transfusion–independent, either spontaneously (about 15%) or after immunosuppressive therapy (about two-thirds). About half of the responding patients will relapse, but again about 80% will respond to a second round of immunosuppression. Thus the great majority of patients can be rendered independent of transfusions. Accordingly, the median survival of patients with acquired PRCA is 14 years. Progression of PRCA to other disorders such as aplastic anemia or leukemia is uncommon but documented: 2 out of 58 patients developed AML in one series.

ACQUIRED AMEGAKARYOCYTIC THROMBOCYTOPENIC PURPURA

This rare condition (about 30 cases reported), as the name implies, is the megakaryocytic counterpart of PRCA. Bone marrow examination reveals normal myeloid and erythroid morphology and numbers, but megakaryocytes are conspicuously absent. Cellularity is normal. Associated conditions include collagen vascular diseases, hepatitis, viral infections (including HIV), and drug use (oxyphenbutazone). Cytogenetic studies should be performed to detect the 5q- syndrome. Patients have responded to ATG, cyclophosphamide, cyclosporine A, lithium, androgens, and prednisone.

AGRANULOCYTOSIS AND OTHER NEUTROPENIC SYNDROMES

Isolated neutropenia in the context of deficient granulocytic precursors in the marrow can be classified as either acquired or intrinsic. Adult cases are generally acquired, and the most common etiology is drug-induced. Pediatric cases are more often inherited, generally in an autosomal or X-linked recessive manner. The presenting symptom is often the development of mouth pain or sore throat; mucositis or oral mucosal ulcers are common because of the important role neutrophils (PMNs) play in normal physiology in the protection and maintenance of the mucosa. Destruction of cells of granulocytic series is often evident *both* in the bone marrow and in the periphery in many of these syndromes, and thus, strictly speaking, some of the conditions discussed in this section do not fulfill the stringent criteria for bone marrow failure syndromes. They are reviewed here for the sake of completeness. Isolated neutropenias can be classified by the diagnostic scheme presented in Table 7-3. Selected types are discussed below.

ACQUIRED NEUTROPENIA

Drug-Induced.

1. Epidemiology: This is a rare syndrome of older patients (>50 years old;

TABLE 7-3. *DIFFERENTIAL DIAGNOSIS OF ISOLATED NEUTROPENIA*

Secondary Neutropenia

Drug induced neutropenia

Toxin induced neutropenia

Secondary to specific infectious agents

    Viruses, including viral hepatitis, Epstein-Barr virus, human immunodeficiency virus-1

    Bacteria, especially typhoid fever

    Rickettsia

    Protozoa

Secondary to overwhelming infection

    Sepsis

    Disseminated mycobacteria

Collagen vascular autoimmune diseases

    Systemic lupus erythematosus

    Felty's syndrome

Starvation and kwashiorkor

Alcoholism

"Normal" Variation

Ethnic and familial neutropenia

Benign chronic neutropenia

Primary Hematologic Diseases

Autoimmune neutropenia*

Isoimmune neutropenia

Pure white cell aplasia*

Large granular lymphocytosis/T-γ-lymphoproliferative disease*

Myelodysplasia

Postchemotherapy, irradiation*

Cyclical neutropenia*

Agranulocytosis*

Chronic idiopathic neutropenia

Inherited/Intrinsic Conditions

Cyclic neutropenia

Kostmann's syndrome–Infantile agranulocytosis

Schwachman–Diamond–Oski syndrome

Reticular dysgenesis

Dyskeratosis congenita (Zinsser-Cole-Engman syndrome)

Chédiak-Higashi syndrome

Myelokathexis/Neutropenia with tetraploid leukocytes

* *Conditions in which the absolute neutrophil count is likely to be <500/μL.*

TABLE 7-4. *IMMUNE VERSUS TOXIC AGRANULOCYTOSIS*

	IMMUNOLOGIC	TOXIC
Paradigm drug	Aminopyrine	Phenothiazine
Time to onset	Days to weeks	Weeks to months
Clinical	Acute, often explosive symptoms	Often asymptomatic or insidious onset
Rechallenge	Prompt recurrence with small test dose	Latent period, high doses required
Laboratory	Leukoagglutinins, other antibody tests positive	Evidence of direct or metabolite-mediated toxicity to cells

probably due to the increased frequency and variety of drug use in this population) with a 2:1 female:male predilection.

2. Etiology/pathophysiology: Drugs can mediate suppression *via* immune mechanisms or by direct toxicity to progenitors of the granulocytic lineage in the bone marrow. Table 7-4 illustrates some of the cardinal features of these two mechanisms. The immune nature of neutropenia has been demonstrated by rechallenge of a recovered patient with the offending drug, aminopyrine, earlier this century: the neutrophil count dropped precipitously within hours. A similar result was obtained upon injection of serum from an affected patient into a normal volunteer. Drugs of many classes have been imputed; the list of common offenders is similar to that for AA and includes aminopyrine derivatives, antithyroid drugs, macrolides, procainamide, phenothiazines, β-lactams, and NSAIDs (Table 7-5).

3. Diagnosis: Sudden neutropenia in the context of a drug with known granulocytic suppressive actions is generally sufficient for presumptive diagnosis; a bone marrow examination should be performed.

4. Management: Recovery of granulopoiesis may take as little as 2 or more than 21 days after discontinuation of the drug. Recovery may be accelerated by growth factors such as G- or GM-CSF.

5. Prognosis 10% of patients may succumb despite optimal management. The offending agent (and, in some cases, related drugs as, for example, with propylthiouracil and methimazole) should not be readministered to the recovered patient.

Autoimmune Neutropenia

1. Epidemiology: In contrast to drug-induced agranulocytosis, this is largely a disease of infants and children. In older patients, an autoimmune disorder such as systemic lupus erythematosus (SLE) or rheumatoid arthritis (RA) may coexist. This is a chronic condition that, by definition, may become evident only with prolonged follow-up.

2. Etiology (Table 7-6): By definition, no drug is implicated. Neutrophil-specific antibodies (to antigens denoted NA1, NA2, NB1, ND1, ND2, etc.) have been demonstrated in some patients but are not required for diagnosis. As implied by the presence of these antibodies to mature blood elements, this condition represents an autoimmune process directed primarily against mature granulocytes that may also involve the latest stages of granulocytic maturation in the bone marrow.

TABLE 7-5. *DRUGS ASSOCIATED WITH AGRANULOCYTOSIS IN THE INTERNATIONAL APLASTIC ANEMIA AND AGRANULOCYTOSIS STUDY*

DRUG	RR	EXCESS RISK
Cinepazide	∞	*
Sulfasalazine	∞	*
Antithyroid drugs	97	5.3
Macrolides	54	6.7
Procainamide	~50	3.1
Aprindine	~49	2.7
Dipyrone	16	0.6
Cotrimoxazole	16	1.7
Thenalidine	~16	2.4
Carbamazepine	11	0.6
Digitalis glycosides	2.5–9.9	0.1–0.3
Indomethacin	6.6	0.4
Troxerutin	6.0	0.3
Sulfonylureas	4.5	0.2
Corticosteroids	4.1	*
Butazones	3.9	0.2
Dipyridamole	3.8	0.2
Beta-lactams	2.8	0.2
Propranolol	2.5	0.1
Salicylates	2.0	0.06

RR = multivariate relative risk estimate.
Excess risk expressed as number of cases per 10^6 users in one week. To calculate excess risk in case-control studies, use the following information: overall incidence (I), relative risk (RR), proportion of exposed cases (P_e), etiologic fraction (EF), which is $(RR - 1/RR) P_e$.
Step 1. Calculate baseline incidence: $I_B = I \cdot (1 - EF)$.
Step 2. Calculate total incidence among exposed: $I_T = I_B \cdot RR$.
Step 3. Calculate excess incidence among exposed: $I_E = I_T - I_B$ or $[(RR) I (I(1 - EF)] - [I(1 - EF)]$ or $(RR - 1) I (1 - EF)$.
* = Excess risk not calculated due to absence of exposed controls or, in the case of corticosteroids, confounding of causal relationship by the diagnosis of rheumatoid arthritis.

TABLE 7-6. *HUMORAL IMMUNE-MEDIATED (?) NEUTROPENIA*

Agranulocytosis

Pure white cell aplasia

Autoimmune neutropenia

Felty's syndrome

Systemic lupus erythematosus

3. Diagnosis
   a. Symptoms: Patients may be asymptomatic or suffer recurrent skin infections, otitis media, upper respiratory tract infections, diarrhea, or bouts of cryptogenic fever.
   b. Physical findings: Hepatosplenomegaly is noted in only half of patients.
   c. Bone marrow examination reveals normal or increased cellularity with late maturation arrest. Neutrophil precursors appear "frozen" at a particular stage of maturation since no representatives of later maturational stages are evident. Histiocyte phagocytosis of myeloid cells may be prominent.

4. Management: Many patients eventually recover spontaneously. Hence the decision to treat is based on the severity of symptoms. Corticosteroids and IV IgG have been used successfully. Splenectomy generally produces only transient resolution of neutropenia (with exceptions, see later) but puts the patient at permanent risk for overwhelming septicemia. In patients with underlying autoimmune disorders (e.g., SLE or RA), cytotoxic agents can be effective.

5. Special clinical problems
   a. Primary splenic neutropenia. hypercellular marrow with abundant *early* myeloid elements; responds to splenectomy.
   b. Felty's syndrome. Neutropenia, splenomegaly, and rheumatoid arthritis (frank myeloid *hypo*plasia is rare). Methotrexate or splenectomy can be effective: a quarter of patients will not respond to the latter, and another one-third will experience recurrence of neutropenia.

Isoimmune Neutropenia. This is the granulocytic equivalent of Rh hemolytic disease. The mother becomes sensitized to paternal neutrophil-specific alloantigens and generates antibodies to the fetus granulocytes that cross the placenta.

1. Incidence: Approximately one in 500 live births
2. Diagnosis: As infants can present with sepsis, and since sepsis itself can produce neutropenia in infants, it can be difficult to separate cause and effect. Late myeloid arrest is characteristic of the syndrome. Antineutrophil antibodies may be detectable in the serum of mother and child, and specific for paternal neutrophils.
3. Differential diagnosis: Congenital disorders should be considered if the patient does not recover
4. Management: Most infants recover within 12–20 weeks without any serious infections. Standard antibiotic regimens should be administered for presumed infections. The safety and/or efficacy of CSFs have not been evaluated in this syndrome.

Pure White Cell Aplasia (PWCA). This very rare syndrome is occasionally associated with thymoma, sometimes long after its excision. Virtually all myeloid elements are absent from the marrow. Humoral and cellular inhibitors of *in vitro* myelopoiesis have been demonstrated. If present, a thymoma should be removed. Patients without a thymoma have responded to thymectomy, splenectomy, plasmapheresis, IV IgG, cyclophosphamide, azathioprine, and cyclosporine.

Large Granular Lymphocytosis (LGL) (Tγ Lymphocytosis) with Neutropenia. Splenomegaly is common, and in the not infrequent association with rheumatoid arthritis, constitutes Felty's syndrome. Large granular lymphocytes are seen on peripheral smear examination (Fig. 4-9C). Maturation arrest specific to the myeloid lineage is seen on examination of the bone marrow. There are three subtypes described:

1. T-LGL leukemia (CD3$^+$). This is a clonal disorder of T cells, as determined by T-cell receptor rearrangement studies, that is subacute in presentation. Corticosteroids, G-, and GM-CSF are occasionally effective in patients requiring treatment for recurrent infection. Low-dose methotrexate and cyclosporine are two therapies that appear promising.
2. NK-LGL leukemia (CD3$^-$). Clonality is defined by the presence of a uniform cytogenetic abnormality. Presentation is acute and only 2 of 11 patients responded to combination chemotherapy. Most patients were dead within months of presentation.
3. NK-LGL lymphocytosis (CD3$^+$ or CD3$^-$). These patients have been shown to have *poly*clonal proliferation of LGLs on the basis of X-linked polymorphism analysis, suggesting a reactive disorder. The clinical course of this syndrome is much more chronic and may not require treatment.

Chronic Idiopathic Neutropenia. As the name implies, this is a diagnosis of exclusion. Neutrophil counts typically range from 200–500/μL. Marrow reserve is demonstrable, with a hydrocortisone stimulation test, in contrast to, for example, drug-induced agranulocytosis. Bone marrow examination in general is notable only for late maturation arrest. Treatment with G-CSF, corticosteroids, splenectomy, and cytotoxic agents should be given only to patients with recurrent infectious complications.

Neutropenic Conditions. Neutropenic conditions without significantly decreased bone marrow granulocytic elements (by definition, these are not bone marrow failure syndromes, but are discussed here for the benefit of the complete workup of patients presenting with neutropenia).

1. Benign familial leukopenia. The inheritance pattern is autosomal dominant and, as the name implies, is not associated with increased infections. The neutrophil count ranges from 2,100 to 2,600/μL. The bone marrow is normocellular. Increased incidence in Yemenite Jews, West Indians, and American and African blacks has been noted. No therapy is required for this nondisease.
2. Chronic (benign) neutropenia of infancy and childhood. This diagnosis is often made only retrospectively. It usually presents in the first year or two of life, typically by virtue of a blood count during an infection, which is not always characteristic for neutropenia. The neutrophil count at birth, if determined, is normal. The bone marrow is normo- to hypercellular, morphology is normal, and myeloid maturation arrest, if present, is usually late. Minor oral, vaginal, or rectal ulcers may be seen. Infections respond well to antibiotics, and, by definition, are not severe. Virtually all patients recover by age 4 years. Failure to fulfill these criteria of benignity should prompt further investigation. Corticosteroids, IV IgG, and G-CSF have been used successfully to raise the neutrophil count but should be used only in infections, not chronically, in this self-resolving syndrome.

3. (Post-)Infectious neutropenia. This phenomenon is most commonly encountered in sepsis of neonates, the elderly, or any debilitated patient, and is multifactorial in etiology. It is generally easily recognized on clinical grounds. If a bone marrow examination is performed it will typically reveal hypercellularity with or without late myeloid arrest. Implicated microorganisms, in addition to the usual bacteria associated with sepsis, include varicella, measles, rubella, EBV, CMV, hepatitis A and B, influenza, mycobacteria, rickettsia, and brucella.

4. Metabolic diseases. Neutropenia in the setting of apparent normal myeloid maturation can be seen with ketoacidosis (associated with hyperglycemia, orotic aciduria, methylmalonic aciduria, and hyperglycinuria) and glycogen storage diseases type Ib. Defects in neutrophil function have also been detected in some patients. Infections can be serious. CSFs have been successfully employed.

INHERITED/INTRINSIC NEUTROPENIAS

Cyclic Neutropenia. Recurring neutropenia with a periodicity of every 15–35 days, classically every 21 days.

1. Presentation: Recurrent fevers or infections in a child, which are found to reflect the severity of the neutropenia. Cases presenting in adulthood may be related to large granular lymphocytosis.
2. Inheritance: Autosomal dominant with variable expression. Associated findings: Monocyte, lymphocyte, reticulocyte, and platelet counts may also exhibit cyclic fluctuations.
3. Associated findings: Monocyte, lymphocyte, reticulocyte, and platelet counts may also exhibit cyclic fluctuations.
4. Diagnosis: Requires twice weekly neutrophil counts for at least eight weeks.
5. Bone marrow examination: Myeloid hypoplasia that parallels the severity of the neutropenia.
6. Management: G-CSF therapy shortens the neutrophil nadir and reduces the frequency of infection, but does not affect cycling of other blood elements.
7. Prognosis: The severity of the clinical manifestations tends to diminish with age.

Kostmann's Syndrome—Infantile Agranulocytosis.
1. Presentation: Severe, recurrent, pyogenic infections, generally by age 6 months
2. Inheritance: Autosomal recessive
3. Associated findings: Occasional mental retardation, microcephaly, cataracts, or short stature
4. Bone marrow examination: Myeloid hypoplasia with arrest at the promyelocyte stage
5. Management: G-CSF is quite promising.
6. Leukemia: One or 2% of patients develop myeloid leukemias (in the pre-G-CSF era)

Shwachman-Diamond-Oski Syndrome. The combination of neutropenia with pancreatic insufficiency defines the syndrome. Hematopoietic manifestations may also include anemia (15%) or thrombocytopenia (9%), which may even antedate neutropenia.

1. Presentation: Recurrent infections with steatorrhea in the first few years of life. Steatorrhea may be subtle and evident only on determination of fecal fat.
2. Inheritance: Autosomal recessive.
3. Associated findings: Short stature (60%), mental retardation (15%), metaphyseal dysostosis (30%), myocardial fibrosis.
4. Diagnosis: Exocrine pancreatic insufficiency must be documented. Sweat chloride should be determined to rule out cystic fibrosis.
5. Bone marrow examination: Normal or decreased cellularity and myeloid maturation; the erythroid series may be hyperplastic.
6. Management
   a. Neutropenia responds to G-CSF but should be reserved for patients with serious infections or a recurrent history thereof.
   b. Anemia may respond to prednisone or androgens.
   c. Pancreatic insufficiency responds to enzyme replacement.
7. Prognosis: Pancytopenia eventually develops in about a quarter of patients, leukemia in about 5%. Median age at death in Shwachman-Diamond-Oski syndrome patients is over 35 years, but less than half of that in the 25% of patients that develop pancytopenia, and less than 10 years in the 5% of patients that develop leukemia.

Reticular Dysgenesis. Reticular dysgenesis consists of the triad of (1) congenital agranulocytosis, (2) lymphopenia, and (3) absent cellular and humoral immunity. Inheritance is recessive, possibly X-linked. Infants present with infections in the first month or two of life. Lymph nodes, tonsils, and thymus are conspicuously absent. Anemia and, in one case, thrombocytopenia may also be present. Bone marrow is hypocellular, with absence of myeloid and lymphoid elements. Erythroblasts may be diminished or dysplastic. Bone marrow transplant, if performed prior to development of serious infectious morbidity, can be curative. Death within 4 months is otherwise inevitable.

Dyskeratosis Congenita (Zinsser-Cole-Engman Syndrome). Defined by the triad of (1) reticulated hyperpigmentation of the face, neck, and shoulders; (2) mucous membrane leukoplakia, and (3) dystrophic nails. Autosomal dominant and recessive modes of inheritance have been reported but X-linked recessive is the predominant mode. Five to 15% of patients develop squamous cell or adenocarcinomas, predominantly of the oropharynx and gastrointestinal tract. Neutropenia or AA develop in the second decade of life in about half of patients. Androgens, often combined with prednisone, can mitigate cytopenias. Bone marrow transplants are associated with high early morbidity.

Chédiak-Higashi Syndrome. Oculocutaneous albinism, progressive neurologic impairment, and giant cytoplasmic granules define this autosomal recessive disorder. These granules are found in many cells, including the granulocytic series, and are presumed related to a granulopoietic defect accounting for the severe neutropenia in this syndrome. Pancytopenia may evolve. Marrow transplantation may be curative. (See Chapter 4.)

Myelokathexis/Neutropenia with Tetraploid Leukocytes. This syndrome generally presents in childhood with recurrent severe infections. Binucleate cells of the granulocytic series become more numerous with each stage of maturation, such that two-thirds of the bands and virtually all the mature neutrophils are tetraploid. Early precursors appear normal. Only rare tetraploid cells enter the circulation, thus accounting for the neutropenia. Many functional abnormalities of the neutrophils in these patients have been documented. G-CSF therapy appears beneficial.

INHERITED BONE MARROW FAILURE SYNDROMES

Inherited bone marrow failure syndromes almost always present in childhood, with symptoms referable to cytopenias or with characteristic physical anomalies. Bone marrow failure, which may not initially be evident, can manifest itself as an isolated cytopenia, or may have already evolved into bi- or tri-cytopenias by the time it is recognized.

Fanconi Anemia. The classical phenotype of Fanconi anemia (FA) includes the following: familial aplastic anemia (autosomal recessive pattern of inheritance), short stature, absent or hypoplastic thumb or radius, microcephaly, café au lait and hypopigmented spots. This constellation of findings has been supplanted as a means of diagnosis by the *in vitro* test of clastogen-induced chromosomal breaks. (See later.) The spectrum of clinical manifestations also may include hypertelorism, abnormal gonadal development, various skeletal abnormalities, deafness, and gastrointestinal and cardiovascular defects. Since nearly one-third of FA patients present with no obvious physical abnormalities, all patients less than 30 years old presenting with cytopenias and a hypocellular marrow should undergo chromosome breakage studies with diepoxybutane (DEB) or mitomycin C (MMC). These agents presumably accentuate the DNA repair defect that is a consequence of the genetic defect in this autosomal recessive disorder.

The hematologic manifestations of FA can range from normal blood counts with subtle elevations in hemoglobin F to severe pancytopenia and complete dependence on transfusion. Likewise, the bone marrow picture can range from mild to profound hypocellularity. The first line of supportive therapy is androgens, with response rates of about 50%. The erythroid lineage usually responds first (within 1–2 months), followed by the granulocytic lineage; last, and least reliably, the platelets may plateau only after a year. Most patients relapse if androgens are discontinued. Bone marrow transplantation from a suitably matched donor is currently the only curative therapy, with up to two-thirds surviving 5 years. The usual high dose chemotherapy regimens given before bone marrow transplantation must be attenuated because of the sensitivity of the FA hematopoietic cells to cytotoxic therapy. (See Chapter 8.) Gene therapy with engineered autologous marrow may prove beneficial in the future as well.

FA patients who do not succumb to cytopenias are at significant risk of developing malignancies, including leukemia (usually myeloid), preleukemia, and carcinoma (in particular, squamous and hepatocellular). The overall incidence of malignancy may approach 20%. Epithelial tumors are not uncommon following bone marrow transplantation, although not always life-threatening.

Diamond-Blackfan Anemia. Isolated congenital failure of erythropoiesis is termed *Diamond-Blackfan anemia* (DBA). The diagnostic criteria are (1) reticulocytopenia with macrocytic or normocytic anemia, (2) normal marrow cellularity with isolated erythroid hypoplasia, and (3) normal or near-normal leukocyte and platelet counts. Most cases are sporadic, although autosomal recessive and autosomal dominant patterns of inheritance have been documented in different kindreds. The patient usually presents to medical attention within the first 6 months of life, and only rarely after age 1 year. Physical anomalies are the exception, occurring in up to 25% of patients, depending on the level of scrutiny. The first line of therapy is prednisone. More than 50% of patients will respond, but many may require prolonged treatment, with the predictable attendant morbidity in this pediatric population. Long-term transfusional support is of course indicated in refractory patients, which in turn obligates long-term iron chelation therapy with deferoxamine. Fifteen to 20% of all DBA patients, however, will ultimately exhibit spontaneous remissions. Long-term complications include iron overload, sepsis, and myeloid leukemias, each of which can prove fatal.

Transient Erythroblastopenia of Childhood. As its name implies, transient erythroblastopenia of childhood (TEC) involves abrupt but transient suppression of erythropoiesis. This suppression is the hallmark of this condition, but definitive diagnosis can often be made only retrospectively. A viral infection of the erythroid lineage is the likely etiology, although studies for parvovirus are rarely positive. The syndrome consists of isolated anemia, reticulocytopenia, and, on bone marrow exam, profound hypoplasia of the erythroid lineage—the same criteria as for DBA. As with DBA, the myeloid and megakaryocytic lineages are not significantly affected. The prospective distinction between the two syndromes is made on clinical grounds. TEC patients are typically older at presentation, generally greater than 2 years old. An antecedent history of a viral infection is suggestive of TEC (although, of course, children with DBA contract viruses as well, sometimes just prior to presentation). If investigations of parameters of stress erythropoiesis are performed during the acute, *reticulocytopenic* phase of TEC, such markers are generally absent in TEC; thus if they are present, this favors a diagnosis of DBA. These markers include increased mean corpuscular volume, hemoglobin F levels, and I antigen levels. During recovery, however, these markers of stress erythropoiesis may increase and prove less useful in delineating between TEC and DBA. The return of the reticulocyte, however, effectively rules out DBA, unless the patient has been treated with steroids. Thus if the clinician has a high index of suspicion for TEC, the patient may simply be observed and, if the diagnosis is correct, recovery will ensue within 1–2 months. Hemoglobin levels of as low as 5 g/dL are often well tolerated, and thus transfusional support is only rarely necessary.

Thrombocytopenia Absent Radii. The characteristic physical anomaly in this rare syndrome—absent (bilateral) radii, with thumbs present—is distinct from the situation in Fanconi anemia, in which thumbs are absent. Infants present in the first weeks of life either on the basis of the dramatic physical abnormality or due to hemorrhagic manifestations. The mode of inheritance is autosomal recessive. Bone marrow examination shows normal myeloid and erythroid lineages, with absent, hypoplastic, or immature megakaryocytic development. Anemia with reticulocytosis may result from bloody diarrhea, which has been attributed to cow's milk and may improve with elimination from the diet. A leukemoid reaction with markedly elevated white counts is not uncommon. The only therapy of proven efficacy is platelet transfusions. If patients survive the first year, which most do, the long-term outlook is excellent, with platelet counts typically plateauing above 100,000/μL.

Amegakaryocytic Thrombocytopenia. Amegakaryocytic thrombocytopenia is the hypomegakaryocytic counterpart of Diamond-Blackfan anemia. By definition, radii are not absent, and physical anomalies are the exception. The thrombocytopenic infant generally presents within the first few months of life, and bone marrow examination reveals an isolated dearth of megakaryocytes. The mode of inheritance is recessive, autosomal in some cases, and X-linked in others. Corticosteroids and/or androgens may prove salutary, although median survival is only 5 years. Many patients will evolve to aplastic anemia. Bone marrow transplantation has been successfully performed.

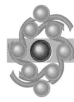

CASE PRESENTATION

A 28-year-old man visits his internist because he feels weak. A few weeks before admission, the patient noted headaches, malaise, myalgia, fever, and chills. Two to 3 days ago a fine macular papular rash was present diffusely and he experienced arthralgia. For approximately 1 week he noted weakness and fatigue, and over the past several days he has been unable to perform usual activities of daily living without feeling short of breath. There has been no recent fever, sweats, or chills. On physical examination, he appears to be a pale young man but in no acute distress. His respiration rate, however, is 22, and his pulse rate is 100 and regular. He is afebrile. The physical exam is significant for pallor of skin and mucous membranes. There is no rash and no lymphadenopathy. The lungs are clear. Heart is normal. Abdomen is benign. Extremities are normal. Rectal examination shows stool that is brown without occult blood. Neurologic system is intact. Urinalysis shows no red blood cells or bilirubin. The CBC shows the hemologbin to be 5 g./dL and hematocrit 15% with an MCV of 93 fL. The white count is 4,500/μL, with a normal differential count; platelet count is 320,000/μL. Review of the peripheral smear shows normal appearance of platelets and white cells. Red cells appear normochromic and normocytic. No polychromasia is noted.

Question 1. What is the next step?

Answer. The patient is more closely questioned about gastrointestinal genitourinary or mucous membrane–associated blood loss. He is asked about dark urine in an attempt to learn whether there had been a hemolytic event in the past with bilirubinuria. No new information was forthcoming from this questioning.

Question 2. What should be done next?

Answer. A reticulocyte count is obtained as well as LDH, haptoglobin, bilirubin, and urine for hemosiderin. These tests showed the reticulocyte count to be zero. The other tests showed no abnormalities.

Question 3. How do you interpret these results?

Answer. The patient is not responding appropriately to his anemic stress by sending out young cells from the marrow (reticulocytes), nor is there evidence of hemolysis from the lab testing. The normal LDH, bilirubin, and haptoglobin indicate there has been no recent hemolytic event, and the normal urinary hemosiderin shows that in the recent past there has been no hemolysis with resulting hemosiderin taken up by renal tubular cells that were then sloughed in the urine and tested for iron pigments.

Question 4. What is the next step?

Answer. Bone marrow examination was performed. The cellularity was normal. Platelet precursors and white blood cells precursors were within normal limits. However, there were very few red cell precursors of any kind. There were some giant pronormoblasts that contained intranuclear inclusions of loose amorphous pink material. Additionally, analysis of blood (DNA dot-blot hybridization analysis) for B19 parvoviral genome was positive and testing for HIV was also positive.

Question 5. What is the likely diagnosis?

Answer. This man is likely to be suffering from B 19 parvovirus infection in the setting of HIV infection.

Question 6. How can this patient's anemia be treated?

Answer. The patient was given a transfusion of red cells. Intravenous immunoglobulin was also administered.

Follow-up:

The patient underwent studies for CD-4 counts and viral load. Appropriate therapy for HIV was begun. Over the next 2 weeks, reticulocytosis developed and the patient had temporary elevation in his hematocrit. However, a chronic program of immunoglobulin infusion was needed to keep the patient's hematocrit at a reasonable level.

SELECTED READING

Alter BP, ed. *Perinatal Hematology.* New York: Churchill Livingstone, 1989.
This monograph represents a comprehensive cataloging of the epidemiology, genetics, clinical presentation, natural history, laboratory parameters, and management of the bone marrow failure syndromes, generally constitutional, that present in early life.

Hoffman RH, et al., eds. *Hematology: Basic Principles and Practice,* 2nd ed. New York: Churchill Livingstone, 1995.
This general hematology textbook discusses virtually all the bone marrow failure syndromes described in this chapter, affecting both pediatric and adult populations. Some helpful diagnostic and therapeutic flow charts are provided, although they do not represent the sole approach to these patients.

Schroeder-Kurth TM, Auerbach AD, Obe G, eds. *Fanconi Anemia: Clinical, Cytogenetic, and Experimental Aspects.* New York: Springer-Verlag; 1989.
This is a thorough compilation of the clinical spectrum of Fanconi anemia (FA), with regard to anatomic anomalies, hereditary patterns, age of presentation, and response to therapies. The latest data on the molecular basis of FA, and attenuated transplant regiments, however, are understandably not present in this 1989 monograph.

Young NS, Alter BP. *Aplastic Anemia, Acquired and Inherited.* Philadelphia: WB Saunders; 1994.

This is a thorough treatise that includes much laboratory data on the pathophysiology and molecular mechanisms of bone marrow failure syndromes, as well as the role of more modern therapeutic modalities such as growth factors in their management.

Young N, Keisu M, eds. Drug related blood dyscrasias workshop. *Eur J Haematol* (Supplement 60), 1996;57.

This monograph addresses primarily acquired aplastic anemia (AA). Clinical, epidemiologic, pathophysiologic, and therapeutic discussions cover both the drug-related and the idiopathic varieties of AA. Possible mechanisms of benzene-induced AA (a classic model of drug-induced aplasia) as well as the pharmacology of drug-induced dyscrasias in general are covered in detail.

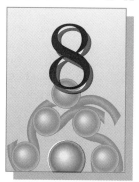

CHAPTER

8

Stem Cell Transplantation

Mitchell E. Horwitz and Cynthia E. Dunbar

INTRODUCTION

HISTORY

Fifty years ago, the hematologic effects seen in patients exposed to irradiation at Hiroshima and Nagasaki stimulated research into possible radioprotective effects of bone marrow. During the 1950s and 1960s, scientists found that hematopoiesis could be completely restored by intravenous infusion of bone marrow cells. Clinicians were quick to realize the potential benefits of bone marrow transplantation (BMT), both to correct inborn and acquired bone marrow failure syndromes and to "rescue" patients from otherwise lethal myeloablative effects of high-dose radiation and chemotherapy used to treat cancer.

The initial trials involved allogeneic transplantation (the transfer of marrow from donor to recipient to permanently replace all hematopoietic cells) as opposed to autologous transplantation (the reinfusion of a patient's own previously stored marrow cells after myeloablative chemo/radiotherapy). The primary hurdle in allogeneic transplantation was a lack of understanding of immunologic barriers involved in both rejection of the donor's marrow by the recipient and graft-versus-host disease (GVHD), the reaction against the recipient's tissues by the donor's immunologically competent lymphocytes. Characterization of the HLA (human leukocyte antigen) system in the mid-1960s allowed clinicians to attempt matched allogeneic BMT between sibling donor/recipient pairs. Nobel laureate E. Donnell Thomas moved the field rapidly forward with research into tolerable radiation and chemotherapy myeloablative regimens, as well as pharmacologic methods for the prevention of GVHD. By the late 1970s, allogeneic BMT had evolved from a highly experimental and usually fatal procedure into an accepted treatment of aplastic anemia, immune deficiency disorders, and many forms of leukemia, with some evidence that these previously untreatable disorders could be cured.

Despite the development of potent immunosuppressive agents such as cyclosporine and broad-spectrum antimicrobials, survival after allogeneic BMT has not changed greatly since the early 1980s. This may in part result from the broader application of the procedure in higher-risk patients. Encouraging results of dose intensification in leukemias and lymphomas and the development of better conditioning regimens has refocused interest on autologous transplantation. Since 1990 more autologous than allogeneic transplants have been performed each year.

OVERVIEW OF TRANSPLANTATION CONCEPTS AND PROCEDURES

As described in Chapter 1, the hematopoietic stem cell (HSC) is defined as a cell capable of reconstituting the entire hematopoietic and lymphoid system of an irradiated recipient. Theoretically, this could be achieved with just one cell, but in the clinical setting, infusion of at least $1–3 \times 10^8$ nucleated bone marrow cells per kilogram recipient body weight ensures durable and rapid engraftment. Only a tiny fraction (less than 1 in 100,000) of nucleated bone marrow cells are HSCs. They are morphologically indistinguishable from lymphocytes but have a characteristic cell surface protein composition, including $CD34^+$, HLA class II^-, and $CD38^-$. They lack lineage markers such as CD4, surface immunoglobulin, and glycophorin.

Bone marrow cells for transplantation are aspirated from the posterior iliac crests through hollow needles inserted repeatedly into the marrow cavity. This procedure is usually done under general anesthesia in the operating room. A total of 15–20 mL of liquid marrow per kilogram of recipient weight is collected and filtered to remove bony fragments and cell clumps before either further processing or immediate reinfusion into the recipient. Marrow harvesting is well tolerated, and the risks to the donor include only those of general anesthesia and, very rarely, significant bleeding from the sites or nerve damage due to misplaced needles.

During the past 5–6 years, alternative sources of HSCs have been discovered and introduced clinically. Treatment of cancer patients with cytokines such as G-CSF or GM-CSF alone or following high-dose chemotherapy stimulates a large number of primitive cells to leave the marrow cavity and move into the bloodstream, where they can be easily collected via one or more apheresis procedures. Mobilized peripheral blood has almost completely replaced marrow as a source of cells for autologous transplantation and appears to contain true long-term repopulating hematopoietic stem cells. Advantages include ease of collection, more rapid engraftment after transplantation, and potentially less tumor contamination. More recently, studies utilizing peripheral blood progenitor cells (PBPCs) mobilized from normal sibling donors treated with G-CSF have been initiated, with promising results thus far.

A third potentially useful source of HSCs is umbilical cord blood, which appears to contain more concentrated primitive cells than marrow. Up to 250 mL can be collected at the time of delivery without detriment to the mother or newborn. Unrelated allogeneic transplantation may be revolutionized by cord blood banking, but cord blood collections may not contain enough HSCs to reliably engraft adult recipients.

The actual transplantation procedure simply involves infusing the cell concentrate through a large-bore intravenous line. Even many medical personnel are surprised to learn that the cells are not actually reinjected into the marrow cavity and that marrow transplants are performed by internists or pediatricians with training in hematology and oncology, not surgeons! The dimethylsulfoxisole solution used to cryopreserve autologous BM or PBPCs can cause immediate moderate pulmonary and systemic toxicity, but fresh allogeneic reinfusions are very well tolerated. The HSCs home to the marrow cavities via poorly understood mechanisms, and within 10–25 days production of first neutrophils, then platelets and red cells should occur. This signifies engraftment of donor stem cells.

ALLOGENEIC TRANSPLANTATION

OVERVIEW

Allogeneic transplantation is a treatment option for a growing number of acquired and genetic diseases (Table 8-1). Because of high treatment-related morbidity and mortality, the majority are performed on patients with life-threatening acquired hematologic diseases, primarily leukemia or aplastic anemia. As morbidity and mortality associated with the procedure decreases, allogeneic transplantation for chronic, nonfatal congenital diseases such as sickle cell anemia will become more commonplace. There are several potential advantages for allogeneic transplantation as compared with autologous transplantation for malignancies. Allogeneic transplantation provides the recipient with hematopoietic stem cells from a normal donor, eliminating the risk of reinfusion of viable tumor cells that could contribute to relapse. In some tumors, most notably chronic myelogenous leukemia, there is also convincing evidence for an immunologic antitumor effect conferred by the donor cells.

TABLE 8-1. *APPLICATIONS FOR ALLOGENEIC TRANSPLANTATION*

Acquired Diseases
Acute myeloid leukemia
Chronic myeloid leukemia
Aplastic anemia
Myelodysplastic syndrome
Multiple myeloma*
Adult acute lymphoblastic leukemia*
Lymphoma*

Genetic Diseases
Thalassemia
Congenital immunodeficiency disorders
Fanconi anemia
Sickle cell anemia*
Storage disorders*

---

* Clear cut indication not yet defined.

DONOR SELECTION

Matching for proteins (antigens) of the major histocompatibility complex (MHC) is the basis for selection of an appropriate allogeneic donor. In humans, these antigens are called the human leukocyte antigen system A (HLA) and are present on virtually all nucleated cells in the body. These proteins bind and present peptides from other proteins to T cells, and MHC-dependent interactions are central to almost all types of immune responses. (See Chapter 4.) Foreign HLA proteins can be recognized and distinguished from self and provoke a potent immune response. Allogeneic transplantation replaces the effector arm of the immune system (T and B cells) with donor cells, as well as monocytes and macrophages that are important in presentation of foreign antigens to lymphoid cells. Shared HLA types between the donor and recipient decrease both the risk of immediate rejection of the donor graft by recipient lymphocytes and the risk of recognition and attack of host tissues by engrafted donor-derived lymphocytes, a process termed *graft-versus-host disease* (GVHD).

Most allogeneic donors are HLA-matched siblings. Matched sibling donors share the same HLA type I antigens A, B, and C as well as type II antigens DR, DQ, and DP. Because the genes for HLA proteins are all found on the short arm of chromosome 6, each sibling receives one chromosome (haplotype) of HLA genes from each parent and has a 25% chance of sharing HLA haplotypes with the patient. Complete HLA-matched sibling transplants have a very low rate of graft rejection, but GVHD remains a problem because of differences between donor and recipient in poorly characterized minor histocompatibility antigens *not* found on chromosome 6. Syngeneic transplantation, when donor and recipient are identical twins, has no risk of graft rejection or GVHD.

Only 25–30% of patients otherwise eligible for allogeneic transplant have an HLA-identical sibling. For patients without a matched sibling, transplantation from a partially matched parent, other relative, or HLA-matched unrelated donor can be considered, and the increased risks of GVHD and other posttransplantation complications must be weighed against the potential benefits. Over the past 10 years, large registries of HLA-typed individuals willing to donate marrow for unrelated recipients have been set up, allowing greatly increased numbers of matched unrelated donor (MUD) transplants. In the United States the National Marrow Donor Program (NMDP) has accrued well over 1 million potential donors. Unfortunately, only 60% of patients find appropriate matches through the registries, and for some the 3–6 months required to identify a donor and collect marrow may make transplantation impossible. Donors have been especially difficult to find for non-Caucasian patients as a result of underrepresentation of some ethnic groups in the registries and increased genetic diversity. The long-term survival after MUD or partially matched transplants as compared with matched sibling transplants is significantly lower as a result of higher incidence of graft rejection, infection, and GVHD, especially in adult patients.

PRETRANSPLANT CONDITIONING

Once an indication for allogeneic transplant is established and a suitable donor is identified, pretransplant conditioning of the patient begins. Goals of conditioning depend on the underlying disease being treated. However, irrespective of the underlying disease, the conditioning regimen must immunosuppress the recipient sufficiently to prevent rejection of the allograft and myelosuppress the recipient enough to allow engraftment of the donor stem cells. When malignancy is involved, it should also provide maximum tumor cell kill within the constraints of toxicity to organs other than the bone marrow. Examples of primarily immunosuppressive conditioning regimens used in nonmalignant disorders include cyclophosphamide plus antithymocyte globulin, total lymphoid irradiation, or a combination of relatively low-dose busulfan for myelosuppression and cyclophosphamide for immunosuppression. Such regimens have been used to transplant patients with thalassemia major and aplastic anemia with relatively low toxicity (only 5–15% transplant-related mortality in young patients using a fully matched sibling donor).

Total body irradiation (TBI) in combination with a cytotoxic agent or agents is commonly used for conditioning patients with malignancies. Benefits of TBI include excellent whole-body antineoplastic activity and strong myelo- and immunosuppression. Cyclophosphamide is the agent most frequently paired with TBI. Other agents, such as etoposide, cytosine arabinoside, and melphalan, have also been effectively added to or substituted into TBI-based conditioning regimens to try and increase antitumor effects. Cyclophosphamide and busulfan combinations have also been used in malignant disease as an equally efficacious alternative to TBI-containing regimens.

DONOR HEMATOPOIETIC STEM CELL PROCUREMENT AND TRANSPLANTATION

Procurement of adequate numbers of HSCs is essential for successful and durable engraftment. Grafts containing a very large number of such CD34+ cells have lower rates of graft rejection and lower rates of early posttransplant infectious complications. Bone marrow harvesting is very safe, with major complication rates in normal donors of 0.1%, primarily related to general anesthesia risk. Donors are hospitalized for at most one night following harvest and can expect to be back to normal activity and work schedules within 1 or 2 weeks. The vast majority of allogeneic transplants currently use donor bone marrow as a source for HSCs, but over the next several years donor PBPC grafts will most likely replace marrow. For PBPC harvesting, donors are treated for 4–6 days with subcutaneous G-CSF or other cytokines, and peripheral blood cells are collected by apheresis, yielding 3–10 times more CD34$^+$ cells in the graft than can be obtained with marrow. Cord blood grafts are also increasing in frequency, and cord blood banks may prove a valuable source of unrelated donor stem cells if these transplants prove safe and effective in both adults and children.

ALLOGRAFT ENGINEERING

Early allogeneic transplantation was performed by simply infusing unmanipulated marrow into a peripheral vein. Filtration was soon instituted to eliminate thrombotic complications from particulate material. As indications for allogeneic transplant broaden and understanding of complications improve, pretransplant manipulation of the graft is becoming more common. In the setting of donor/recipient red cell incompatibility, donor RBCs and/or serum are removed from the graft to prevent immediate lysis of donor or recipient RBCs by isohemagglutinin. T-cell depletion of marrow has been shown to decrease the incidence of GVHD, but this beneficial effect is not without costs. Graft failure or rejection occurs more commonly using T-cell-depleted marrow, and infectious complications such as cytomegalovirus disease are more common because of delayed immune recovery. In addition, the graft versus leukemia (GVL) effect may be lost along with the GVHD. This translates into an increased incidence of leukemic relapse, especially in myeloid leukemias. Such refinements as determining the optimal degree of T-cell depletion or adding back T cells after engraftment and recovery from the acute toxicity of conditioning are being actively pursued to try and overcome these problems. In addition, specific T-cell subset depletion, for instance of CD8 but not CD4 positive T-cells, may decrease GVHD without abrogating GVL. In patients being transplanted for nonmalignant disorders, T-cell depletion is an attractive approach as long as adequate conditioning is given to prevent graft rejection.

TRANSPLANTATION TIMELINE

This section is designed to serve as a guide to the management of patients undergoing transplantation. It is organized chronologically as a step-by-step outline of expected events and complications associated with the procedure, and Figure 8-1 summarizes much of this information. Day 0 is always defined by the infusion of the autologous or allogeneic HSCs into the patient. Before engraftment, complications in autologous and allogeneic transplant patients are very similar. After engraftment,

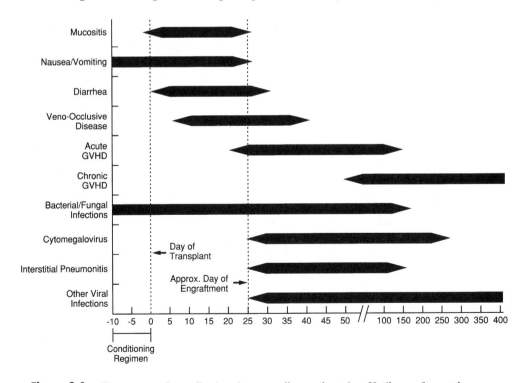

Figure 8-1. Time course of complications in stem cell transplantation. Until engraftment the complications for patients undergoing autologous and allogeneic transplantation are similar. After engraftment, the complications are generally limited to allogeneic recipients. The bars represent the time period where each complication may occur but should serve only as a general guide. Patients with severe graft-versus-host disease have much more prolonged immunosuppression and may develop serious bacterial, fungal, and viral infections even after the period of greatest risk shown in the figure.

autologous transplantation recipients have few problems, and thus the subsequent sections apply only to allogeneic patients.

Initiation of Conditioning Therapy Through Engraftment

Infection Prophylaxis. Infectious complications are a major concern, beginning with the initiation of conditioning therapy. White blood cell counts approach their nadir at day 0 or soon thereafter, resulting in a period of extreme susceptibility to bacterial and fungal infections. Even after normalization of the neutrophil number, patients remain profoundly immunocompromised, especially after allogeneic transplantation. Antibiotic and environmental prophylaxis have, in some cases, proven effective in decreasing infectious complications. Positive-pressure laminar-air-flow rooms equipped with high-efficiency particulate air (HEPA) filters are now found in most transplantation units and are effective in removing most airborne bacterial particles and fungal spores.

Oral fluoroquinolones are commonly used as antibacterial prophylaxis. Norfloxacin, a poorly absorbed quinolone can be used for gut decontamination. The mainstay of antifungal prophylaxis consists of fluconazole therapy. Some studies have demonstrated effectiveness of fluconazole in reducing the incidence of both invasive and superficial candidal infections. However, *Aspergillus* and resistant candidal species are not sensitive to fluconazole and continue to be problematic. Most centers discontinue bacterial and fungal prophylaxis after neutrophil engraftment. *Pneumocystis carinii* prophylaxis is also given to both allogeneic and autologous recipients for 3 months or more using either week-end oral trimethoprim-sulfamethoxazole or monthly aerosolized pentamidine. Antiviral prophylaxis is targeted at the herpesviruses: herpes simplex virus, varicella zoster virus, and cytomegalovirus (CMV). Herpes simplex and zoster reactivation are prevented by low-dose intravenous acyclovir. The optimal anti-CMV prophylactic regimen is still evolving. If both donor and recipient are CMV seronegative, steps should be taken to prevent primary infection by use of CMV-negative or filtered blood products. For recipients who are seropositive, high-dose acyclovir prophylaxis may help to prevent reactivation. In addition, there is good evidence to support the use of weekly intravenous gamma globulin as CMV prophylaxis for seropositive patients or seronegative patients transplanted with cells from a seropositive donor. Although myelosuppressive effects preclude its routine prophylactic use, ganciclovir has also been considered in high-risk patients.

Infectious Complications. Despite optimal prophylactic measures, infectious complications are a major source of morbidity and mortality in stem cell transplantation. Clinicians typically rely on fever as a prime indication of an infections process. Although fever in an immunocompromised patient should never be ignored, it is likely that a significant fraction of the febrile episodes in a transplant patient result not from an active or identifiable infection but from mucositis, GVHD, or other causes of inflammation.

Bacteria. Bacterial infections are the predominant concern in the pre-engraftment period. Not only is the patient profoundly neutropenic, but new portals of entry result from disruptions of skin, mucous membranes, and gastrointestinal (GI) surfaces because of conditioning agents. Bacteremias occur in 15–50% of patients. The source is usually endogenous, arising from the GI tract or indwelling catheters. Gram-positive bacteremias predominate, probably as a result of use of prophylactic antibiotics with gram-negative activity. Some centers give prophylactic ceftazidime or other intravenous broad-spectrum coverage as soon as the patient becomes neutropenic; others wait until the first fever occurs. Vancomycin is also often given with the first neutropenic fever.

Other common sites of bacterial infection in the pre-engraftment period include the skin, lungs, sinuses, and GI tract. Weekly chest films and screening sinus films or computed tomography (CT) scans can be helpful for early detection. Typhlitis is a fulminant necrotizing infection of the bowel wall with gram-negative organisms, candidal species, and/or clostridia. Patients typically complain of abdominal pain, nausea, and vomiting. If ultrasound or CT scan is suggestive of bowel wall thickening or inflammation, surgical intervention may be indicated. Mortality rates for typhlitis have been reported to be 50–100%. Bacterial pneumonia can occur, but a typical lobar infiltrate is very rare. The diagnosis of diffuse infiltrates in the pre-engraftment period can be difficult, as fluid overload, pulmonary hemorrhage, and early radiation or CMV pneumonitis are all in the differential. In a febrile patient with pulmonary infiltrates, empiric broadening of antibiotic coverage to include double anti-gram-negative therapy and antifungal treatment with amphotericin is often instituted prior to obtaining results from bronchoalveolar lavage, which is frequently nondiagnostic.

Fungi. Up to 30% of recipients develop fungal infections in the pre-engraftment period. Candidal species, primarily albicans, and *Aspergillus* species are the most common fungal isolates. In practice, documentation of fungal infection can be difficult. When recurrent febrile episodes persist for more than 3–7 days despite broad-spectrum antibacterial coverage, empiric antifungal therapy with amphotericin should be instituted, even in patients already receiving prophylactic fluconazole. Candidal infections can manifest as an erythematous, macular skin rash; fungemia; or visceral infection. Rising liver enzymes, especially alkaline phosphatase, and typical liver lesions on CT scan or magnetic resonance imaging (MRI) suggest hepatosplenic candidiasis. Treatment of invasive candidal infections in the pre-engraftment period is relatively ineffective, and persistent infection is an extremely poor prognostic sign. Oral and esophageal superficial infection can be prevented by good oral hygiene, prophylactic fluconazole, and oral antiseptic rinses and antifungal troches.

Aspergillus pneumoniae is the most common and dreaded fungal complication. Inhalation of aspergillus spores that escape HEPA filtration or pre-existent colonization of the patient is the initiating event. Aspergillus can also present as a sinus, skin, or central nervous system infection. Diagnosis of aspergillus infection can be quite difficult, with the characteristic nodular or cavitary appearance and/or the halo sign, which is a zone of low attenuation surrounding a pulmonary mass found on CT scan, often lacking. Biopsy of the affected tissue is the only means of confirming the diagnosis, and in a compromised patient with a low platelet count this may be impractical. High-dose amphotericin must be instituted if aspergillus is seriously suspected.

Viral Infections. Viral infections in the pre-engraftment period are less commonly problematic than they are after transplantation, at least in allogeneic recipients. Reactivation of herpes simplex virus (HSV) occurs in 85% of patients who are not prophylaxed with acyclovir. Gingivostomatitis from HSV-1 is the most common manifestation, and these painful lesions lead to decreased oral intake. They also provide portals of entry for bacterial and fungal superinfection. Other potential viral pathogens include adenovirus and respiratory syncytial virus. Early CMV infection or reactivation can occur and is very serious, but the peak incidence is after engraftment, and will be discussed later.

Gastrointestinal Complications. High-dose chemotherapy, TBI, and such antibiotics as imipenem, ganciclovir, and amphotericin can produce severe nausea and vomiting. Mucositis occurs 5–14 days after initiation of the conditioning regimen and correlates with the period of severe neutropenia. The rapidly dividing cells that line the GI tract are killed or damaged by the conditioning agents, and superinfection of the ulcers with bacteria, fungus, HSV, or CMV exacerbates the problem. Healing of these lesions is delayed until neutrophils return. Symptoms include pain, nausea, vomiting, and diarrhea. With very severe mucositis, airway compromise due to sloughing and hemorrhage of perilaryngeal or submental tissue can occur. Any patient with even a suspicion of this complication should be placed in a monitored setting with the capability of performing an emergency tracheostomy. Adequate analgesia is the most important component of mucositis treatment, and patient-controlled narcotics should be provided as soon as moderate to severe symptoms occur. Oral rinses such as chlorhexidine may decrease superinfection and should be used throughout the neutropenic period. Total parenteral nutrition is invariably instituted as oral intake decreases secondary to the complications just described.

Inflammation and sloughing of the intestinal mucosa impairs the absorptive capacity of the large and small bowels. Although this is the most common reason for diarrhea, clinicians must maintain a constant awareness that other, more dangerous causes may develop concurrently. *Clostridium difficile* infection resulting in pseudomembranous colitis, even without prolonged broad-spectrum antibiotics usage, is very frequent. Screening for *Clostridium difficile* toxin should be done whenever there is an abrupt increase in the stool volume, especially if it is bloody and accompanied by fever.

Liver Abnormalities. Mild elevations in liver enzymes and bilirubin are common in the pre-engraftment period. The reasons are multifactorial and include drug effects, total parenteral nutrition-related cholestasis, and infections. More serious is hepatic veno-occlusive disease (VOD), an often fatal complication of the conditioning regimen. Occurring in 10–20% of allogenic and autologous transplantation recipients, symptoms usually begin between days 7 and 14, and consist of the triad of hepatomegaly, jaundice, and ascites or unexplained weight gain. In addition, right upper quadrant pain mimicking an acute abdomen has been described. There is a broad range in the severity of symptoms. The differential diagnosis includes GVHD or hepatitis due to infection or drug effects. An increased bilirubin in the absence of significant elevations in transaminases and alkaline phosphatase helps distinguish early VOD from these other possibilities. If diagnostic confirmation is needed, transvenous measurement of hepatic venous pressure as well as transvenous liver biopsy can be performed, but in practice this is rarely indicated. Although the pathophysiology of VOD is unclear, damage to the endothelium of liver venules and thrombosis is always seen histologically. Decreased levels of endogenous anticoagulants such as protein C are seen, as are changes in multimer patterns of von Willebrand factor (Chapter 6), but most of these perturbations are thought to be secondary to the liver damage, not primary to the etiology of the condition.

Other than supportive care, there is no standard treatment for VOD. Patients with suspected VOD should be maintained as close as possible to their baseline weight via sodium and fluid restriction, along with aggressive diuresis. Some trials have shown a benefit for anticoagulation or replenishment of endogenous anticoagulants, but results have not been consistent, and there are obvious risks to anticoagulation of these patients. The mortality rate of VOD has been reported as high as 50% but may actually be lower since many mild cases may not have been included. Poor prognosis is related to the onset of multiorgan failure, especially hepatorenal syndrome. The risk of developing VOD is increased by very intensive conditioning regimens, increased recipient age, and pretransplant liver compromise of any etiology.

Supportive Care. Transfusion of blood products during the pre-engraftment period is unavoidable. On average, the allogenic transplant recipient will require up to 10–15 U of packed RBCs, and as many as 150 U of platelets. Autologous transplant patients typically require much less blood product support. Because of profound immunosuppression, steps must be taken to prevent transfusion-related GVH, which occurs when viable lymphocytes in the blood product react against recipient antigens. Leukodepletion filters remove up to 99% of leukocytes, and irradiation renders the remaining leukocytes inactive. If both the donor and recipient are CMV negative, primary CMV infection from blood products must be prevented, either by use of CMV negative donors or leukodepletion filters. It is standard practice at most transplant centers to maintain the hemoglobin between 8 and 10 g/dL.

Platelet support may be difficult in many transplantation recipients, because of pretransplant allosensitization resulting from prior transfusions. Unlike RBCs, platelets possess HLA class I antigens and are very immunogenic. Transfusion of at least partially HLA-matched platelets may be necessary to increase the platelet count. Other factors which lead to platelet refractoriness include hypersplenism, fever, and sepsis. There is little disagreement that patients with platelet counts of less than $5,000/\mu L$ are at increased risk for spontaneous bleeding and should be transfused. Clinical judgment dictates when patients above $5,000/\mu L$ should be transfused. Active bleeding, fever, or use of invasive monitoring devices are all reasons to aim for a higher platelet count.

In autologous transplantation, the use of mobilized peripheral blood cells instead of marrow has shortened engraftment time to the degree that treatment with myeloid-stimulating cytokines such as G-CSF or GM-CSF may not further significantly shorten time to neutrophil engraftment. Ongoing studies with new cytokines such as thrombopoietin and interleukin 11 may define a role for shortening platelet recovery times. In allogeneic transplantation there are no definitive guidelines for the use of hematopoietic growth factors (HGFs) after transplantation. There is good evidence that high levels of endogenous growth factors are present during the pre-engraftment period. There has also been ambivalence on the part of clinicians to give HGF to patients with myeloid leukemias because of the theoretical concerns of stimulating the malignant clone, but in practice, an increased relapse rate of myeloid leukemia with HGF use has not been documented. Despite its questionable efficacy in the early transplantation period, it is common practice to use HGFs in the setting of delayed engraftment.

Engraftment. Although there is great patient-to-patient variability in time to engraftment, evidence of donor hematopoiesis usually is seen by day 12–23 in allogeneic marrow transplantation recipients. In PBPC autologous transplants, neutrophil recovery can occur as early as day 7–9. Monocytes are often the first cells to be detected in the peripheral blood emerging from a recovering marrow. Neutrophil and then platelet and red cell production should follow shortly thereafter.

There are many possible causes of delayed engraftment. These include graft rejection in allogeneic recipients and low HSC numbers in donor or autologous grafts. T-cell depletion, tumor purging, overwhelming infection, or marrow suppressive medications such as ganciclovir may also delay or compromise engraftment. Hematopoietic cytokines may be able to speed recovery, but in some instances a second graft or a boost with donor PBPCs or more marrow is necessary.

Engraftment Through Day 100

Acute Graft-Versus-Host Disease.

Pathophysiology. When immunologically competent T-lymphocytes derived from the donor react against antigens expressed on recipient tissues, GVHD is initiated. The onset and clinical constellation of GVHD are quite variable and depend on many factors, some of which are poorly understood. The constellation of symptoms and signs commonly seen in the first 100 days characterize acute GVHD (aGVHD), whereas manifestations after day 100 are usually very different and characterize a distinct chronic GVHD syndrome. Patients who are not adequately prophylaxed against GVHD can begin to manifest symptoms within a week or two of donor cell infusion.

Incidence. GVHD occurs to some degree in up to 80% of allogeneic transplantation recipients. Factors that predispose patients to aGVHD are shown in Table 8-2. The most reliable predictor for the development of aGVHD is HLA incompatibility. Multiparous female donors are more likely to cause GVHD because of HLA alloimmunization during pregnancy or delivery, and risk of GVHD increases over age 30. Increased donor age may also be a risk factor. Polymorphisms of HLA proteins may account for much of the more severe aGVHD seen with matched unre-

---

TABLE 8-2. *RISK FACTORS FOR ACUTE GRAFT VS HOST DISEASE*

Recipient
- Increased age
- Infection with DNA viruses (HSV, VZV, CMV)
- Intensive conditioning
- Low progenitor cell dose

Donor
- Previous transfusions
- Previous pregnancies
- Increased age

Donor-recipient matching
- Sex mismatch
- HLA-A, B, DR mismatch
- Unrelated donor

278

lated transplants. Infection and inflammation may potentiate or initiate aGVHD, because of cytokine release and stimulation of donor lymphocytes to react with antigens at the site of inflammation.

Clinical Manifestations. Clinical manifestations of aGVHD primarily occur in the skin, liver, and GI tract. One or many organ systems can be affected by aGVHD, and a transplant physician soon learns that "typical" GVHD with all the organ manifestations occurring simultaneously in a nonambiguous clinical setting is rare! A maculopapular skin rash is usually the first sign of aGVHD and is commonly localized on the extensor surfaces of the limbs, as well as on the face, neck, and trunk. In severe aGVHD, the rash becomes confluent and may progress to bullae or desquamation. Skin biopsy can help distinguish aGVHD from drug reactions or viral exanthems.

GI tract manifestations typically follow the skin rash and primarily include watery voluminous diarrhea, which can be bloody in severe cases. Other symptoms include crampy abdominal pain and ileus. The diagnosis of GI aGVHD is established after careful consideration of the time of onset and other potential causes of the symptomatology. The differential diagnosis includes residual effects of conditioning; infections from such agents as *Clostridium difficile* , CMV, common enteric pathogens, or drug effects. Direct visualization and biopsy via endoscopy can be useful in establishing a diagnosis.

The onset of liver aGVHD is heralded by laboratory evidence of cholestasis, which results from the preferential attack of cytotoxic T cells on small interlobular and marginal bile ducts. Although elevation of the bilirubin and alkaline phosphatase predominate, liver parenchymal involvement with elevation of SGOT and SGPT are also commonly observed. The differential diagnosis of liver aGVHD includes viral hepatitis, veno-occlusive disease, and toxic drug effects. Cyclosporine liver toxicity in particular can confuse the picture. Liver biopsy is rarely required to make the diagnosis,

GVHD Prophylaxis. All allogeneic (but not autologous or syngeneic) transplantation recipients receive some sort of GVHD prophylaxis. The two most effective methods of GVHD prophylaxis are T-lymphocyte depletion of donor cells, or treatment of the recipient with immunosuppressive drugs. The three commonly used immunosuppressive drugs are cyclosporine, methotrexate, and prednisone or other corticosteroids. Combination therapy with at least two agents is given with non-T-depleted grafts, but the exact regimen and the use of two versus three drugs is determined by individual centers and patient characteristics. Cyclosporine is the cornerstone of most prophylactic regimens, and is begun at the time of marrow infusion or just before (Day 0). Levels should be checked at least weekly, and adjusted to maintain therapeutic blood levels. GVHD prophylaxis is continued for 3–6 months posttransplantation. GI tract decontamination with antibiotics and HEPA-filtered environment may also decrease GVHD by decreasing the incidence of initiating infectious events.

Treatment. Treatment strategies for aGVHD build on the prophylactic immunosuppressive regimen already in place. The same agents used for GVHD prophylaxis are also used for treatment of aGVHD. The decision to treat is often based on the grading system shown in Table 8-3. Mild skin GVHD alone does not require treatment, but any significant GI involvement or level 2 or greater skin injury should trigger an aggressive attempt to interrupt the process. In general, immunosuppressive agents are added in a stepwise fashion according to clinical response. High-dose

TABLE 8-3. *ORGAN-SPECIFIC CLASSIFICATION OF ACUTE GRAFT VERSUS HOST DISEASE*

LEVEL OF INJURY	SKIN	LIVER (BILIRUBIN)	INTESTINAL TRACT
1	Maculopapular rash <25% of body surface	2–3 mg/dL	500–1000 mL liquid stool/day
2	Maculopapular rash 25–50% of body surface	>3–6 mg/dL	>1000 and <1500 mL liquid stool/day
3	Generalized erythroderma	>6–15 mg/dL	>1500 mL liquid stool/day
4	Generalized erythroderma with bullae and desquamation	>15 mg/dL	Severe abdominal pain with or without ileus

CLINICAL GRADE	LEVEL OF INJURY		
	Skin	Liver	Intestinal Tract
I	1 or 2	0	0
II	1–3	1	1
III	2 or 3	2 or 3	2 or 3
IV	2–4	2–4	2–4

methylprednisolone is commonly used in conjunction with cyclosporine. Once signs and symptoms abate, the dose is tapered down over several weeks. Steroid-refractory aGVHD has a very poor prognosis, and second-line agents such as anti-thymocyte globulin or experimental immunosuppressives should be instituted for serious (grade III or IV) aGVHD after 1 week of unresponsiveness to high-dose steroids. Patients with significant GI involvement require careful fluid and electrolyte management. Bowel rest should be instituted, and p.o. intake should be advanced gradually once diarrhea abates. Pain medication for abdominal cramping may be required. Antidiarrheals such as loperamide or octreotide have little utility in most cases.

Prognosis. The prognosis of aGVHD is highly dependent on the clinical grade. If the patient progresses to grade IV aGVHD despite aggressive immunosuppression, mortality is almost 100% and often results from superinfections complicating the aggressive immunosuppression rather than direct organ failure from aGVHD. Immune dysfunction appears to result from aGVHD itself as well as from the treatment. Marrow suppression with subsequent increase in transfusion requirements, especially platelets, is common in severe GVHD. Patients with severe aGVHD are more likely to develop chronic GVHD.

Cytomegalovirus. In the general population, 50–70% are seropositive (possess antibodies) for cytomegalovirus (CMV), indicating prior primary CMV infection and latency of the virus within a small percentage of leukocytes or other reservoirs. The profound immunosuppression experienced by patients undergoing allogeneic transplantation is accompanied by reactivation and release of this latent virus in up to 70% of allogeneic transplantation recipients at risk (either seropositive recipients or seronegative recipients receiving cells from a seropositive donor). This is much rarer in autologous recipients.

Clinical Manifestations. Posttransplantation CMV reactivation can be asymptomatic, and detected on routine screening for active viral replication. When CMV reactivation becomes symptomatic, it is termed *CMV disease.* CMV disease occurs in approximately 25–35% of allogenic transplantation recipients. The peak incidence occurs at days 50–60, but CMV disease can occur much early or later, especially in patients with preexisting profound immunosuppression or persistent GVHD. CMV disease can manifest as a typical viral infection, with fever and chills, malaise, and myalgias. Whether through direct infection of early hematopoietic precursor cells or through stimulation of inhibitory cytokine release, it also commonly causes worsening cytopenias. It can also be organ specific, presenting in the lung as interstitial pneumonitis or in the GI tract as diffuse intestinal ulceration accompanied by diarrhea or abdominal pain. Liver enzyme elevations are often present. CMV retinitis is rare.

CMV-associated interstitial pneumonitis is the most common and most feared CMV disease manifestation. An estimated 15–30% of allogeneic transplant recipients will develop CMV pneumonitis, and up to 90% of these patients will die of the disease. Patients present with fever, dyspnea, and a nonproductive cough, with hypoxemia in all but the mildest cases. Although diffuse interstitial infiltrates are most typical, there is variability in the radiographic findings. Complicating the picture further is the extensive differential diagnosis for this constellation of symptoms in allogeneic transplant recipients. This includes diffuse alveolar hemorrhage, pulmonary edema, idiopathic interstitial pneumonitis, acute respiratory distress syndrome (ARDS), or other infectious etiologies.

Diagnosis. Recent advances in diagnostic techniques should reduce life-threatening complications of CMV infection. Instead of delaying treatment until actual CMV disease develops, detection of replicating CMV in peripheral blood leukocytes or rapid culture of virus from certain body fluids allows institution of treatment prior to significant organ damage. It is now common to screen patients once or twice per week in the early postengraftment period. Surveillance of the blood leukocytes for CMV-specific antigens provides a quick, sensitive method for diagnosis of early infection. Rapid "shell-vial" (CMV assay) 24–48-hour CMV culture techniques are also sensitive and detect early viral antigen expression in a monolayer of indicator cells co-cultured with blood leukocytes from the patient. The significance of positive throat or urine cultures is unclear, but positive blood or pulmonary lavage cultures should trigger institution of treatment, as should a positive blood antigen test. If all noninvasive testing is negative but pulmonary infiltrates develop in a patient 30–100 days after transplantation, bronchoscopy and bronchoalveolar lavage (BAL) should be performed in an attempt to make a diagnosis. Empiric anti-CMV treatment is prudent even if no cultures are positive, because of the high frequency and mortality of CMV pneumonitis.

Treatment. Documented CMV infection or disease is usually treated with ganciclovir, in combination with very-high-dose IVIG. Daily ganciclovir is generally continued for at least 10 days, and then a maintenance regimen of 3–4 times per week is continued until day 100–120. Bone marrow suppression almost always occurs with ganciclovir therapy, and in patients with early reactivation or tenuous grafts this drug may not be tolerated. Foscarnet is an effective alternative with little associated bone marrow suppression but has significant renal toxicity. Once pulmonary disease develops, treatment is very ineffective, and patients that require intubation for pneumonitis have a survival rate of less than 1–2%.

Other Infections. The newly engrafted allogeneic transplant recipient remains immunocompromised and susceptible to many of the same organisms outlined in the pre-engraftment section. Reasons for this include ongoing GVHD prophylaxis, residual mucositis, and varying degrees of aGVHD. Indwelling catheters remain in place through day 100 and contribute to frequent episodes of Gram-positive bacterial infections. The incidence of *Pneumocystis carinii* is low with adequate prophylaxis but remains a concern, as does toxoplasmosis. Reactivation of tuberculosis must be considered in transplant recipients who develop pulmonary infiltrates with a history of a positive PPD or origination from a high-risk area. Patients who are highly immunocompromised due to MUD or haplotype-matched grafting, rigorous T depletion, or prolonged intensive aGVHD therapy are at risk for Epstein-Barr virus–associated lymphoproliferation.

Idiopathic Interstitial Pneumonitis. When diffuse interstitial pulmonary infiltrates develop without an identifiable cause, the etiology is considered idiopathic. Five to 10% of allogeneic transplant patients will develop idiopathic interstitial pneumonitis (IIP). IIP is clinically indistinguishable from CMV-associated interstitial pneumonitis, and some previous series may have included patients with CMV that would have been detected by modern assays. The lung damage in IIP is most likely a sequela of the toxic effects of the conditioning regimen, especially TBI and busulfan. Supportive care is the standard treatment for IIP, and some patients may respond to high-dose steroids.

Post Day 100

Chronic Graft-Versus-Host Disease. Although chronic graft-versus-host disease (cGVHD) is classically defined as occurring after day 100 of allogeneic transplantation, findings consistent with the syndrome can occur earlier. It is most common for cGVHD to evolve from aGVHD, but aGVHD is not a prerequisite. Other risk factors for the development of cGVHD are degree of donor/recipient matching and increasing recipient age.

Pathophysiology. The pathology of cGVHD differs from that of aGVHD and resembles an autoimmune/connective-tissue disorder. The underlying mechanisms are poorly understood, but T cells in cGVHD are inappropriately activated, and widespread inflammation and collagen deposition result. Diagnosis of cGVHD is usually made quite definitively by the clinical presentation. Skin or liver biopsy can help in the diagnosis of atypical presentations of the disease.

Clinical Manifestations. The clinical features and grading of cGVHD are shown in Table 8-4. The skin is involved in 80% of cases. Lichen planus is seen with papulosquamous dermatitis, plaques, and vitiligo. If unchecked, skin cGVHD will progress to scleradermoid induration, joint contractures, and chronic skin ulceration. Dry mouth and eyes are also common symptoms, and frequent ophthalmologic exams with Schirmer's testing for tear formation are important to detect early cGVHD that could damage vision. cGVHD may also affect the liver, with chronic hyperbilirubinemia, pruritus, and symptoms of malabsorption. Other, more nonspe-

TABLE 8-4. *GRADING OF CHRONIC GVHD*	
TYPE OF DISEASE	**EXTENT OF DISEASE**
Limited	Localized skin involvement and/or liver dysfunction
Extensive	Generalized skin involvement
	Localized skin involvement or liver dysfunction plus any one of the following:
	Chronic aggressive hepatitis, bridging necrosis, or cirrhosis
	Ocular sicca
	Mucosalivary gland involvement
	Involvement of other target organs

cific GI manifestations—such as anorexia, nausea, weight loss, early satiety, and difficulty swallowing—may occur. Restrictive pulmonary disease is one of the most serious forms of cGVHD, and periodic PFTs are performed in most posttransplant patients. cGVHD itself, as well as immunosuppressive treatments used in response to it, weaken the immune system and further delay immune reconstitution. Patients with cGVHD that remain on steroid or cyclosporine treatment past day 100 should continue to receive prophylactic drugs for *Pneumocystis carinii, Herpes simplex,* and even candidal esophagitis.

Treatment. The same immunosuppressive medications used to treat or prevent aGVHD are also used for cGVHD. Limited disease often responds to prednisone. More extensive or refractory cGVHD may require the addition of cyclosporine. Azathioprine and thalidomide have also been used in this setting. PUVA (psoralen and ultraviolet A radiation) is an effective modality for the treatment of refractory cutaneous cGVHD.

Immune Reconstitution. Early in the posttransplant period, evidence of donor cellular and humoral immunity can be demonstrated. This phenomenon is likely related to the transfer of mature donor T- and B-lymphocytes. As these mature cells disappear, they are replaced by naive lymphocytes derived from transplanted hematopoietic stem cells. As naive donor T-lymphocytes are reeducated in the presence of recipient antigens, tolerance develops. Reconstitution of humoral and cellular immunity in the transplant recipient is highly dependent on the presence of GVHD. In patients without evidence of cGVHD, T-lymphocyte-dependent immunity (cellular immunity) is reestablished by 4–6 months after transplantation. Humoral immunity requires appropriate communication between an antigen-specific T-lymphocyte and the antibody producing B-lymphocyte. In recipients of non-T-depleted marrow, normal antibody production is reestablished by 7–9 months. Immune reconstitution is delayed or prevented by active GVHD and GVHD treatment.

Other Late Complications of Transplantation. Table 8-5 lists other late complications of transplantation. The major risk factors appear to be conditioning regimen related, or secondary to tissue damage from GVHD or chronic immunosuppression in allogeneic recipients. Since many patients are within the reproductive age range, fertility is a significant concern. Ovarian function returns to normal in 15% of postpubertal women, and testicular function returns to normal in 25% of men. Radiation dose in the conditioning regimen was found to be the most important predictor of fertility. Because patients with malignant diseases are more likely to receive high doses of TBI, the fertility rate in this population tends to be lower.

Late hypothyroidism and growth hormone deficiency can occur. The latter is most important in the pediatric population. Early growth hormone supplementation can augment bone growth and prevent short stature. Cataract formation is the most common ophthalmologic complication, and results from TBI and/or prolonged glucocorticoid therapy. Other ocular pathology can result from cGVHD, including corneal scaring or perforation.

Bone disease may result from glucocorticoid therapy, usually for the treatment of GVHD. Avascular necrosis of bone is the most serious complication, but generalized osteoporosis is also of great concern if prolonged glucocorticoid therapy is necessary.

Salivary gland dysfunction often results from TBI and GVHD, causing sicca syndrome (which includes dry mouth or xerostomia), followed by dental decay and frequent oral infections. Both pre- and posttransplantation dental care by a dentist experienced in treating transplant patients is very beneficial.

There is a significant risk of developing a new malignancy following allogeneic or autologous transplantation. The conditioning regimen can provide a carcinogenic insult, followed by a prolonged immunocompromised state with decreased antineoplastic immune surveillance. The Fred Hatchinson Cancer Research Center in Seattle reviewed 4,294 patients who underwent autologous or allogeneic transplant and found 82 patients with secondary malignancies. Lymphoproliferative disorders were the most common malignancies, many of which were EBV-related. Ten percent or more of autologous transplant recipients surviving long term develop

TABLE 8-5. *LATE EFFECTS OF ALLOGENEIC TRANSPLANTATION*

Pulmonary
    Infection
    Chronic lung disease

Endocrinologic
    Infertility
    Premature menopause
    Hypothyroidism

Ophthalmic
    Sicca syndrome
    Cataracts

Oral
    Sicca syndrome
    Dental decay
    Periodontal disease

Musculoskeletal
    Avascular necrosis
    Osteoporosis (with chronic steroid therapy)

General
    Secondary malignancy
    Autoimmune phenomena
    Psychosocial effects

secondary myelodysplasia or leukemia, presumably because of pretransplant damage to residual bone marrow stem cells.

Efficacy of Allogeneic Transplantation. The outcome of allogeneic transplantation depends on the underlying disease and on donor and recipient characteristics. Allogeneic transplant for acute myelocytic leukemia (AML) is most effective when undertaken while the patient is in remission. When it is performed during first remission, 40–70% of long-term survivors appear to be cured. When it is done at the time of relapse or during subsequent remissions, these rates drop to 20–40%, because of increased relapse. Transplant-related mortality is also increased in these later-stage patients. Since 20–25% of AML patients treated with chemotherapy alone may be cured and 20–40% of those who relapse after conventional chemotherapy can then be cured with allogeneic transplant, the timing of transplant is often controversial, and there is an emphasis on identifying patients at high risk of relapse in first remission and transplanting them immediately.

Fifty to 75% of chronic myelogenous leukemia (CML) patients survive long term and are presumed cured after HLA matched related donor allogeneic transplants performed during chronic phase; thus all patients younger than age 60 with an HLA-matched family donor should be considered for the procedure. Results in accelerated phase and blast crisis are much less favorable, but those patients have very short life expectancies with any other therapy.

Large-scale clinical trials are needed to better define the role of allogeneic transplantation in the treatment of the other hematologic malignancies, such as multiple myeloma, lymphoma, acute and chronic lymphocytic leukemia, and myelodysplastic syndromes.

There is an established indication for allogeneic transplantation for the treatment of lethal immunodeficiency states such as severe combined immunodeficiency (Chapter 4), Wiskott-Aldrich syndrome (Chapter 5), or Chédiak-Higashi syndrome (Chapters 4 and 7). Patients with acquired severe aplastic anemia under the age of 30 with a matched sibling donor should be transplanted as initial therapy, but the relative roles of transplant versus immunosuppression in older patients with this disorder remain controversial (Chapter 7). Patients with thalassemia major with no organ damage from iron overload should probably be transplanted before age 10 if they have a matched sibling donor (Chapter 3).

AUTOLOGOUS TRANSPLANTATION

OVERVIEW

The dose-limiting toxicity of many chemotherapeutic agents and of irradiation is bone marrow suppression. The doses of many of these agents can be significantly escalated if followed by rescue with stored hematopoietic stem cells. For autologous transplantation to be beneficial, the malignancy should have a dose-dependent response to chemotherapy and/or irradiation, meaning that the higher doses possible with HSC rescue can kill more tumor cells without significantly increasing treatment-related morbidity and mortality. Since autologous transplantation does not involve replacement of the entire hematopoietic and immune systems with those from another individual, many of the complications that occur after allogeneic transplantation are not an issue, such as graft rejection, graft-versus-host disease, and infectious complications related to prolonged suppression of T-cell immunity. However, the lack of any graft-versus-tumor effect and the likely reinfusion of tumor cells with the graft are two reasons that autografts may result in a higher relapse rate than allografts for most malignancies.

HEMATOPOIETIC STEM CELL PROCUREMENT

Before 1990, bone marrow was the source of HSCs for the vast majority of autologous grafts. Marrow from these often heavily pretreated cancer patients was sometimes difficult to collect, and often required 4 weeks or more to engraft and maintain hematopoiesis. During this prolonged period of cytopenias, the complication rate from infections and bleeding was relatively high, with procedure-related mortality rates of 10% or greater. More recently, mobilized PBPCs have almost completely replaced marrow as a source of stem cells for autologous transplantation. The discovery that the number of circulating primitive cells could be increased 100-fold or more by prior treatment with hematopoietic cytokines with or without chemotherapy decreased the number of aphereses necessary to collect an adequate graft. Besides the comparative ease of collection, these grafts tend to "take" much more quickly, with hematopoietic recovery as soon as 9–14 days after transplantation. This rapid recovery has decreased the morbidity and mortality from the procedure, and some centers even perform these procedures in the outpatient setting, with patients admitted only if they develop a neutropenic fever or other complication. The upper age limit for autologous transplantation has been increasing, with reports of good results in patients as old as 70.

AUTOGRAFT ENGINEERING

After autologous BM or PBPCs are collected, further processing steps are sometimes carried out to try and "purge" the graft of residual tumor cells, using methods designed to eliminate tumor cells selectively, such as antitumor monoclonal antibodies, cytotoxic agents, physical separation based on size or density, or positive selection of hematopoietic progenitor and stem cells. The need for purging has been a source of much controversy, with little definitive data, because of the lack of large randomized controlled trials or large registry studies. Using sensitive molecular and immunohistochemical methods, it is often possible to detect tumor cells in BM or PBPC collections, even if the sample is morphologically free of tumor cells. This is true even in solid tumors such as breast cancer. Logically, one would expect that reinfusing these cells would lead to relapse and that removing tumor cells from the graft would be beneficial. But reengraftment of tumor cells after transplantation is probably a relatively inefficient process, and animal models as well as some clinical trials suggest that residual tumor in the patient surviving the conditioning chemo/radiotherapy is much more likely to be the primary source of relapse. However, genetic marker studies using viral vectors to permanently mark autologous grafts have shown that at least some relapsing tumor cells originate from the graft in childhood leukemia and neuroblastoma.

There are two major practical problems with purging. First, lack of knowledge about tumor and stem cell biology makes it difficult to identify the best method of selecting the normal hematopoietic elements away from tumor cells. Second, many of the purging approaches, especially those employing treatment of the graft with cytotoxic agents such as 4HC or IL-2, appear to damage hematopoietic cells and delay engraftment, increasing the morbidity and mortality of the procedure. More recently, interest has focused on using "positive" instead of "negative" selection procedures. Instead of trying to kill or physically remove tumor cells from the graft, immunoselection of HSCs is performed utilizing antibodies that bind to cell surface proteins, such as CD34, that are not found on most tumor cells but are found on HSCs. CD34-selected BM and PBPC grafts, despite containing less than 1–2% of starting cell numbers, have been shown to produce prompt engraftment and be significantly depleted of some types of tumor cells.

CONDITIONING AND TRANSPLANTATION

After processing, the graft is cryopreserved and the patient undergoes conditioning therapy with myeloablative doses of chemo/radiotherapy. The regimen is chosen based on activity of the agents against the specific tumor being treated. It is also important to design a regimen that is dose-limited by myelotoxicity, not by other organ damage. For instance, cisplatin is rarely used in autologous transplantation because renal toxicity is dose-limiting before lethal myelotoxicity. After completion of the regimen and enough time to allow complete metabolism or excretion of the active forms of the chemotherapeutic agents, the BM or PBPC graft is thawed and reinfused intravenously.

The preengraftment period that follows closely resembles that of allogenic transplantation previously discussed. (See the earlier section entitled "Allogeneic Transplantation.") Once engraftment has occurred, patients tend to feel better rapidly and may be back to full performance status by 6–12 weeks after the transplant. Unlike patients who have undergone allogeneic transplantation, autologous transplantation patients do not experience late complications such as aGVHD or viral or fungal infections. Long-term toxicities such as cataracts, thyroid dysfunction, and infertility may result from TBI, and recent studies suggest that up to 10% of patients may develop secondary myelodysplasia several years after the graft.

APPLICATIONS AND EFFICACY

The goals of autografting vary, depending on the specific malignancy and clinical situation. In acute leukemias and in some lymphomas, cure or at least very prolonged disease-free survival has been reported in a significant fraction of patients. In multiple myeloma, cure does not appear possible after an autograft, but results from a randomized trial suggest that autografts produce significantly longer disease-free intervals than conventional chemotherapy. In breast cancer, cure is very unlikely in patients transplanted for stage IV metastatic disease (widespread visceral or bony metastatic disease), and any survival benefit from the procedure has been difficult to demonstrate. However, it may be that the most promising application in breast cancer is the use of autografting as an intensive consolidation treatment in patients with high-risk stage II or III disease (lymph node metastatic disease ± large primary tumor).

It is very important to realize that almost every application of autografting is controversial. Very few randomized controlled trials have been performed comparing autografting to standard therapy, and comparison to historical controls has been fraught with misinterpretation because of improvements in supportive care over time and patient selection bias. Thus very inconsistent criteria have been used by insurance companies regarding coverage of these expensive procedures ($50,000–$150,000), and often political or legal wrangling has determined application of these procedures in different disease categories or individual patients. The next 5 years will determine whether the enormous increase in the application of autografts in these and other clinical situations is justified, and then policy makers and economists will need to argue whether they are cost effective. In the meantime, whenever possible, patients undergoing autologous transplantation should be enrolled in well-designed clinical trials with close follow-up and expeditious reporting of the results.

CASE PRESENTATION

A 35-year-old male with a history of chronic myelogenous leukemia (CML) in chronic phase is referred for allogeneic bone marrow transplantation. His younger brother is found to be a 6 out of 6 HLA antigen match. Pretransplant testing of both the patient and his donor show evidence of prior cytomegalovirus (CMV) infection.

The patient is admitted to the transplant unit. Norfloxacin and fluconazole are started for antibacterial and antifungal prophylaxis. Intravenous acyclovir is also started for herpes simplex and CMV prophylaxis. High-dose cyclophosphamide is infused through a central venous catheter on *DAYS -7 and -8* before the transplant. He then receives total body irradiation 1200 rads on *DAYS -6 through -1*. During conditioning, the patient complains only of mild intermittent nausea and lethargy. Cyclosporine and methotrexate are given as graft-versus-host disease prophylaxis.

On *DAY 0*, the donor undergoes a bone marrow harvest under general anesthesia. Later that day, the donor marrow is infused uneventfully through the central venous catheter into the recipient.

By *DAY 4* after the transplant, the patient is complaining of dysphagia, diarrhea, and nausea. Physical exam is significant for redness and some sloughing of the oral mucous membranes, but no thrush or ulcerations are noted. The patient is now pancytopenic, and transfusion of irradiated, leuko-depleted blood products is required to maintain a platelet count above $10,000/\mu L$ and hemoglobin above 8 g/dL.

On *DAY 10*, a temperature of 38.8°C PO is noted. Physical exam is significant only for the previously noted mouth findings. On *DAY 14*, review of the clinical data flow sheets reveals a net positive fluid balance, and a 2-kg weight gain for 2 consecutive days. Physical exam reveals icteric sclera, right upper quadrant tenderness, and shifting dullness consistent with ascites. A cyclosporin level was checked, and found to be in the therapeutic range. Fluid restriction, and a potassium-sparing diuretic, Aldactone, are added. The weight gain and hyperbilirubinemia do not change significantly.

CBC on *DAY 22* was significant for an increase in WBC count to $500/\mu L$. Peripheral smears show predominantly monocytes and a few mature neutrophils. The next 6 days are marked by a steadily increasing WBC count, and a decrease in transfusion requirements. Concurrent with this is a significant improvement in the patient's sense of well-being. The intermittent fever spikes cease. Dysphagia begins to resolve, and with this comes increased oral intake.

Diarrhea, while still present, is decreased in frequency and volume. On _DAY 28_ the absolute neutrophil count reaches $1,000/\mu L$, and antibiotics are discontinued. The patient is discharged from the hospital. Discharge medications include cyclosporine for GVHD prophylaxis, and trimethoprim/sulfamethoxazole three times per week for pneumocystis pneumonia prophylaxis.

The patient is followed closely as an outpatient. On _DAY 50_, evidence of CMV reactivation (positive CMV antigen) is noted on a weekly screening test. The patient denies fever, shortness of breath, diarrhea or dysphagia, and the blood counts remain stable. Chest X-ray remains clear. Twice-daily ganciclovir infusions are started and weekly infusions of intravenous immunoglobulin continue as a supplement to the recovering immune system. One week later, CMV antigen is no longer detected in the blood. Full-dose ganciclovir is stopped after 10 days and is replaced by a thrice-weekly maintenance dose.

DAY 120 post transplant, routine blood tests reveal an elevated SGOT, SGPT, and alkaline phosphatase. An erythematous skin rash is also noted on his back. Oral prednisone is prescribed for treatment of presumed chronic graft-versus-host disease, and the symptoms slowly resolve. Prednisone is later tapered off.

ONE YEAR POST TRANSPLANT, the patient is feeling well. He is off all medications and has returned to work. Blood counts are normal, and the bone marrow examinations shows no evidence of residual leukemia.

Question 1. The dysphagia, diarrhea, nausea, and mucous membrane sloughing described on day 4 of the transplant are characteristic of mucositis. How is mucositis best managed?

Answer. Narcotic analgesia should be used as needed to control pain. Chlorhexidine antiseptic mouth rinses can be used to help prevent superinfection. Parenteral nutrition should be added as p.o. intake declines. The diarrhea associated with mucositis is usually refractory to medical intervention. Careful attention to fluid status is necessary to prevent dehydration and electrolyte abnormalities.

Question 2. The patient develops fever on day 10. What are the potential sources of infection?

Answer. Bacterial infections are most common at this stage of bone marrow transplantation. The most likely sources are the gastrointestinal tract, lungs, sinuses, skin, and the central venous catheter. It is quite common that the source of infection is never identified.

Question 3. How should the fever be worked up?

Answer. All fevers that occur in a neutropenic patient should be taken seriously. Empiric broad-spectrum antibacterial antibiotic coverage, such as ceftazidime, should be started without delay. A careful review of systems, and physical exam focusing on the most common sources listed above is next. Blood cultures, urinalysis, and a chest X-ray should also be performed. If fevers persist for more than 3–4 days despite adequate antibacterial coverage, empiric antifungal treatment with amphotericin must be added.

Question 4. What is in the differential diagnosis for the symptoms describe on day 14?

Answer. The patient has likely developed a mild form of hepatic veno-occlusive disease. The differential includes toxic hepatitis from drugs such as cyclosporine, an infectious hepatitis, or acute graft-versus-host (GVHD) disease involving the liver. <u>DAY 14</u> is early for GVHD, and this condition is not normally associated with ascites, RUQ pain, or weight gain.

Question 5. What are the potential complications that may arise from CMV reactivation?

Answer. CMV-associated interstitial pneumonitis is the most feared complication of CMV reactivation. The liver and the gastrointestinal tract may also be targets. CMV infection, as well as ganciclovir, which is commonly used to treat it, often cause bone marrow suppression. Granulocyte colony stimulating factor can be used to increase the neutrophil count in this setting, or foscarnet can be used as an alternative to ganciclovir.

Question 6. Is chronic graft-versus-host disease likely to be a recurrent problem in this patient?

Answer. The prognostic factors demonstrated by this patient suggest that he will not have recurrent problems with chronic GVHD. Favorable prognostic factors include limited extent of disease, the lack of significant acute GVHD earlier in his course, onset of chronic GVHD after <u>DAY 100</u>, and a complete response to the administered therapy.

SELECTED READING

Almici C, Carlo-Stella C, Wagner JE, Rizzoli V. Umbilical cord blood as a source of hematopoietic stem cells: from research to clinical application. *Haematologica* 1995;80:473–479.
Stem cell transplantation utilizing umbilical cord blood (UCB) as the donor source is now being performed. This review outlines the advantages of UCB as well as its limitations.

Appelbaum FR, Clift R, Radich J, Anasetti C, Buckner CD. Bone marrow transplantation for chronic myelogenous leukemia. *Semin Oncol* 1995;22:405–411.
This review summarizes the results of bone marrow transplantation for the treatment of chronic myelogenous leukemia (CML). Included in the discussion is a review of the efficacy of mismatched family member transplants and matched unrelated donor transplants for CML. More conventional matched sibling transplantation is also discussed.

Appelbaum FR, Fisher LD, Thomas ED. Chemotherapy versus marrow transplantation for adults with acute nonlymphocytic leukemia: a five-year follow-up. *Blood* 1988;72: 179–184.
This single-institution prospective study demonstrates the advantages of allogeneic bone marrow transplantation over conventional chemotherapy for the treatment of acute nonlymphocytic leukemia. The study brings to light the importance of age and prognostic factors of the tumor when considering treatment options.

Barrett J, Treleaven J. *Bone Marrow Transplantation in Practice.* New York: Churchill Livingstone; 1992.
This is a clinically oriented textbook, covering both autologous and allogeneic bone marrow transplantation. The first section of the book discusses the role of bone marrow transplantation in the treatment of malignant and nonmalignant disorders. The second section discusses the practical aspects of this procedure.

Cheson BD. Chemotherapy and bone marrow transplantation for myelodysplastic syndromes. *Semin Oncol* 1992;19:85–94.
A review of the published experience of bone marrow transplantation for the treatment of myelodisplastic syndrome is provided. While BMT is the only curative treatment for myelodysplasia, transplant-related mortality, and disease relapse is more common when compared to de novo leukemia, perhaps because of the increased age and extensive prior treatment history in this patient population.

Fennelly D, Vahdat L, Schneider J, et al. High-intensity chemotherapy with peripheral blood progenitor cell support. *Semin Oncol* 1994;21:21–25.

The infusion of peripheral blood progenitor cells (PBPC) is an effective means of facilitating delivery of high doses of chemotherapy. Data reported here from Memorial Sloan-Kettering Cancer Center demonstrate a significantly shorter period of neutropenia when PBPC support is used after a regimen consisting of carboplatin, etoposide, and cyclophosphamide. In a separate study, PBPCs were used to facilitate two rapidly cycled courses of high-dose chemotherapy.

Ferrara JLM, Deeg HJ. Graft-versus-host disease. *N Engl J Med* 1991;324:667–674.

This review article covers the basics of acute and chronic graft versus host disease. It includes details of the clinical presentation, pathophysiology, and approaches toward prophylaxis and treatment, as well as hypotheses regarding the role of cytokine release in the etiology of acute GVHD.

Lu L, Shen RN, Broxmeyer HE. Stem cells from bone marrow, umbilical cord blood and peripheral blood for clinical application: current status and future application. *Crit Rev Oncol Hematol* 1996;22:61–78.

Information is provided on the potential uses of umbilical cord blood. It also reviews the concept of gene transfer into hematopoietic stem cells as a treatment modality for genetic diseases.

Miller AM. Hematopoietic growth factors in autologous bone marrow transplantation. *Semin Oncol* 1993;20:88–95.

This paper reviews the published experience using G-CSF, GM-CSF, and erythropoietin in the setting of autologous stem cell transplantation. The neutropenic period is clearly shortened with the use of G-CSF or GM-CSF. The beneficial effects of erythropoietin are well defined.

Momin F, Chandrasekar PH. Antimicrobial prophylaxis in bone marrow transplantation. *Ann Intern Med* 1995;123:205–215.

This comprehensive review outlines numerous prophylactic antimicrobial regimens.

Purdy MH, Shpall EJ. The role and methodology for purging tumor from autologous bone marrow and peripheral blood progenitor cells. *Med Oncol* 1994;11:47–51.

Evidence of tumor contaminating stem cells collected from patients with cancer is summarized. The methods that have been utilized to rid the stem cell sample of tumor include the chemotherapeutic agent 4-HC, and positive selection of stem cells using the CD34 antigen.

Sable CA, Donowitz GR. Infections in bone marrow transplant recipients. *Clin Infect Dis* 1994;18:273–284.

This is an excellent review which discusses individually, the important infectious complications which arise during and after bone marrow transplantation.

Shulman HM, Hinterberger W. Hepatic veno-occlusive disease: liver toxicity syndrome after bone marrow transplantation. *Bone Marrow Transplant* 1992;10:197–214.

This review makes clear that there is still much to be learned about what causes VOD, and summarizes current approaches to manage this often fatal complication.

Storb R, Anasetti C, Appelbaum F, et al. Marrow transplantation for severe aplastic anemia and thalassemia major. *Semin in Hematol* 1991;28:235–239.

The risk/benefit ratio must be readdressed when considering transplantation of nonmalignant diseases. This is especially the case with thalassemia major. This issue, and others are discussed in this review.

Wingard JR. Viral infections in leukemia and bone marrow transplant patients. *Leukemia and Lymphoma* 1993;11:115–125.

The primary focus of this review is herpes simplex and cytomegalovirus infections. A variety of treatment approaches are outlined.

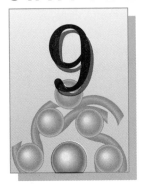

Hematologic Malignancies

Lawrence N. Shulman

THE MOLECULAR BASIS OF THE HEMATOLOGIC MALIGNANCIES

All the diseases described in this chapter are the result of the malignant transformation of hematopoietic cells that leads to their clonal dysregulated growth. As shown in Fig. 9-1, all hematopoietic cells arise from stem cells that, under normal circumstances, undergo both self-replication to assure the continued production of blood cells throughout the life of the person and differentiation to mature progeny that are equipped to carry on the functional needs of the organism. This carefully balanced and regulated growth normally results in an appropriate number of mature progeny while not exhausting the primitive stem cells and has sufficient flexibility to respond to stress, such as infection or hemorrhage. (Chapter 1)

It should also be noted that it is the mature progeny—red blood cells, white blood cells, and platelets—that are programmed for cell death. Stem cells are not, since they must preserve themselves for the life of the organism. This fact will influence the phenotype of hematologic malignancies. In the myeloproliferative disorders, for instance, there is increased self-renewal of early stem cells, and maintained differentiation, with increased differentiation along certain cell lines (such as the red cell line in polycythemia vera). In acute myelogenous leukemia, self-renewal of blasts is preserved but differentiation is lost, and therefore there is an accumulation of blast forms without the production of their mature progeny.

Chromosomal damage to hematopoietic stem cells is characterized by abnormal and clonal growth. As will be described, the chromosomal abnormalities that are associated with these diseases are being identified in increasing numbers. Our knowledge of how these chromosomal abnormalities—such as the t(9;22) bcr-abl translocation in chronic myelogenous leukemia or the t(15;17) in acute promyelo-

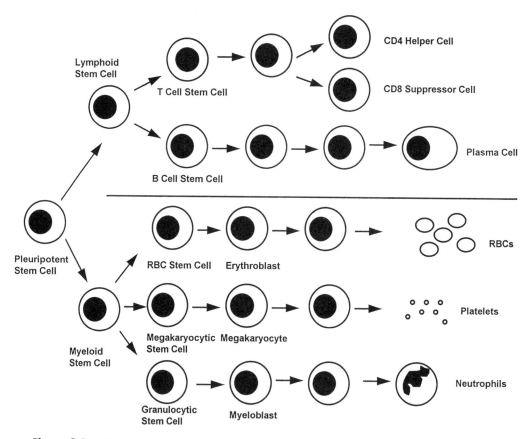

Figure 9-1. Hematopoietic development, grossly simplified, for the myeloid and lymphoid compartments.

cytic leukemia—affect cellular growth and malignant transformation are now being elucidated. It is likely that in the coming years we will have a much better understanding of the molecular events that lead to these malignancies and will be able to use that knowledge to prevent and treat them.

The leukemias are subdivided into the acute leukemias and the chronic leukemias. The acute leukemias are characterized by the production of immature blast cells without maturation, resulting in the rapid replacement of the normal hematopoietic elements of the bone marrow. The acute leukemias can be derived from myeloid or lymphoid lineage. Left untreated, the acute leukemias are rapidly fatal because of neutropenia, resulting in infection, and thrombocytopenia, leading to hemorrhage. The chronic leukemias are, when untreated, more indolent diseases. Chronic myelogenous leukemia initially represents both increased proliferation of myeloid progenitor cells and maintained differentiation to mature cell products (red blood cells, white blood cells, and platelets). Chronic lymphocytic leukemia is really an indolent non-Hodgkin's lymphoma with peripheral blood involvement and will be discussed in the lymphoma section of this chapter.

THE ACUTE LEUKEMIAS

Pathophysiology and Classification. Acute myelogenous leukemia (AML) and acute lymphoblastic leukemia (ALL) comprise the acute leukemias. Both diseases are characterized by the malignant and clonal proliferation of immature blast precursors that have largely lost the potential to differentiate. Manifestations of each derive from the ability of the leukemic blasts to replace normal elements in the bone marrow, leading to pancytopenia, and the infiltration of other tissues, such as the gums and meninges.

Acute Myelogenous Leukemia. AML constitutes a group of diseases characterized by the proliferation of malignant blasts derived from precursors of the myeloid compartment. The malignant blasts include myeloblasts, promyeloblasts, monoblasts, erythroblasts, and megakaryoblasts. All these cells are progeny of a common myeloid stem cell, and under normal circumstances they both replicate in a process of self-renewal and differentiate into the mature functional cellular components of blood: red cells, neutrophils, monocytes, and platelets (Fig. 9-1). Since the word *myeloid* is sometimes used to denote only the neutrophil line, this group of leukemias has, in the past, been called the acute nonlymphocytic leukemias, but acute myelogenous leukemia is now the favored term. The French-American-British (FAB) working group has proposed a classification for AML as shown in Tables 9-1 and 9-2. M1, M2, and M3 subgroups represent different stages of differentiation of myeloblasts. MO AML can be determined to be of myeloid origin by cell surface markers such as the myeloid marker CD33, but blasts in this disorder lack myeloid enzyme production, so that myeloperoxidase histochemical stains are negative. M1–M3 subgroups have increasing degrees of primary granulation, with M3 representing acute promyelocytic leukemia. M4–M5 AML are monoblastic leukemias with and without myeloid elements, respectively. M6 AML is erythroleukemia and M7 represents megakaryoblastic leukemia. As shown in Table 9-2, these subtypes can be distinguished by morphology, histochemical staining, karyotype, and immunophenotypic analysis. These techniques also help to distinguish AML from ALL when morphology is ambiguous.

TABLE 9-1. *THE FRENCH-AMERICAN-BRITISH (FAB) CLASSIFICATION OF ACUTE MYELOGENOUS LEUKEMIA*

MO: Acute undifferentiated leukemia

M1: Acute myeloblastic leukemia without differentiation

M2: Acute myeloblastic leukemia with some granule formation

M3: Acute promyeloblastic leukemia

M4: Acute myelomonocytic leukemia

M5: Acute monocytic leukemia

M6: Erythroleukemia

M7: Megakaryoblastic leukemia

Adapted from Bennett JM, Catovsky D, Daniel M-T, et al. Proposals for the classification of the acute leukemias. Br J Haematol 1976;33:329–331.

TABLE 9-2. *HISTOCHEMICAL, IMMUNOPHENOTYPIC, AND CHROMOSOMAL CHARACTERISTICS OF THE ACUTE LEUKEMIAS*

DISEASE	HISTOCHEMISTRY	IMMUNO-PHENOTYPE	CHROMOSOMAL ABNORMALITIES
AML, M0	All negative	CD13, CD33, CD34	
AML, M1,2	Myeloperoxidase Sudan black	CD13, CD33	t(8;21)
AML, M3	Myeloperoxidase Sudan black	CD13, CD33	t(15;17)
AML, M4	Myeloperoxidase Nonspecific esterase	CD13, CD33 CD11b, CD14	Inv 16
AML, M5	Nonspecific esterase	CD11b, CD14	
AML, M6	PAS	CD13, CD33	5q⁻, 7q⁻
AML, M7	Factor VIII antigen	CD13, CD33, CD41	
ALL, T-cell type	PAS	CD3, CD5, CD7	
ALL, pre–B-cell type	PAS	CD10, CD19	t(9,22)

AML arises from a single cell that has undergone chromosomal damage resulting in the clonal expansion of a malignant clone that has a reduced capacity to differentiate into mature progeny. Because of their need to self-replicate and produce cells throughout a person's life, blasts are not programmed to die. Mature progeny (red cells, neutrophils, platelets) have a finite lifespan with programmed cell death. In AML, blasts continue to replicate without differentiation and therefore accumulate in the bone marrow and other tissues. AML blasts do not grow more quickly than normal blasts, but because there is no differentiation, they accumulate, crowding out normal elements of the bone marrow, with resulting deficiencies of red blood cells, mature white blood cells, and platelets.

Most cases of AML have no known cause, but a number of etiologic agents have been identified. Radiation is a weak but significant leukemogen. Certain chemotherapy agents, such as alkylating agents and topoisomerase II inhibitors are leukemogenic, as are solvents such as benzene. AML can also arise from previous hematologic disorders, such as polycythemia vera, myeloid metaplasia, paroxysmal nocturnal hemoglobinuria, and myelodysplasia.

Distinctive chromosomal abnormalities have been associated with AML blasts and certainly play an important role in leukemogenesis. Identification of these chromosomal abnormalities is important because they also have prognostic significance. Certain abnormalities are pathognomonic of a particular subtype of AML, such as the t(15;17) seen in essentially all cases of M3 acute promyelocytic leukemia (APML). Some portend a good prognosis, such as the t(8;21) translocation, or inversion of chromosome 16; and others, such as deletions of the long arms of chromosomes 5 and 7, have a poor prognosis. Elucidation of the molecular events associated with these translocations and deletions will undoubtedly help greatly in our understanding of the pathogenesis of AML and may impact on therapy, as it already has for M3 APML, as described later. All patients with newly diagnosed AML should have cytogenetic studies performed on their leukemic blasts from either the bone marrow or peripheral blood.

Acute Lymphoblastic Leukemia. ALL can be of the pre-B or T-cell type. (See Chapter 4 for lymphoid physiology.) In each case immature lymphoblasts are produced that do not further differentiate into mature lymphoid progeny. There are two classifications of ALL, the FAB classification, which is morphologic, and an immunologic classification, as shown in Tables 9-2 and 9-3. The FAB classification is not widely used and does not reflect the important immunologic origin of the ALL subtypes. It is important to know, though, because it is now recognized that lymphoblastic-appearing cells of the L3 variety often represent a closely related disease, small noncleaved cell non-Hodgkin's lymphoma or Burkitt's lymphoma. (See later.) Many now feel that this is a distinct entity and requires different therapy than ALL. It therefore must be distinguished from ALL, and the immunologic classification is very helpful in this regard.

Approximately 70% of patients with ALL demonstrate lymphoblasts of the *pre-B-cell type.* These cases were referred to as "null cell" ALL in the past because the cells did not demonstrate surface immunoglobulin and were not recognized as early B cells before immunophenotypic and gene rearrangement studies became available. It is now known that these blasts will bear the early B-cell antigen CD19 and will have rearrangements of their immunoglobulin genes, confirming they are of B-cell lineage. The remaining cases of ALL are composed of T-lymphoblasts *(T-cell type),* demonstrating early T-cell antigens as well as rearrangements of the T-cell receptor genes.

As noted earlier, most cases previously referred to as true B-cell ALL, morphologically of the L3 variant, are composed of cells that are in a later phase of B-cell differentiation, expressing cell surface immunoglobulin and CD20, and are now classified as small noncleaved cell non-Hodgkin's lymphoma (Burkitt's lymphoma). These cells often contain the t(8;14) chromosomal translocation and are now usually treated with regimens that are different from those used with ALL.

Chromosomal abnormalities have also been associated with ALL. The most important is the t(9;22) translocation known as the Philadelphia chromosome. Initially described in chronic myelogenous leukemia and thought to be pathognomonic of that disease, the abl gene from chromosome 9 is translocated into the breakpoint cluster region (bcr) of chromosome 22, giving rise to one of two bcr-abl aberrant protein kinases, the p210 or p190 types. The p210 type is more common in chronic myelogenous leukemia and the p190 type is more common in ALL. Only about 5% of children with ALL have blasts containing this abnormality, but more than 30% of

---

TABLE 9-3. *THE CLASSIFICATION OF ACUTE LYMPHOBLASTIC LEUKEMIA*

Pre–B Cell (Null cell) (L1 or L2 morphology)*
   75% of cases: Ia + (HLA-DR), B4 + (CD19), CALLA + (CD10)

T-Cell (L1 or L2 morphology)*
   20% of cases: Leu 1 + (CD5), Leu 9 + (CD7)

B-Cell (L3 morphology)*
   5% of cases: Ia +, surface immunoglobulin present. The L3 variety (of the French-American-British [FAB] classification) has very poor prognosis, similar or identical to small non–cleaved-cell lymphoma (also referred to as Burkitt's lymphoma). Patients with this disease are usually treated on protocols for small non–cleaved-cell lymphoma rather than on ALL protocols.

---

* FAB morphology for ALL.
L1: *Relatively small size, regular nuclear shape, high nuclear/cytoplasmic ratio; inconspicuous nucleoli.*
L2: *Heterogeneous size, lower nuclear/cytoplasmic ratio.*
L3: *Large homogeneous cells, nuclei with fine chromatin, nucleoli prominent; basophilic cytoplasm with prominent vacuoles.*

adults with ALL have blasts with this translocation. This is of clinical significance since patients with ALL whose blasts bear this translocation have a poor prognosis. It is also important to note that standard metaphase cytogenetics are difficult to perform on ALL cells since they frequently do not divide in tissue culture. Molecular probes are available to identify the bcr-abl translocation and should be used as part of the evaluation of all patients with newly diagnosed ALL.

Diagnosis. The diagnosis of AML or ALL requires the identification of leukemic blasts either in the peripheral blood or in the bone marrow. When blasts are identified in the peripheral blood, examination of the bone marrow is essentially always performed to confirm infiltration with leukemia. In the case of AML, more than 30% of hematopoietic cells are blasts, a standard criterion for the diagnosis of AML (in distinction from myelodysplastic syndromes, as discussed later).

Often the blasts can be identified as being of myeloid or lymphoid origin by morphology. Myeloblasts are larger than lymphoblasts and have very fine nuclear chromatin and large distinct nucleoli. Lymphoblasts are smaller, with less cytoplasm and less prominent nucleoli. Not infrequently, a patient's blasts may not be clearly myeloid or lymphoid, and further evaluation is required. In practice, in all cases the diagnosis is confirmed with cytochemical stains and immunophenotypic analysis (Table 9-2). Myeloid blasts of the M1–M4 type will stain with myeloperoxidase; those of the M4–M5 type, with nonspecific esterase; some of the M6 type, with PAS; and those of the M7 variety, for the factor VIII antigen. ALL blasts will not stain with myeloperoxidase or nonspecific esterase, but they sometimes demonstrate large PAS-positive granules. Immunophenotypic analysis will show myeloid blasts to be positive for CD33 and other myeloid antigens, whereas ALL blasts will bear CD19 and CD10 (CALLA). As mentioned earlier, cytogenetics should always be performed and can help to distinguish difficult cases, but results are often not immediately available and may not help in the initial diagnostic work-up of the patient.

Clinical Features. Patients generally present with manifestations of pancytopenia. They may demonstrate pallor, fatigue, or shortness of breath secondary to anemia. Bleeding may occur as a result of thrombocytopenia, and infection may be a manifestation of neutropenia. Often the symptoms may seem minor and difficult to separate from common complaints such as fatigue and lingering viral-type symptoms. The situation becomes clarified when a complete blood count is performed. Anemia and thrombocytopenia are almost always present. The white blood count can be high or low, but the differential count is almost always abnormal, with a decrease in the number of neutrophils. Circulating blasts in the peripheral blood are usually present, but in both AML and ALL the white blood count can be low without identifiable circulating blasts, and in this case only a bone marrow examination will suggest the diagnosis of acute leukemia. When circulating blasts are present, morphologic, histochemical, and immunophenotypic analysis can usually be rapidly performed on the peripheral blood.

Therapy of Acute Myelogenous Leukemia. Left untreated, patients with AML will rapidly die of either uncontrolled infection or bleeding. The basis of treatment is to administer intensive chemotherapy, rendering the bone marrow hypoplastic—devoid of leukemic blasts as well as normal cells, which should therefore permit the regrowth of normal hematopoietic lineages. The most commonly used regimens include the combination of an anthracycline drug (daunorubicin or idarubicin) and Ara-C (cytarabine). With this treatment approximately 65% of patients will enter remission. The remission rates are higher for younger patients, approaching 80% for those in their 20s, but is only about 50% for patients over the age of 60 years. Remission must be distinguished from cure. Remission only reflects the absence of visible leukemic blasts, but if, after the induction of an initial remission, no further therapy is administered, very few patients will remain in remission and truly be cured. The administration of postremission intensive therapy improves the durability of remission and cure rate. However, even with the addition of intensive consolidation therapy, only 30–40% of patients are cured by standard chemotherapy. Bone marrow transplantation (BMT), autologous and allogeneic, may improve the cure rates when utilized for patients in first remission, as shown in Fig. 9-2. (See also Chapter 8.) In the study depicted, patients were induced into remission with an intensive regimen including 3 days of daunorubicin and 7 days of continuous-infusion Ara-C (standard induction therapy), followed by an additional 3 days of high-dose Ara-C. The complete remission rate was 89% in this study. Patients entering remission underwent allogeneic transplantation if they had an HLA-matched sibling or autologous transplantation if they did not. These data suggest that both allogeneic and autologous transplantation improved overall survival for these patients, and when used in this manner, 55% of patients remain in long-term remission. For patients with relapsed AML, allogeneic transplantation remains the only potentially curative therapy. (See Chapter 8.)

Acute promyelocytic leukemia (APML–M3 subtype) is unique in that, in essentially all cases, the t(15;17) translocation is present. This translocation involves the retinoic acid receptor α gene on chromosome 17. It has been shown that oral administration of all-trans retinoic acid can induce differentiation of APML cells and can lead to a histologic and cytogenetic remission. Unfortunately, the remissions are not durable, and standard chemotherapy is required as well. The finding, though, that treatment with this all-trans retinoic acid (a substance clearly related to the observed retinoic acid receptor gene abnormality) can cause differentiation and suppression of the malignant clone is an essential component of current therapy for this disease.

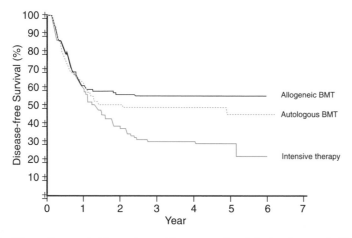

Figure 9-2. Disease-free survival for patients with acute myelocytic leukemia treated with intensive induction chemotherapy, followed by consolidation with standard chemotherapy, autologous BMT, or allogeneic BMT. Note there is an advantage to the use of BMT. (Used with permission, from Zittoun RA, et al. Autologous or allogeneic bone marrow transplantation compared with intensive chemotherapy in acute myelogenous leukemia. *N Engl J Med* 1995;332:217.)

Therapy of Acute Lymphoblastic Leukemia. The choice of therapy for patients with ALL is highly dependent on both patient age and cytogenetics of the leukemic blasts. Children with ALL whose leukemic blasts do not contain the Philadelphia chromosome t(9;22) can be treated with regimens including doxorubicin, vincristine, prednisone, and L-asparaginase, resulting in a 90–95% complete remission rate. Prolonged maintenance therapy is administered over 2 years, including prophylactic treatment to the central nervous system, and 80–90% of children will remain in remission and presumably are cured. Children with ALL containing the Philadelphia chromosome have an extremely poor prognosis and should be treated with more intensive therapy, possibly including BMT. (Chapter 8.)

Adults with ALL do not do well with the therapy administered to children. They require much more intensive treatment, and even so only 35–50% of patients will be cured with standard chemotherapy. Survival depends upon age, as shown in Fig. 9-3, with patients under 30 years faring well, but older patients having an inferior survival. Adults with T-cell ALL have a slightly better prognosis than those with B-lineage ALL, as shown in Fig. 9-4. As indicated earlier, patients with true B-cell ALL (L3) are treated with regimens for small noncleaved cell non-Hodgkin's lymphoma (Burkitt's lymphoma). As is the case in children, adults with Philadelphia chromosome positive ALL have an extremely poor prognosis and should be offered BMT in first remission if an acceptable donor is available. (Chapter 8.) This is also true for patients whose leukemic blasts demonstrate other, less common, poor-prognosis chromosomal abnormalities. As with children, central nervous system prophylaxis is a necessary component of any treatment regimen.

MYELOPROLIFERATIVE DISORDERS

Pathophysiology and Classification. As is the case with the acute leukemias, the myeloproliferative disorders are a group of diseases characterized by clonal and abnormal growth. In the myeloproliferative disorders, though, there is both increased replication of precursor cells and maintained differentiation. Therefore mature progeny continue to be produced and cytopenias are usually not a problem early on. The proliferative thrust is different in the various myeloproliferative disorders, with red cell production increased most dramatically in polycythemia

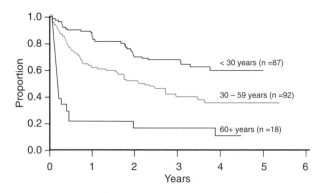

Figure 9-3. Survival for adults with acute lymphoblastic leukemia treated with intensive chemotherapy. Note that younger patients have superior survival when compared to older patients. (Used with permission, from Larson RA, Dodge RK, Burns CP, et al. A five-drug remission induction regimen with intensive consolidation for adults with acute lymphoblastic leukemia: Cancer and Leukemia Group B study 8811. *Blood* 1995;85:2025.)

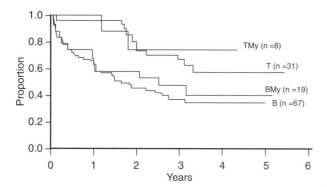

Figure 9-4. Survival based on immunophenotype for adults with acute lymphoblastic leukemia treated with intensive chemotherapy. (Used with permission, from Larson RA, Dodge RK, Burns CP, et al. A five-drug remission induction regimen with intensive consolidation for adults with acute lymphoblastic leukemia: Cancer and Leukemia Group B study 8811. *Blood* 1995;85:2025.)

vera, platelet production in essential thrombocythemia, granulocyte production in chronic myelogenous leukemia (CML), and megakaryocytic production in myeloid metaplasia. Splenomegaly is frequently present, since the spleen becomes a site of extramedullary hematopoiesis. Relative increases and decreases in blood counts and other important clinical distinguishing features are shown in Table 9-4.

All these diseases are clonal malignant disorders arising from an early stem cell, with all three hematopoietic cell lines involved in each. In the case of CML there is proof that the malignant cell is a very early stem cell that has retained the ability to differentiate along the lymphoid as well as myeloid pathways. These data are derived from the observation that when CML progresses to the blast phase, in one-third of patients the blasts will have a lymphoid phenotype.

Diagnosis. The diagnosis of a myeloproliferative disorder is suggested by either an abnormal blood count or a splenomegaly on physical examination. If the patient is polycythemic, with an elevated hematocrit, the physician must distinguish between *polycythemia vera* (the myeloproliferative disorder) and secondary polycythemia due to abnormal hemoglobin, erythropoietin-producing tumors, or other abnormalities, such as congenital heart disease leading to chronic hypoxia, as shown in Table 9-5 and described in Chapter 3. The bone marrow is hypercellular, but this is nonspecific and as shown in Table 9-6 is not included in the diagnostic criteria for P. vera.

The diagnosis of *essential thrombocythemia* begins with an attempt to eliminate other disorders where there are increased numbers of platelets, especially secondary or "reactive thrombocytosis," as discussed in Chapter 5. Patients with polycythemia vera who are iron deficient may demonstrate thrombocytosis but not erythrocytosis because of their lack of iron. Isolated thrombocytosis can also be the presenting sign of CML in a minority of patients. The absence of the Philadelphia chromosome will rule out CML in most cases. Essential thrombocytosis must also be distinguished from causes of reactive thrombocytosis, the most common of which are nonhematologic malignancy, infection, and iron deficiency. In essential thrombocytosis, the bone marrow may be normal or hypercellular. Megakaryocytes are often increased and may be large and morphologically abnormal.

Myeloid metaplasia is characterized by bone marrow fibrosis, presumably caused by abnormal megakaryocytic growth with release of fibroblast growth factors, and by extramedullary hematopoiesis, most markedly in the spleen, which can grow to enormous size. Patients are usually anemic, and the white blood count can be low or elevated. Initially, the platelet count can be elevated, but may be low in late phases of the disease.

Chronic myelogenous leukemia is a malignant clonal disorder, characterized by the Philadelphia chromosome t(9;22) where the abl gene from chromosome 9 is translocated into the breakpoint cluster region of chromosome 22. There are two prominent clinical phases of the disease: the *chronic phase*, when there is an increase in production of mature granulocytes and platelets, as well as a modest anemia, and a *blast transformation phase*, when the early blast precursors lose their ability to differentiate and the disease takes on the phenotype of acute leukemia of either the myeloid or lymphoid type.

Clinical Features and Therapy. The clinical features and therapy are quite different for the different disorders and will be dealt with separately.

Polycythemia Vera. Polycythemia vera is characterized by an increased red blood cell mass and increased hematocrit, and white blood cell count, as well as thrombocytosis in most cases (see Tables 9-5 and 9-6). The prime manifestations of the disease include hyperviscosity, with resulting thrombosis and/or hemorrhage due to both blood sludging in the microvasculature and abnormal platelet function. The elevated hematocrit itself is sufficient to account for many of the hyperviscosity symptoms, as well as some thrombotic episodes. The hematocrit, therefore, should be maintained below 45%, which can be readily accomplished by phlebotomy. With repeated phlebotomy, iron deficiency will ensue, which will decrease red cell production. However, even when the hematocrit is well controlled, thrombosis and hemorrhage can occur and lead to morbidity. This is due in part to platelet abnormalities that can lead to spontaneous thrombosis and/or hemorrhage. Treatment with antineoplastic agents such as chlorambucil, radioactive phosphorus, or hydroxyurea can reduce the platelet count and reduce the risk of thrombosis and hemorrhage. These agents will often reduce the need for phlebotomy as well. Unfortunately, treatment with chlorambucil and radioactive phosphorus leads to an increased risk of transformation to acute myelogenous

TABLE 9-4. *THE MYELOPROLIFERATIVE DISORDERS*

DISORDER	RBC	WBC	PLTS	FIBROSIS	SPLENOMEGALY	LAP	Ph[1]
Polycythemia vera	+ + +	+ +	+ +	+/−	+	Inc	−
Essential thrombocythemia	+/−	+/−	+ + +	+/−	+/−	nl/Inc	−
Myeloid metaplasia	+/−	+ +	+ + +	+ + +	+ + +	nl/Inc	−
Chronic myelogenous leukemia	−	+ + +	+ + +	+ + +	+ + +	Dec	+

LAP = leukocyte alkaline phosphatase; Ph[1] = Philadelphia chromosome; Inc = increased; Dec = decreased; nl = normal.

TABLE 9-5. *THE DIFFERENTIAL DIAGNOSIS OF POLYCYTHEMIA*

Primary polycythemia
  Polycythemia vera

Secondary polycythemia
  Congenital cyanotic heart disease
  Malignancy
    Hepatocellular carcinoma
    Renal cell carcinoma
  Lung disease with hypo-oxygenation
  High-affinity hemoglobin
  Low oxygen tension, high altitude
  Renal cysts

Pseudo-polycythemia
  Stress polycythemia
  Intravascular volume contraction

leukemia. This transformation to AML will occur in 1–3% of patients treated with phlebotomy only, but treatment with chlorambucil and radioactive phosphorus increases this risk. It is unclear whether treatment with hydroxyurea will also increase the risk of transformation to AML. In some patients increasing bone marrow fibrosis will lead to a "burned-out" phase of polycythemia vera and eventual pancytopenia.

Essential Thrombocythemia. Essential thrombocythemia (ET) is associated with very high platelet counts and can manifest itself as either thrombosis or hemorrhage. Patients are usually not significantly anemic and may or may not have an elevated white blood count. Many patients do not appear to require any therapy, and they remain asymptomatic in spite of a very high platelet count. Others have life-threatening thrombosis and/or hemorrhage. The ideal treatment for ET is unknown. Some patients are successfully treated with aspirin, and others, with hydroxy-

TABLE 9-6. *THE DIAGNOSTIC CRITERIA OF POLYCYTHEMIA VERA**

Major Criteria

Increased red cell mass

Splenomegaly

Normal oxygen saturation

Minor Criteria

Thrombocytosis: >400,000/μL

Leukocytosis: >12,000/μL

Elevated leukocyte alkaline phosphatase

Elevated serum B_{12} or B_{12} binding protein

Adapted from Berlin NI. Diagnosis and classification of the polycythemias. Sem Hematol 1975;12:339.
* All three major criteria or two major and two minor criteria are necessary to make diagnosis.

urea. Some patients continue to have severe thrombotic episodes in spite of these treatments. One study randomized patients with essential thrombocythemia to either treatment with hydroxyurea or observation only. Those patients treated with hydroxyurea had a significantly lower incidence of thrombosis. Because of a concern that long-term treatment with hydroxyurea may be leukemogenic and because of the variability of the disease, patients must be managed in an individualized manner.

Myeloid Metaplasia. Myeloid metaplasia is a disease with heterogeneous manifestations usually characterized by marked bone marrow fibrosis and massive splenomegaly caused by extramedullary hematopoiesis. Patients often have significant discomfort from the splenomegaly, as well as hypermetabolic symptoms. Anemia can be severe, and the white blood count can be either increased or decreased. Neutropenia can result in infection. The platelet count can also be increased or decreased, and when severely decreased can result in increased bleeding. Treatment options for myeloid metaplasia are unsatisfactory. If the patient is young and has a bone marrow donor, allogeneic BMT can be curative. The bone marrow fibrosis will resolve after transplantation, demonstrating that it results from growth factors produced by the abnormal hematopoietic clone. Otherwise, treatment consists primarily of supportive care with transfusions and antibiotics. Hydroxyurea and other antineoplastic agents can help control symptoms but can also lead to severe pancytopenia. Splenectomy can also result in pancytopenia, and on occasion leads to development of extramedullary hematopoiesis in the liver, which can cause significant liver dysfunction.

Chronic Myelogenous Leukemia. Patients with CML generally present in the *chronic phase* with a high white blood count, thrombocytosis, anemia, splenomegaly, and hypermetabolic symptoms. In the *chronic phase* mature neutrophils are produced, as well as functional platelets. This phase of disease can be easily controlled with hydroxyurea or α-interferon. Both will reduce the white blood count and platelet count, as well as the splenomegaly and hypermetabolic symptoms; as a result, patients will feel quite well. Treatment with hydroxyurea does not eliminate the leukemic clone, but merely controls proliferation. Cytogenetic analysis of the bone marrow will reveal that all cells contain the Philadelphia chromosome, even if the blood counts return to normal. Treatment with α-interferon will sometimes suppress the leukemic clone, so that the Philadelphia chromosome positive cells cannot be found by standard metaphase cytogenetics. Some have also suggested that treatment with α-interferon reduces the rate of transformation to blast crisis.

Unfortunately, in all cases treated with either hydroxyurea or α-interferon there is an inevitable progression to "*blast transformation,*" where the leukemic progenitors lose the ability to differentiate and the bone marrow becomes replaced with myeloblasts in two-thirds of patients, or lymphoblasts in one-third of patients. Blast transformation is extremely difficult to control and is generally fatal in several months.

The only potentially curative therapy for CML is allogeneic BMT. This therapy is most effective when used early in the course of the disease and is much less effective if used during blast transformation, as shown in Fig. 9-5. All patients less than 55 or 60 years of age with an appropriate bone marrow donor should undergo allogeneic BMT relatively early in the course of the disease. The anemia associated with this disorder is called refractory because no standard therapy seems capable of reversing it. Iron metabolism abnormalities are sometimes seen and manifested by ringed cytoplasts.

MYELODYSPLASTIC SYNDROMES

Pathophysiology and Classification. The myelodysplastic syndromes are a heterogeneous group of disorders characterized by abnormal growth of the myeloid bone marrow components. As is the case with AML and the myeloproliferative disorders, the primary affected cell is an early stem cell, and this is also a clonal, neoplastic disease. In most cases there is reduced production of granulocytes, red blood cells, and platelets, with resulting pancytopenia. On occasion, the white blood count is high, with an increase in mature but dysplastic neutrophils. In many cases the neutrophils produced are qualitatively abnormal, functioning poorly as antibacterial and antifungal cells.

These diseases are sometimes referred to as the refractory anemias since no standard anemia therapy, such as iron replacement or B_{12} or folate replacement, will correct the defect.

Because of the variability of the myelodysplastic syndromes the FAB group developed a classification for these diseases, as shown in Table 9-7. As can be seen, more advanced stages of disease are characterized by an increase in the percentage of blasts found in the bone marrow. This reflects the progression to acute myelogenous leukemia, which eventually occurs in many patients with myelodysplasia. Clonal chromosomal abnormalities are frequent in the bone marrow cells of patients with myelodysplasia, and with time these cells develop additional chromosomal abnormalities, leading to further loss of the ability to differentiate into mature progeny and resulting in increasing numbers of myeloblasts until AML ensues. Abnormalities of the long arms of chromosomes 5, 7, and 20, as well as trisomy 8 are common in this population of patients. Myelodysplasia is known to occur after treatment with alkylating agents, radiation, solvent exposure, and other primary hematologic disorders such as polycythemia vera, but most cases have no known etiologic agent.

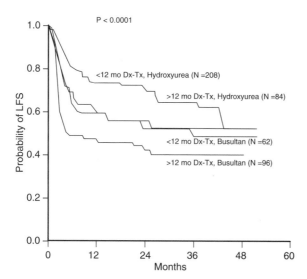

Figure 9-5. Survival for patients with chronic myelogenous leukemia, treated with either hydroxyurea or busulfan, followed by BMT. Note that patients treated with hydroxyurea fared better than those treated with busulfan, and those patients treated earlier in the course of their disease also fared better. (Used with permission, from Goldman JM, et al. Choice of pretransplant treatment and timing of transplants for chronic myelogenous leukemia in chronic phase. *Blood* 1993;82:2235–2238.)

Clinical Features and Therapy. Clinical features develop as a result of pancytopenia and include symptoms from anemia, bleeding from thrombocytopenia, and infection from neutropenia. Even if the neutrophil count is not very low, infection is often a problem, since neutrophils from these patients often function poorly. Splenomegaly is rare.

Red blood cell and platelet transfusions as well as antibiotics are needed support for these patients. Rarely, the anemia can be improved by use of high dosages of pyridoxine. "Differentiating agents" such as retinoids and low-dose Ara-C have had little impact on this disease. Hematopoietic growth factors such as G-CSF and erythropoietin have also been tried with variable success. In some patients these cytokines may decrease transfusion requirements or numbers of infections, but inevitably the disease progresses and becomes increasingly difficult to control. Antileukemic therapy has been used, particularly when patients transform to frank AML, but unfortunately, the remission rate is low, and many patients die during a prolonged hypoplastic period after administration of the therapy.

Allogeneic BMT can be curative in patients with myelodysplasia, but many of the patients are too old for allogeneic transplantation or do not have an acceptable donor.

THE LYMPHOMAS

The lymphomas are neoplastic transformations of cells that reside predominately in lymphoid tissues. The malignant lymphomas are divided into Hodgkin's disease and the non-Hodgkin's lymphomas. Both usually involve malignant growth of lymph nodes and the spleen, though extranodal tissues can be involved as well. The origin of Hodgkin's disease remains unknown, but the non-Hodgkin's lymphomas arise from various normal lymphoid cells that have undergone malignant transformation. The distinction between Hodgkin's disease and the non-Hodgkin's lymphomas is useful because the natural history, prognosis, and therapy of the two groups of diseases differ. The non-Hodgkin's lymphomas, though, are in themselves a heterogeneous group of diseases.

Hodgkin's Disease

Hodgkin's disease is a malignancy of uncertain etiology with a malignant cell, the Reed-Sternberg cell, of unclear origin. Despite our lack of understanding of the basic pathophysiology of the disease, it is one of the most successfully treated malignancies. It was one of the first neoplasms to be cured with combination chemotherapy, even when in an advanced stage. The Reed-Sternberg cell has no obvious normal counterpart in white cell ontogeny, as has been demonstrated in other lymphoproliferative disorders (such as the pre-B cell in ALL). In addition, the Reed-Sternberg cell is present in only small numbers in affected lymph nodes and is surrounded largely by benign polyclonal T cells that presumably represent a reaction to the malignant cell. There are four histologic subtypes of Hodgkin's disease: lymphocyte predominant, nodular sclerosis, mixed cellularity, and lymphocyte depleted. Nodular sclerosis is the most common variety, particularly in young adults. Primarily a disease of young adults, more commonly affecting upper socioeconomic families, there has been a long search for a viral etiology. Epstein-Barr virus has been found in the nuclei of Reed-Sternberg cells in about 25% of patients, but the significance of this is unknown and the genesis of this disease remains largely a mystery.

TABLE 9-7. *THE FRENCH-AMERICAN-BRITISH CLASSIFICATION OF REFRACTORY ANEMIAS (MYELODYSPLASIA)*

RA:	Refractory anemia (<5% blasts in bone marrow)
RArs:	Refractory anemia with ringed sideroblasts (<5% blasts in bone marrow)
RAEB:	Refractory anemia with excess blasts (5–10% blasts in bone marrow)
RAEBT:	Refractory anemia with excess blasts in transformation (10–30% blasts in bone marrow)

Adapted from Bennett JM, Catovsky D, Daniel M-T, et al. Proposals for the classification of the myelodysplastic syndromes. Br J Haematol 1982;51:189–199.

Clinical Features and Treatment. Hodgkin's disease usually presents in cervical, supraclavicular, or mediastinal lymph nodes. Less commonly, the pelvic nodes are the first site of involvement. Hodgkin's disease progresses in a step-wise fashion to contiguous nodal areas. Eventually, dissemination occurs with involvement of the liver, bone marrow, and other extranodal sites. Patients may present with an asymptomatic enlarged neck lymph node, with symptoms related to mediastinal adenopathy, or, when the disease is advanced they may develop symptoms, including fevers, night sweats, and weight loss, which are referred to as *B symptoms.*

When a biopsy confirms the diagnosis of Hodgkin's disease, a staging work-up should follow, including CT scans of the chest, abdomen, and pelvis; a gallium scan; and bone marrow biopsies. The staging system most frequently used for patients with Hodgkin's disease is shown in Table 9-8. Staging is critical for patients with Hodgkin's disease since it dictates therapy. Patients who have disease confined to sites above the diaphragm can be cured in the majority of cases with radiation therapy alone, and those who relapse are often cured with "salvage" chemotherapy. If disease is present on both sides of the diaphragm (stage III disease), then chemotherapy is required to maximize cure rate.

When the disease is minimal and appears by radiologic evaluation to be confined to sites above the diaphragm (mediastinum, cervical, etc.), a staging laparotomy can be considered. Approximately 30% of patients who appear after radiologic staging to have stage II disease may have disease discovered in the abdomen at laparotomy. The most common site of occult involvement below the diaphragm is the spleen, and splenic involvement is almost always missed on radiologic staging. An alternative to staging laparotomy is to treat the patient with chemotherapy, which will treat disseminated disease.

Radiation therapy alone can cure most patients with very localized disease without bulky masses. When disease is advanced, either stage III or IV, particularly if there is extranodal spread, such as bone marrow involvement, then combination chemotherapy is the primary therapy and is curative in a majority of patients. In the 1960s, therapy with the acronym of MOPP (**n**itrogen **m**ustard, vincristine, [**O**ncovin®] **p**rocarbazine, and **p**rednisone) was shown to be curative in approximately 50% of patients with advanced disease. This was a major advance, but the therapy was difficult to administer because of side effects, bone marrow suppression, and the fact that treatment was associated with long-term complications, including sterility in all males and many females, and the development of myelodysplasia and AML. ABVD (doxorubicin [**A**driamycin®], **b**leomycin, **v**inblastine, and **d**acarbazine) was introduced in the late 1970s and is now known to yield higher cure rates than MOPP. In addition, it is not sterilizing and is not associated with the development of myelodysplasia or AML. Some patients develop pulmonary toxicity from the bleomycin or cardiac toxicity from the doxorubicin, but these complications are rare.

The development of "second cancers" after the treatment for Hodgkin's disease has become a major focus of investigators (Fig. 9-6). As mentioned, myelodysplasia and AML have been seen in 3–5% of patients treated with MOPP chemotherapy and are seen at higher rates in patients who are more than 40 years of age at the time of treatment. Chemotherapy-induced AML usually occurs 2–9 years after treatment, after which the risk disappears. Radiation therapy appears to predispose patients for the development of tumors within the radiation ports, including lung cancers, gastrointestinal cancers, sarcomas, and breast cancers. These solid tumors tend to develop 10–20 years after treatment, and continue to increase in frequency with longer follow-up. Current studies are investigating ways to maintain the high cure rate of Hodgkin's disease while reducing long-term morbidity and mortality, particularly from second cancers.

Non-Hodgkin's Lymphoma.

The non-Hodgkin's lymphomas represent a wide spectrum of histologic, immunologic, and clinical entities. They are all clonal, malignant proliferations of lymphoid cells of either B- or T-cell type.

Pathophysiology and Classification. The etiology of most cases of non-Hodgkin's lymphoma is unknown. Some etiologic agents have been identified, such as Epstein-Barr virus in some lymphomas that develop in immunocompromised patients with HIV infection or patients receiving immunosuppressive therapy after solid organ transplantation. Abnormal lymphoid cells may circulate in the peripheral blood, and it is common for the non-Hodgkin's lymphomas to disseminate by the hematogenous route. Patterns of spread are variable among the different types of lymphomas, and the proliferative thrust of the disease is very variable. Some are very indolent and others grow extremely rapidly.

The field of non-Hodgkin's lymphomas has been troubled by inconsistent nomenclature. Several classifications are presently in use, adding to the confusion about these diseases. One of the more common classifications is the "Working Formulation" based on recommendations of a National Cancer Institute–sponsored workshop, which was published in 1982 and is shown in Table 9-9. This classification

---

TABLE 9-8.   *LYMPHOMA STAGING SYSTEM*

Stage I: Involvement of one lymph node group on either side of the diaphragm. *E* refers to direct invasion of local structures or one extranodal site as only manifestation of disease

Stage II: Involvement of 2 or more lymph node groups on one side of the diaphragm; can include spleen if the other nodal groups are infradiaphragmatic

Stage III: Involvement of nodal groups on both sides of the diaphragm; can include the spleen

Stage IV: Involvement of extranodal sites such as bone marrow or liver
  A: No symptoms
  B: Fever, night sweats, weight loss (>10% body wt), +/− pruritis

Adapted from Carbone PP, et al. Report of the committee on Hodgkin's disease staging. Cancer Res 1971;31: 1860.

is easy to use and has received wide acceptance. It does not, though, reflect our present understanding of immunology. Nowhere are T- or B-cell diseases distinguished in this classification. In addition, many lymphomas were omitted entirely, such as mycosis fungoides and multiple myeloma. More recently, a new classification has been proposed that divides the lymphomas into B- and T-cell disorders. It is much more inclusive than the "Working Formulation," but it is also much more complicated. This nomenclature is shown in Table 9-10. (The **R**evised **E**uropean–**A**merican Classification of Lymphoid Neoplasms [REAL]).

Clinical Features and Treatment. Most of the non-Hodgkin's lymphomas present with involvement of the lymph nodes, but extranodal involvement can be prominent and sometimes the only manifestation of the disease. A complete description of all the lymphomas is beyond the scope of this chapter, but a few examples will be cited.

Follicular, small cleaved cell lymphoma is a low-grade, indolent lymphoma, and among the most common of the lymphomas (Table 9-9). Patients without organ compromise (such as ureteral obstruction) can often be followed for long periods of time without treatment. When treatment is required because of symptomatology or organ compromise, relatively gentle chemotherapy can be administered, often with good control of the disease. Alkylating agents and purine analogs such as fludarabine have been shown to be effective at inducing remissions in this disease. Unfortunately, these agents are not curative, and the lymphoma will recur with time. High-dose chemotherapy and BMT are being investigated as a potentially curative therapy for these patients, though it appears that most patients will relapse after

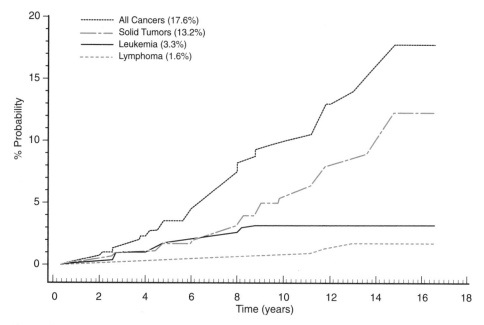

Figure 9-6. Development of second cancers in patients treated for Hodgkin's disease at Stanford. Note that the risk of developing acute myelogenous leukemia occurs between 3 and 9 years, but the risk of developing a solid tumor continues to increase with time. (Used with permission: Tucker MA, et al. Risk of second cancers after treatment for Hodgkin's disease. *N Engl J Med* 1988; 318:76.)

transplantation. A minority of patients may be cured with this therapy, but longer follow-up will be necessary to truly understand its role in this disease.

Another common lymphoma is *diffuse large-cell lymphoma.* As opposed to follicular small cleaved cell lymphoma, large-cell lymphoma is faster growing, and if left untreated is rapidly fatal. On the other hand, about 50% of patients appear to be cured with combination chemotherapy. One of the most commonly used regimens at present is CHOP (**c**yclophosphamide, **h**ydroxyldaunomycin [doxorubicin], vincristine, [**O**ncovin®] **p**rednisone). This regimen is well tolerated and appears as good for most patients as more complicated and more intensive regimens. Five prognostic factors have been shown to be predictive of relapse in these patients after treatment with intensive therapy: age of more than 60 years, stage III/VI, elevated LDH, poor performance status, and extranodal involvement. The more of these risk factors present at the time of diagnosis, the less likely the patient is to do well with treatment. Patients with a poor prognosis may benefit from more intensive, investigational treatments.

Chronic lymphocytic leukemia (CLL) is one of the low-grade lymphomas and is synonymous with well-differentiated lymphoma in the Working Formulation. It is an indolent disease in most patients. It is not, though, curative with standard chemotherapy, and the role of BMT in this disease is uncertain. Patients with CLL usually have significant bone marrow involvement and eventually develop lymphadenopathy and splenomegaly. With progressive bone marrow involvement, anemia and thrombocytopenia will develop. Anemia and thrombocytopenia may also occur as a result of autoantibody production, which causes immunologic destruction, a frequent com-

---

TABLE 9-9. *THE WORKING CLASSIFICATION OF NON-HODGKIN'S LYMPHOMA*

Low Grade

Small lymphocytic (CLL) (diffuse well differentiated)

Plasmacytoid lymphocytic (Waldenstrom's)

Follicular small cleaved

Follicular mixed

Intermediate Grade

Follicular large cell

Diffuse small cleaved

Diffuse mixed

Diffuse large cell

High Grade

Immunoblastic

Lymphoblastic

Small non—cleaved (Burkitt's and non-Burkitt's)

Adapted from The Non-Hodgkin's Lymphoma Pathologic Classification Project. National Cancer Institute sponsored study of classifications of non-Hodgkin's lymphoma: summary and description of a working formulation for clinical usage. Cancer 1982;49:112.

TABLE 9-10. *THE REVISED CLASSIFICATION OF NON-HODGKIN'S LYMPHOMA*

B CELL

1. Precursor B-cell neoplasms
   a. Pre–B-cell lymphoblastic leukemia/lymphoma

2. Peripheral B-cell neoplasms
   a. B-Cell CLL/small lymphocytic lymphoma
   b. Lymphoplasmacytoid lymphoma/immunocytoma
   c. Mantle cell lymphoma
   d. Follicle center lymphoma, follicular
         Small cell, mixed small- and large-cell, large-cell
         Diffuse, predominantly small-cell
   e. Marginal zone B-cell lymphoma
         Extranodal (MALT ± monocytoid)
         Nodal (± monocytoid)
         Splenic (± villous)
   f. Hairy cell leukemia
   g. Plasmacytoma/myeloma
   h. Diffuse large B-cell
         Primary mediastinal B-cell subtype
   i. Burkitt's lymphoma

T CELL

1. Precursor T-Cell Neoplasms
   a. T-cell Lymphoblastic Lymphoma/Leukemia

2. Peripheral T-Cell and NK-Cell Neoplasms
   a. T-Cell CLL/prolymphocytic
   b. Large granular lymphocyte leukemia (T-cell and NK-cell)
   c. Mycosis fungoides/Sezary syndrome
   d. Peripheral T-cell lymphoma
         Mixed medium and large-cell, large-cell, lymphoepithelioid
   e. Angioimmunoblastic T-cell lymphoma (AILD)
   f. Angiocentric lymphoma
   g. Intestinal T-cell lymphoma (± enteropathy)
   h. Adult T-Cell lymphoma/leukemia (HTLV-1)
   i. Anaplastic large-cell lymphoma (ALCL − CD30 +), T and null cell

Adapted from Harris N, et al. A revised European-American classification of lymphoid neoplasms: a proposal from the International Study Group. Blood 1995;84:1361.

plication for patients with CLL. The survival of patients with CLL is closely linked to the stage of disease, as shown in Table 9-11.

Therapy for CLL usually consists of oral alkylating agents or purine analogs such as fludarabine. Initially, these agents are effective at controlling the disease, but with time the disease becomes resistant to therapy. CLL should not be treated until it either causes the patient symptoms, the lymphadenopathy is large enough to result in symptoms or organ compromise, or the patient becomes anemic or thrombocytopenic. Therapy of early CLL does not extend life and may lead to an inferior survival because of treatment toxicity.

The most common cause of death is infection, caused by a combination of poor antibody production demonstrated by many patients with CLL, as well as neutropenia either from bone marrow replacement by lymphoma or from bone marrow suppression from chemotherapeutic agents.

Patients with CLL are also prone to develop autoimmune diseases, including autoimmune hemolytic anemia and immune thrombocytopenic purpura (ITP).

Multiple myeloma is a malignancy of plasma cells, which are the end product of B-cell differentiation and the cells that normally produce antibody. In this disease there is a clonal expansion of malignant plasma cells, usually throughout the bone marrow, that results in the manifestations of the disease noted in Table 9-12. Monoclonal immunoglobulin is produced, which can be recognized on serum protein electrophoresis as a sharp peak in the gamma region, and can be characterized and quantitated by monoclonal antibodies using immunofixation or immunoelectrophoresis techniques. Usually the monoclonal protein is IgG, but it can also be IgA; less frequently, the malignant cells produce light chains only. When the monoclonal antibody produced is IgM, the disease is referred to as Waldenstrom's macroglobulinemia, which has different clinical features than multiple myeloma. As is the case with CLL, though high levels of monoclonal protein are produced, patients with myeloma do not make specific antibodies to antigen challenge, and this defect leads to infection as the prime cause of morbidity and mortality in this disease. In addition, the myeloma cells produce an "osteoclast activating factor" that causes bone resorption, osteoporosis, lytic bone lesions, and pathologic fractures. Renal failure is also common because of the effects of the monoclonal protein, particularly excess light chains, on the renal tubules. Hypercalcemia can occur as well and can worsen renal failure.

The diagnosis of myeloma is made by the identification of a monoclonal immunoglobulin in the serum or urine and by the demonstration of an increased number of monoclonal plasma cells in the bone marrow.

Myeloma is not a curable disease, but treatment with alkylating agents such as melphalan, together with prednisone, will induce a partial remission in about half of the patients. Overall survival, though, remains approximately 24 months, and the utilization of intensive multiagent chemotherapy (six drugs) has not improved treatment results or survival, as shown in Fig. 9-7. BMT has been tried, and though the ultimate efficacy of this treatment is not yet known, it is clear most patients will relapse after transplantation.

TABLE 9-11. *THE RAI STAGING SYSTEM FOR CHRONIC LYMPHOCYTIC LEUKEMIA*

STAGING	SURVIVAL
Stage 0: lymphocytosis only	>150 months
Stage 1: lymphocytosis and lymphadenopathy	100 months
Stage 2: splenomegaly or hepatomegaly	71 months
Stage 3: anemia, Hb <11 g%, or Hct <33%	19 months
Stage 4: thrombocytopenia, platelets <100,000/μL	19 months

Adapted from Rai KR, et al. Clinical staging of chronic lymphocytic leukemia. Blood 1975;46:219.

| **TABLE 9-12.** | *CLINICAL CHARACTERISTICS OF MULTIPLE MYELOMA* |

1. Monoclonal immunoglobulin
   a. IgG in 70% of cases
   b. IgA in 20% of cases
   c. Light chain only in 5% of cases
2. Bone disease
   a. Osteoporosis and lytic bone lesions due to increased bone resorption
   b. Pathologic fractures, particularly in the spine, are common
3. Renal disease
   a. Myeloma proteins (light chains) clog the renal tubules and can be reabsorbed by the renal tubular cells, causing damage.
   b. Hypercalcemia can cause renal damage.
   c. Amyloid can be present in myeloma and cause glomerular damage.
4. Infection
   a. Patients with myeloma produce antigen-stimulated antibodies poorly, leading to an increase in infection, particularly with encapsulated bacteria.
   b. Bone marrow involvement with myeloma cells can cause neutropenia.
   c. Chemotherapy used to treat myeloma can cause neutropenia.

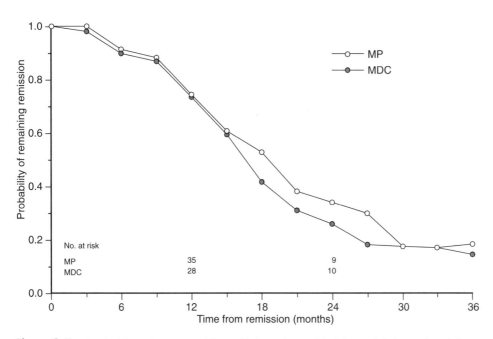

Figure 9-7. Survival for patients treated for multiple myeloma with either melphalan and prednisone (MP) or intensive multidrug therapy (MDC). Melphalan and prednisone provides equal benefit and less toxicity. (Used with permission: Hjorth M, et al. Initial treatment in multiple myeloma: No advantage of multidrug chemotherapy over melphalan-prednisone. *Br J Haematol* 1990; 74:185.)

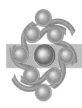

A 26-year-old man finds a swelling in his left neck region. He sees his physician, who finds that he is asymptomatic with no significant clues from medical history, but notes a 3- × 2-cm rubbery, fixed, left anterior cervical lymph node. The patient undergoes biopsy, which reveals nodular sclerosing Hodgkin's disease. A series of diagnostic tests is planned.

Question 1. What would you do next?

Answer. After routine blood work and urinalysis, a chest x-ray would be necessary to look for mediastinal adenopathy and pulmonary parenchymal disease. If abnormalities are noted, a CT scan of the chest would further define things. Additionally, a CT scan of the abdomen and pelvis would be needed to assess lymph node enlargement in these areas.

Question 2. Chest x-ray and CT scan of the chest show a left hilar mass approximately 3-cm in diameter. The routine blood work, urinalysis, and CT scans of the abdomen and pelvis show no abnormalities. Can you begin to treat this patient?

Answer. Because of the possibility of disease below the diaphragm, especially in the spleen (perhaps as high as 30%), many would recommend a staging laparotomy to determine the presence of "occult" disease in the abdomen. This kind of aggressive staging should be undertaken only under the following circumstances: Staging must change the implications for therapy, and therapy must lead to a change in outcome (survival, and disease-free survival are the usual measures of success). If staging revealed no disease below the diaphragm, then radiation therapy alone would be used. If lymphoma were found, then a different radiotherapeutic approach and/or chemotherapy would be considered.

If, because of incomplete staging, subdiaphragmatic lymphoma was initially missed and less intensive therapy delivered, all would not be lost. Even if relapse occurred, it might be possible to "salvage" the patient with additional therapy and obtain good long-term survival. However, most clinicians who diagnose and treat Hodgkin's disease would prefer to "overstage" (stage more comprehensively) and thereby "undertreat" (provide focused therapy that minimizes risks and complications).

In this patient, one standard diagnostic approach would be to perform exploratory laparotomy and splenectomy. If no Hodgkin's disease were found in the abdomen, then treatment with radiotherapy to mantle and upper para-aortic nodes would be given.

Follow-up

CT of the abdomen and pelvis showed no evidence of lymphadenopathy. Gallium scan showed increased activity in the mediastinal region. The patient received vaccines against *Haemophilus influenzae*, *Streptococcus pneumoniae*, *Neisseria meningitidis*. The patient then underwent exploratory laparotomy and splenectomy, and no disease was found. Mantle and upper para-aortic radiation therapy were given. The patient has done well for 5 years after his therapy.

Although this patient has apparently been cured of his illness, he requires comprehensive surveillance for the development of consequences of his illness and its treatment that may take many years to develop. These include the occurrence of hypothyroidism or thyroid carcinoma from the radiation therapy, overwhelming postsplenectomy sepsis from the encapsulated organisms mentioned earlier (despite immunizations). Other bacteria, malaria, and babesia can also cause problems. Additionally, the development of second malignancies, especially in the radiated field, is being found in increasing numbers 5, 10, and 15 years following radiation therapy. Adolescent women are especially prone to develop breast cancer following radiation therapy.

CASE PRESENTATION

A 77-year-old man comes to your office because of an abnormal blood test. He has been in good health lately, although 7 years ago he underwent coronary artery bypass surgery for angina pectoris resistant to drug therapy. He now takes only a calcium channel blocking drug and feels fine. At his annual physical examination 2 weeks ago, blood was drawn. An elevated erythrocyte sedimentation rate and an elevated total protein were found. A subsequent serum protein electrophoresis showed a monoclonal "spike" in the gamma globulin region of 2.6 g/dL; other immunoglobulins (normal gamma globulin range is 0.7–1.7 g/dL) were normal. You are asked to consider the diagnosis of multiple myeloma. The patient is apprehensive because a friend recently died with this illness, succumbing after struggling with bone fractures, bleeding, and infections. On physical examination the patient appears healthy but fearful. Other than a well-healed midsternal incision, you find no abnormalities on your examination.

Question 1. Could this man have multiple myeloma?

Answer. Several criteria need to be met before the label of multiple myeloma can be applied. In this patient, we all hope that the gamma spike (the monoclonal paraproteinemia) indicates that he suffers only from a benign monoclonal gammopathy (BMG), also known as monoclonal gammopathy of unknown significance (or MGUS). Workup now should be directed toward the classification of his illness.

Question 2. What are the next diagnostic steps?

Answer. Review of his blood work from 2 weeks ago reveals that except for the high protein value, all serum chemistries are normal, including the serum calcium. This is good news, because the lack of anemia, azotemia, or hypercalcemia is a favorable sign as we attempt to exclude multiple myeloma. The urinalysis is ordered, with specific instructions to the laboratory to search for light chains (Bence-Jones proteins) even if the dipstick screening test for urine protein shows none. No light chains are found. Further characterization of the serum protein abnormalities is undertaken. Immunoglobulin is of the IgG type with only small amounts of free light chains in the serum but all of the lambda subtype.

Question 3. Is there more to do?

Answer. Yes. To fully reassure the patient (and perhaps first convince yourself), an x-ray series of skull and long bones should be performed. In multiple myeloma, diffuse osteopenia or, more typically, "punched-out lesions" (the bones may look like Swiss cheese) may be seen.

Unlike some other malignancies of bone, where a bone scan (using radioactive technetium) can reveal images not seen on plain x-rays, in multiple myeloma, the bone scan is usually negative (cold) even where there is bony involvement. This is so because the lack of osteoblastic activity and the presence of predominantly osteoclastic activity in most forms of multiple myeloma do not cause neovascularization. Because new tumor-associated blood vessels serve as the basis for uptake of radioactive technetium, resulting in a positive (hot) bone scan, this imagining technique reveals *apparently* normal bones even when bone plasmacytomas are present and plain films show "punched-out" lesions.

Question 4. The x-ray studies are all normal. Can you tell him now that he does not have multiple myeloma?

Answer. To exclude the presence of "smoldering multiple myeloma," where disease would be confined to bone marrow alone, a bone marrow aspirate and biopsy should be performed. This was done and found to be normal, with less than 5% plasma cells seen on specimen review.

Question 5. What is your conclusion?

Answer. The patient's current health and normal CBC, chemistries, x-rays, and bone marrow; the relatively low level of paraprotein; and preserved levels of other immunoglobulins strongly favor BMG here. Additionally, the hospital record of his surgical admission 7 years ago shows that the serum protein was elevated then, suggesting no progressive disease.

Follow-up:

After 3 more years of surveillance, the patient shows no evidence of change in his immunoglobulin level and no clinical signs of development of multiple myeloma. Although approximately 25%–30% of patients with BMG or MGUS progress to full-blown multiple myeloma over 20 years, this man seems to have been spared for now. However, he must live in a state of uncertainty, fearing bony aches and pains that may represent osteolytic lesions and dreading the results of each serum protein electrophoresis that might be the first indication that his disease is becoming more aggressive.

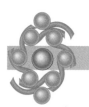

CASE PRESENTATION

A 78-year-old woman visits her primary care physician for a routine examination. She feels generally well but the physician finds several rubbery, soft lymph nodes, measuring 1×2 cm in size in the left cervical region and right axilla. CBC is notable for a WBC of $26,000/\mu L$ with 69% lymphocytes, 13% neutrophils, 10% monocytes, 5% atypical lymphocytes, and 3% eosinophils. Hb = 12.8 g/dL, HCT = 37.5%, platelet count = $353,000/\mu L$.

Question 1. What is the likely diagnosis?

Answer. The picture is compatible with chronic lymphocytic leukemia (CLL).

Question 2. What should be done next?

Answer. The diagnosis can be confirmed by flow cytometric studies for immunophenotypic markers and gene rearrangement studies, but first the peripheral blood smear should be examined.

Question 3. Review of the peripheral smear showed features of typical CLL. What do they include?

Answer. The red cell series is morphologically normal. There is no polychromasia, suggesting that the reticulocyte count will not be elevated. (If polychromasia and an elevated reticulocyte count are seen with anemia, these suggest active blood loss or hemolysis with a bone marrow that can respond to those stresses.) Platelet morphology was fine. There are few neutrophils present. The lymphocytes are in abundance, with most appearing to be small and mature. Several smudge cells are present (fragile lymphocytes in CLL susceptible to disruption during blood smear preparation).

Question 4. What is the typical immunophenotypic pattern seen with CLL?

Answer. Most are of B-cell lineage, but there is the dual expression of B-cell antigens CD19, CD20, CD21, CD24 with a T-cell antigen CD5 on the cell, which is usually diagnostic of B-cell CLL. The coexpression of CD20 and CD5 is especially important diagnostically. In most cases a monoclonal immunoglobulin can be demonstrated on the cell surface. A serum paraprotein and/or hypogammaglobulinemia can sometimes be detected.

Question 5. What events might mark her course in the future?

Answer. Susceptibility to infection, autoimmune thrombocytopenia or hemolytic anemia, progression of lymphadenopathy and splenomegaly, transformation to a more aggressive form of lymphoma may occur.

Question 6. When should the patient receive treatment for CLL?

Answer. The problems mentioned in item 5 could each be a reason to begin therapy. Additionally, a markedly elevated WBC or organ impingement from lymphadenopathy could indicate the need to start medication or radiation therapy.

Follow-up:

From a hematologic standpoint, this patient did quite well. Although the WBC rose modestly, there were none of the feared complications of CLL, including the transition to an aggressive large-cell lymphoma. Unfortunately, 5 years after diagnosis, she died in an auto accident.

SELECTED READING

Canellos GP, et al. Chemotherapy of advanced Hodgkin's disease with MOPP, ABVD, or MOPP alternating with ABVD. *N Engl J Med* 1992;327:1478.

This is a large multi-institutional study of patients with advanced Hodgkin's disease, treated with the three most common chemotherapy regimens, demonstrating that ABVD gave superior results and minimal toxicity and now represents the treatment of choice for these patients.

Canellos GP, Lister TH,Sklar JL. The Lymphomas. Philadelphia:WB Saunders, 1998.
A recent authoritative text on all aspects of lymphoma.

Clavell LA, et al. Four-agent induction and intensive asparaginase therapy for the treatment of childhood acute lymphoblastic leukemia. *N Engl J Med* 1986;315:657.
This paper describes the treatment and results of childhood acute lymphoblastic leukemia, demonstrating that combination chemotherapy leads to a high rate of cure in children with this disease.

Fisher RI, et al. Comparison of a standard regimen (CHOP) with three intensive chemotherapy regimens for advanced non-Hodgkin's lymphoma. *N Engl J Med* 1993;328:1002.
This seminal paper compares CHOP chemotherapy with more complicated and toxic regimens for the treatment of patients with large-cell lymphoma, finding that CHOP is as good as other alternatives, and more tolerable.

Foon KA, Rai KR, Gale RP. KA. Chronic lymphocytic leukemia: New insights into biology and therapy. *Ann Intern Med* 1990;113:525.
This is an excellent review of the biology, pathophysiology, and treatment of CLL.

French Cooperative Group on Chronic Lymphocytic Leukemia. Effects of chlorambucil and therapeutic decision in initial forms of chronic lymphocytic leukemia (Stage A): Results of a randomized clinical trial on 612 patients. *Blood* 1990;75:1414.
This large randomized study demonstrates that treatment of early-stage CLL does not improve survival and that patients should only be treated when their disease advances and there is symptomatology or organ compromise.

Gahrton et al. Allogeneic bone marrow transplantation in multiple myeloma. *N Engl J Med* 1991;325:1267.
This is the largest allogeneic bone marrow transplantation study for patients with myeloma, demonstrating that this treatment has limited benefit for these patients, though some may be helped.

Harris N, et al. A revised European-American classification of lymphoid neoplasms: a proposal from the International Study Group. *Blood* 1995;84:1361.
This manuscript describes a revised classification of the malignant lymphomas that is rapidly gaining acceptance. It provides a comprehensive description of these diseases.

Hjorth M, et al. Initial treatment in multiple myeloma: No advantage of multidrug chemotherapy over melphalan-prednisone. *Br J Haematol* 1990;74:185.
This paper demonstrates that intensive chemotherapy offers no benefit over "gentle" melphalan and prednisone for the treatment of patients with myeloma.

International Non-Hodgkin's Lymphoma Prognostic Factors Project. A predictive model for aggressive non-Hodgkin's lymphoma. *N Engl J Med* 1993;329:987.
This manuscript details prognostic factors for patients with large-cell lymphoma and represents a major advance in our understanding of this disease. The model also has major implications for the treatment of these patients.

Kaplan HS. Hodgkin's Disease: Biology, treatment, prognosis. *Blood* 1981;57:813.
This is an excellent review of the biology and treatment of Hodgkin's disease, written by Henry Kaplan, who revolutionized our treatment approaches to this disease.

Kyle RA. Multiple myeloma: Review of 869 cases. *Mayo Clin Proc* 1975;50:29.
Though 20 years old,this manuscript remains as a significant description of this disease, outlining the clinical characteristics very well.

Larson RA, Dodge RK, Burns CP, et al. A five-drug remission induction regimen with intensive consolidation for adults with acute lymphoblastic leukemia: Cancer and Leukemia Group B study 8811. *Blood* 1995;85:2025.

This manuscript reports a seminal study in the treatment of adult acute lymphoblastic leukemia, demonstrating that with intensive chemotherapy a high percentage of patients can be cured. This was a major advance in the treatment of these patients, and gave new insight into treatment results for patients with specific subgroups of this disease.

Longo, DL, et al. Twenty years of MOPP therapy for Hodgkin's Disease. *J Clin Oncol* 1986;4:1295.

MOPP was the first demonstration that combination chemotherapy could lead to the cure of a disseminated malignancy. With long-term follow-up we were able to see that cure was truly attained in about half of the patients.

Mayer RJ, Davis RB, Schiffer CA, et al. Intensive postremission chemotherapy in adults with acute myeloid leukemia. *N Engl J Med* 1994;331;896.

This paper demonstrates that intensive postremission chemotherapy improves outcome for patients with AML. More than 1,000 patients participated in this study.

Mitus AJ, Miller KB, Schenkein DP, et al. Improved survival for patients with acute myelogenous leukemia. *J Clin Oncol* 1995;13:560.

The manuscript demonstrates that intensive remission induction therapy, followed by either autologous or allogeneic bone marrow transplantation, results in improved survival for patients with AML.

Rai KR, et al. Clinical staging of chronic lymphocytic leukemia. *Blood* 1975;46:219.

This is a seminal paper in our understanding of the biology of CLL and prognosis for patients with this disease.

The Non-Hodgkin's Lymphoma Pathologic Classification Project. National Cancer Institute sponsored study of classifications of non-Hodgkin's lymphoma: summary and description of a working formulation for clinical usage. *Cancer* 1982;49:2112.

This is still the most widely used lymphoma classification, though it is being supplanted by the revised classification of Harris et al.

Tucker MA, et al. Risk of second cancers after treatment for Hodgkin's disease. *N Engl J Med* 1988;318:76.

Since the majority of patients with Hodgkin's disease are now cured of their illness, they are living long enough to suffer the consequences of their treatment. Both chemotherapy and radiation therapy are mutagenic and can cause leukemia and solid tumors in the survivors of this disease. This report of 1,500 patients from Stanford details these effects.

Warrell Jr RP, et al. Differentiation therapy of acute promyelocytic leukemia with tretinoin (All-trans-retinoic acid). *N Engl J Med* 1991;324:1385.

This manuscript is one of the first descriptions of the ability of ATRA to cause acute promyelocytic leukemia cells to differentiate, leading to clinical remission. This is also a prime example of the connection between a chromosomal abnormality and a specific intervention aimed at that abnormality.

Zittoun R, et al. Alternating v repeated postremission treatment in adult acute myelogenous leukemia: A randomized phase III study (AML6) of the EORTC Leukemia Cooperative Study. *Blood* 1989;73:896.

This is a large study comparing standard chemotherapy with allogeneic and autologous bone marrow transplantation for patients with AML. It suggest that the additional intensive treatments that are part of transplantation may improve survival for these patients.

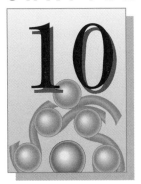

Hematologic Manifestations of HIV Infection

Bharat Ramratnam, Jayanthi Parameswaran,
Timothy P. Flanigan, and James A. Hoxie

The acquired immunodeficiency syndrome (AIDS) is caused by infection with the human immunodeficiency virus (HIV), a retrovirus first identified in 1983. Although HIV has been cultured from many body fluids, infection occurs almost exclusively by sexual contact (homosexual and heterosexual), parenteral inoculation of infected blood or blood products through transfusion or intravenous drug use, and vertical transmission from an infected mother to infant. It is estimated that more than 20 million people have been infected worldwide. In the United States, approximately 40,000 men and women are infected each year, and by 1996 AIDS had become the leading cause of death among men between the ages of 25 and 44.

Several stages of HIV infection have been defined according to particular laboratory and clinical profiles (Fig. 10-1). The mechanisms by which HIV infection produces immunodeficiency remain under intense investigation and likely reflect a complex interplay of viral and host factors. HIV is able to infect a multitude of cells, most prominently CD4 lymphocytes and macrophages. Central to the immune dysfunction in AIDS are both quantitative and qualitative abnormalities in CD4 lymphocytes. Proposed mechanisms for the depletion of these cells include both direct killing and destruction by indirect mechanisms through cellular or humoral responses to HIV. Long before CD4 cells are lost, they lose their ability to stimulate an effective immune response to HIV and other infections.

The hematologic manifestations of HIV infection are wide-ranging and include anemia, leukopenia, thrombocytopenia, and abnormalities in coagulation. The mechanisms are multifactorial and may include the following:

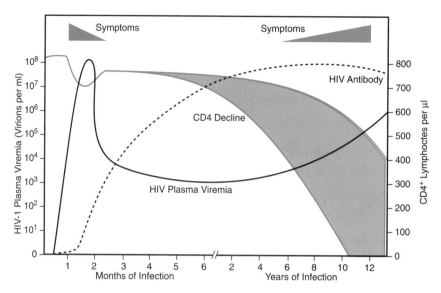

Figure 10-1. Natural history of HIV-1 infection. (Redrawn from Flanigan TP et al. Update of HIV and AIDS in North America. *R I Med* 79(5): 181;1996)

Direct HIV infection of bone marrow cells or other supporting cells required for hematopoiesis;

Dysregulation of the host immune system, leading to destruction or inhibition of hematopoietic cells and the production of abnormal immunoglobulins;

Complications of antiretroviral therapy;

Secondary complications of opportunistic infections, malignancies, and/or therapy for these disorders (Tables 10-1, 10-2).

RED BLOOD CELL ABNORMALITIES

Anemia is common in HIV-infected individuals, and the incidence is increasing with disease progression. When HIV infection is complicated by opportunistic infections, anemia is seen in 75–90% of individuals. However, even in those with early HIV infection, a mild but significant reduction in hematocrit has been reported in 15–20% of patients. The anemia is usually normocytic and normochromic in individuals not taking zidovudine. Macrocytosis occurs in most individuals treated with zidovudine for 2 or more weeks. Zidovudine-related macrocytosis is not due to B_{12} or folate deficiency. Anemia may result from depressed or ineffective erythropoiesis, acute or chronic blood loss, or peripheral destruction of red blood cells.

Depressed or ineffective erythropoiesis in HIV-associated anemia has been suggested by the low or inappropriately normal reticulocyte count. Bone marrow examination often reveals no distinctive histopathologic changes and commonly shows normal to increased numbers of erythroid precursor cells, along with a variable degree of dyserythropoiesis. Drugs, opportunistic infections, malignancies, nutritional deficiencies, and HIV itself have all been implicated in bone marrow suppression.

Many of the drugs used to treat HIV or its complications can suppress erythropoiesis (Table 10-2). Among antiretroviral agents, zidovudine causes macrocytic

TABLE 10-1. *HEMATOLOGICAL MANIFESTATIONS OF SELECTED HIV-RELATED INFECTIONS*

TYPE	DIAGNOSIS	HEMATOLOGIC AND CLINICAL MANIFESTATIONS	TREATMENT
Viral			
B19 parvovirus	Demonstration of IgM antibody to B19 parvovirus (but may be absent in advanced disease) Demonstration of viral DNA by PCR of serum or bone marrow Demonstration of pure red cell aplasia and giant pronormoblasts on bone marrow examination	Infection of red cell precursors causes signs and symptoms of severe anemia Reticulocyte count = 0	Intravenous immunoglobulin Optimize antiretroviral therapy
Cytomegalovirus	Demonstration of intranuclear inclusion bodies in bone marrow or gastrointestinal biopsy specimens Retinal examination	May present with cytopenia, colitis, visual disturbances	Treat with gancyclovir or foscarnet
Bacterial			
Mycobacterium avium intracellulare	Recovery from bone marrow or isolator blood culture and/or demonstration of acid-fast organisms on bone marrow biopsy	Disseminated infection with CD4 < 50 Bone marrow infiltration leading to anemia, neutropenia	Treat active disease with drug combination including a macrolide antibiotic (clarithromycin or azithromycin)
Fungal	Culture from clinical specimens including bone marrow aspirates and/or demonstrate organisms on bone marrow biopsy with appropriate histochemical stains	Cytopenia from bone marrow infiltration in disseminated disease	Antifungal agents including Triazoles (fluconazole, itraconazole) or amphotericin B
Protozoa *Leishmania species*	Culture from blood, bone marrow, liver, lymph node, or spleen. Also histochemical stains	Cytopenias from hypersplenism, bone marrow infiltration and possible autoimmune process	Antimonial compounds and amphotericin B

TABLE 10-2.   *HEMATOLOGIC COMPLICATIONS OF COMMONLY USED MEDICATIONS IN HIV-INFECTED PATIENTS*

MEDICATION—DRUG (INDICATION)	HEMATOLOGIC EFFECT	MANAGEMENT OPTIONS
Antiretroviral agents		
Zidovudine (AZT)	Anemia and macrocytosis	Discontinue Reduce dosage Supplement with EPO Transfusion therapy
Antiviral agents		
Acyclovir (herpes virus infections)	Myelosuppression in high dosages	Discontinue if severe
Foscarnet (CMV)	Anemia and granulocytopenia	Supplement with G-CSF Discontinue Trial of gancyclovir
Gancyclovir (CMV)	Neutropenia common (anemia and thrombocytopenia have also been observed)	Supplement with G-CSF Discontinue Trial of foscarnet
Interferon (hepatitis C, Kaposi's sarcoma, genital warts)	Neutropenia, anemia, or thrombocytopenia	Discontinue if severe
Antiprotozoal agents		
Primaquine (PCP pneumonia)	Hemolytic anemia in G6PD deficiency	Use alternative agent
Trimethoprim/sulfamethoxazole (PCP prophylaxis and treatment)	Myelosuppression	Use alternative agent
Dapsone (PCP prophylaxis and treatment)	Dose-related hemolysis in patients with or without G6PD deficiency, neutropenia	Use alternative agent
Pyrimethamine (toxoplasmosis)	Megaloblastic anemia, thrombocytopenia, neutropenia	Supplement with folinic acid (NOT folic acid) to prevent neutropenia
Pentamidine (PCP)	Anemia	Consider alternative agent
Antibacterial/Mycobacterial Agents		
Rifabutin (MAI prophylaxis)	Neutropenia thrombocytopenia (rare)	Use alternative agent such as a macrolide antibiotic
Rifampin (M TB)	Thrombocytopenia with high-dose intermittent therapy, transient anemia, hemolytic anemia, and leukopenia	Use alternative TB medications
Antifungal agents		
Amphotericin B (for disseminated or resistant fungal infections)	Normochromic, normocytic anemia	Monitor closely Consider replacing with triazole agents or liposomal formulations

CMV, cytomegalovirus; PCP, pneumocystis carinii pneumonia; MAI, Mycobacterium avium intracellulare; G—CSF, granulocyte colony stimulating factor; EPO, erythropoietin; MTB, mycobacterium tuberculosis.

anemia in a dose-dependent manner. When zidovudine was initially used in high doses (>1,000 mg/day), roughly one-third of HIV-infected patients developed severe anemia (hemoglobin level < 8.0 g/dL), particularly those who had advanced stages of HIV infection with a low CD4 cell number (<200/μL). However, at the currently recommended dose (600 mg/day), severe anemia develops less frequently.

Many HIV-related opportunistic infections may inhibit erythropoiesis by infiltrating the bone marrow (e.g., *Mycobacterium avium intracellulare* [MAI]) or by direct cytopathic effects on hematopoietic precursors (e.g., B19 parvovirus). MAI is a nontuberculous mycobacterium that has become a common opportunistic pathogen in persons with AIDS, second only to *Pneumocystis carinii*. MAI infection takes place in the setting of severe immunodeficiency (CD4 usually below 50 cells/μL) and is commonly associated with fever, weight loss, profound anemia, abdominal pain, and diarrhea. Blood cultures are positive in most patients, and organisms can be visualized in bone marrow biopsies with acid-fast stains. Prophylactic medications (azithromycin or rifabutin) reduce the incidence of MAI infection by approximately 50%. Disseminated infection is treated with combination antibiotic therapy that includes a macrolide antibiotic (clarithromycin or azithromycin). However, MAI infection is generally persistent and poorly responsive to therapy.

B19 parvovirus is cytopathic for erythroid progenitor cells in the bone marrow and has been associated with severe aplastic crises in patients with sickle cell anemia and other hemoglobinopathies. Infection in the general population is common, and eradication of the virus is dependent upon adequate production of antibodies against the major viral capsid protein. In patients with advanced HIV infection, the neutralizing antibody response is often inadequate; as a result, parvoviral infections may be persistent and cause a severe hypoproliferative anemia and even pure red cell aplasia. (Chapter 7.) Treatment with intravenous immunoglobulin (IVIG) improves hemoglobin levels and reduces B19 parvovirus viremia by passively providing neutralizing antibodies. Chronic IVIG treatment may be required in some individuals.

Increased peripheral destruction of red blood cells (RBCs) can be seen through immune and nonimmune mechanisms. Polyclonal hypergammaglobulinemia is seen in nearly all HIV-infected patients, and serosurveys have shown a variable incidence (5–20%) of patients with anti-RBC antibodies and a positive direct antiglobulin (Coombs) test. However, the clinical significance of these findings is unclear, given the rarity of immune hemolytic anemia in these individuals. G6PD-deficient HIV-positive individuals may be at risk for hemolysis when exposed to oxidizing medications (e.g., dapsone, primaquine) that are used to prevent or treat opportunistic infections. Severe microangiopathic hemolytic anemia can also be seen in the setting of thrombotic thrombocytopenic purpura, which is now a well-described complication of HIV infection.

Acute or chronic gastrointestinal blood loss may be caused by HIV-related infections (CMV colitis) or malignancies (Kaposi's sarcoma, lymphoma) and underscores the importance of including fecal testing for occult blood when evaluating anemia in the HIV-infected patient.

The diagnostic evaluation of anemia begins with a complete history, physical examination, and laboratory evaluation. As multiple etiologies can be implicated, a thorough and systematic approach is warranted:

Consider acute blood loss: physical examination with orthostatic signs, abdominal examination and stool examination for occult blood.

Review the peripheral smear (Table 3-3) for evidence of macrocytosis (e.g., as seen in patients on zidovudine therapy); schistocytes (e.g., as seen with TTP or DIC), spherocytes (e.g., as in immune-mediated hemolysis); and polychromasia as a surrogate for the reticulocyte count. (However, in patients with HIV infection it should be recognized that the reticulocyte count is frequently inappropriately low for the degree of anemia.)

Order a complete blood count and a reticulocyte count. Obtain isolator blood cultures if the CD4 count is less than 100 and MAI infection is suspected. Other laboratory tests may be ordered if one suspects hemolysis (LDH, haptoglobin, indirect bilirubin) or nutritional deficiencies (RBC folate, vitamin B_{12}). Available evidence does not indicate that decreased iron, vitamin B_{12}, or folate levels contribute significantly to HIV-related chronic anemia, although consideration of these potentially reversible etiologies is always warranted.

Review medications. As mentioned, anemia is a well-known complication of zidovudine therapy. Treatment of zidovudine-related anemia may include discontinuation or reducing the dose, transfusion support, or erythropoietin (EPO). Other drugs that can cause reversible anemia include trimethoprim sulfamethoxazole, dapsone, isoniazid and chemotherapeutic agents used to treat AIDS-associated malignancies (Table 10-2).

Consider a bone marrow examination to exclude infiltrative malignant processes (non-Hodgkin's and Hodgkin's lymphomas) or infections (MAI and parvovirus B19 infection). The presence of giant pronormoblasts with nuclear and cytoplasmic abnormalities on bone marrow examination is pathognomonic for B19 parvovirus infection. (Chapter 7.)

Obtain serum erythropoietin levels. If levels are below 500 U/L consider supplementation with EPO. Several studies have demonstrated improvement of anemia and decreased transfusion requirements in HIV-infected individuals treated with subcutaneous EPO.

Treat the patient, not the CBC. Blood transfusion should be reserved for individuals with significant signs and symptoms of anemia indicative of impaired physiologic function (e.g., poor tolerance of activity, dyspnea, angina, lightheadedness, orthostasis or congestive heart failure).

WHITE BLOOD CELL ABNORMALITIES

Leukopenia is common in HIV-infected individuals and occurs in up to 75% of patients with AIDS. A number of drugs, infections, and neoplastic complications of AIDS can produce leukopenia, although treatable causes are often not found. Leukopenia can involve both lymphoid and myeloid lineages. As noted previously, a progressive decline in the absolute number and percentage of CD4 T-lymphocytes is a characteristic immunologic abnormality of HIV infection. A CD4 count below 200 cells/μL is an important prognostic indicator for the risk of developing severe opportunistic infections.

Granulocytopenia is a common complication of several drugs used to treat HIV or HIV-related infection or malignancy (Table 10-2). However, even when drugs can be implicated as the cause, management decisions are frequently complicated by risks associated with discontinuing medications that are required to treat other medical complications of AIDS. Disseminated infections and malignancies or their treatments can also affect myelopoiesis. The direct effect of HIV on the bone marrow is still under study, and the issue of whether or not myeloid progenitor cells are infected by HIV remains controversial. Although antibodies to neutrophil antigens have been detected in 32% of AIDS patients, the presence of these antibodies has not correlated with presence or absence of neutropenia. Aside from a reduction in absolute numbers, dysplastic changes have also been noted in myeloid cells in the peripheral blood and bone marrow, and functional defects have been reported in the ability of granulocytes to phagocytose and kill intracellular organisms.

The initial approach to the HIV-infected person with leukopenia should center around identifying secondary and potentially reversible causes of myelosuppression. Myelotoxic medications should be reviewed and discontinued or replaced after careful consideration. Certain medications such as ganciclovir and pyrimethamine should only be used with careful monitoring of the neutrophil count (Table 10-2). In patients with depressed CD4 counts (<200 cells/μL) and systemic signs and symptoms of infection, examination of the bone marrow should be considered to exclude mycobacterial or fungal infection or marrow infiltration by neoplasms (e.g., non-Hodgkin's lymphoma). Histochemical stains of bone marrow can be diagnostic of fungal or mycobacterial infection and provide valuable clinical information long before blood cultures are positive.

Several reports have described the use of myeloid colony-stimulating factors in the treatment of HIV-associated leukopenia. A rapid, dose-dependent increase in peripheral blood neutrophils, monocytes, and eosinophils has been observed after treatment with intravenous and subcutaneous GM- and G-CSF. Though responses were transient in initial studies, subsequent work has demonstrated that long-term subcutaneous therapy with these agents can produce a sustained increase in granulocyte counts lasting from weeks to months. Colony-stimulating factors can be useful in improving the leukocyte count in patients with neutropenia secondary to myelosuppressive medications (e.g., individuals with CMV infection receiving ganciclovir or those with HIV-related lymphomas receiving chemotherapy). Although the use of GM- or G-CSF has improved the ability of patients to tolerate myelosuppressive therapy, their effect on HIV replication and HIV-specific therapies is unclear. *In vitro* studies have indicated that GM-CSF can increase HIV viral load, although the clinical relevance of these findings is unclear.

Further study will be needed to determine the cost effectiveness and ultimate impact of hematopoietic growth factors on quality of life, viral load, and survival of HIV-infected persons.

PLATELET ABNORMALITIES

Unlike anemia and leukopenia, which are generally seen in advanced stages of HIV infection, thrombocytopenia may occur at any stage of HIV and can often be the first hematologic abnormality seen. Thrombocytopenia has been reported in 3–8% of asymptomatic seropositive individuals and in 30–45% of patients with AIDS. The degree of thrombocytopenia is generally mild to moderate, with mean counts ranging from 40,000 to 100,000/μL, but severe reductions to levels below 10,000/μL also occur.

Studies on the mechanism of thrombocytopenia in HIV-infected patients have demonstrated decreased platelet survival, alterations in cytokines and growth factors, and, in some patients, the presence of circulating and platelet-associated immune complexes and antiplatelet antibodies. Several studies have also shown that megakaryocytes are susceptible to HIV infection, indicating that an underlying defect in platelet production may also contribute to this disorder.

A number of therapeutic options are available for patients with HIV-related thrombocytopenia, including antiretroviral therapy, IV gammaglobulin, corticosteroids, and splenectomy. However, responses are often partial and there is no single form of therapy that is effective for all patients. Treatment should be considered when platelet counts decrease to less than 50,000/μL or when clinically significant bleeding occurs. Specific forms of therapy are described in the following discussion, and an approach to the management of patients with HIV-related thrombocytopenia is shown in Fig.10-2.

Zidovudine. Zidovudine can improve platelet counts in approximately half of patients with HIV-related thrombocytopenia. Although the mechanism of action is unclear, it seems likely that zidovudine improves platelet production by HIV suppression, given the evidence that megakaryocytes are a

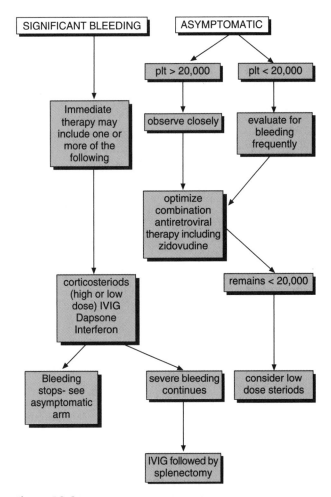

Figure 10-2. Algorithm for management of HIV related thrombocytopenia.

target for HIV infection. Responses in HIV-related thrombocytopenia have also been described for other antiretroviral drugs.

Corticosteroids. Treatment with low-dose corticosteroids may improve the platelet count in 40–80% of individuals, but long-term remissions are uncommon (10–20%). Recently, short-course, high-dose dexamethasone (10 mg po qid × 2–4 days) was shown to increase the platelet count in HIV-infected individuals with clinical bleeding and severe thrombocytopenia that was refractory to other therapies including zidovudine. However, an obvious drawback to the use of corticosteroid therapy in an HIV-infected patient is its potential to induce additional immunosuppression.

IV gammaglobulin. Intravenous gammaglobulin produces a rapid improvement in the platelet count (similar to that seen in classic *immune thrombocytopenic purpura* [ITP]) in a majority of patients (about 90%) and is the treatment of choice in the setting of a medical emergency or as a supportive measure before an invasive procedure. Responses typically last for several days or weeks but are usually transient. Therapy with anti-Rh(D) immunoglobulin may also produce transient or sometimes lasting improvements in the platelet count, presumably as a result of effects on the reticuloendothelial modulation caused by IgG-coated red blood cells.

Splenectomy. Improvements in platelet count after splenectomy have been described in more than 90% of patients. However, the potential morbidity of this invasive procedure in this patient population needs to be considered, especially in view of the large number of noninvasive therapeutic alternatives available.

Other therapies with variable rates of efficacy include splenic irradiation, dapsone, danazol, and interferon-α.

Thrombotic thrombocytopenic purpura (TTP) is a potentially fatal complication of HIV infection that is associated with the formation of platelet microthrombi in the microvasculature. Patients present with thrombocytopenia, fever, neurologic changes, microangiopathic hemolytic anemia, renal abnormalities, and purpura. The pathogenesis of TTP in HIV-infected patients is unknown. Similar to TTP in non-HIV-infected patients this disorder is generally fulminant and requires aggressive and emergent management with plasmapheresis with or without fresh-frozen plasma infusions, antiplatelet agents, corticosteroids, or vincristine. (Chapter 5.)

COAGULATION ABNORMALITIES

Antiphospholipid antibodies have been detected in 20–70% of patients with HIV infection and frequently exhibit activity as lupus anticoagulants (e.g., causing a prolongation of the activated partial thromboplastin time that does not correct following mixing with normal plasma and incubation at 37°C). Despite a prolonged aPTT, a lupus anticoagulant does not predispose to bleeding and is not a contraindication to performing an invasive procedure. (See Chapter 6.) In HIV-negative individuals, a lupus anticoagulant can be associated with an increase in thrombotic events. However, in HIV-infected individuals, this activity is rarely associated with thrombosis.

Acquired protein S deficiency has been reported in 17–73% of HIV-infected patients and, unlike lupus anticoagulants, may predispose some HIV-infected individuals to thrombotic events. In 159 patients studied in three published reports, eight had reduced protein S levels that were associated with thromboembolic complications. The mechanism of protein S deficiency in this patient population is unclear and could reflect decreased synthesis or abnormalities in endothelial cell function.

HEMATOLOGIC MALIGNANCIES

Several malignancies are more common in the setting of HIV infection than in the general population, including non-Hodgkin's lymphoma (NHL), Kaposi's sarcoma. Cervical carcinoma, and (in homosexual men) squamous cell carcinoma of the anus, may occur with increased frequency as well.

Of the hematologic malignancies, NHL is by far the most common and occurs with 200 times greater relative risk in HIV-infected people than in the general population. Unlike opportunistic infections, AIDS-associated lymphomas can occur in individuals with only a mild reduction in CD4 cell number. However, NHL is usually a late complication of HIV infection. Patients commonly present with extranodal disease that most frequently involves the gastrointestinal tract, bone marrow, and central nervous system. Responses to various chemotherapeutic regimens have ranged from 24% to 56%, but the median survival is often poor, at 4–7 months. There is also an increased incidence of Hodgkin's disease, which commonly presents in an advanced stage (III and IV) and with an increased frequency of extranodal involvement.

Primary CNS lymphoma is a late complication of HIV infection and tends to occur in patients with CD4 cell counts below 50 cells/μL. Radiation therapy can produce clinical improvement, but survival times remain short in most individuals, who often die of opportunistic infections.

The therapy of AIDS-associated lymphomas is complicated by the immunosuppressive effects of the underlying HIV infection as well as systemic chemotherapy, which is frequently poorly tolerated. These lymphomas are characteristically aggressive, with unfavorable histologies. Response to low- or moderate-dose combination chemotherapy appears to be similar to that seen with standard-dose chemotherapy. The use of hematopoietic growth factors can improve the ability of patients to tolerate chemotherapy; however, the overall effect of these agents on survival is unclear. It is likely that future approaches for the treatment as well as the prevention of HIV-associated neoplasms will incorporate strategies directed at reversing the immunosuppressive effects of HIV infection.

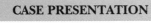

CASE PRESENTATION

A 32-year-old HIV positive woman presents to the Emergency Room with a one month history of dizziness and shortness of breath. Past medical history was significant for gastrointestinal bleeding from endoscopically proven gastritis, but there was never significant anemia. Eight years prior to this visit, she was diagnosed with HIV infection contracted through injection drug use. Medications on admission included Zidovudine, 3TC, trimethoprim/sulfamethoxazole (TMP/SMX). A recent CD4 count was 90 cells μL. In the Emergency Room she was pale and appeared ill. Oral temperature was 37°C. Blood pressure was 120/80 and arterial pulse was regular at 80/min. Pertinent findings on physical examination were pallor, anicteric sclera, nontender abdomen with no hepatosplenomegaly; no lymphadenopathy was present. There was no

blood in the stool. Laboratory testing initially revealed a hemoglobin of 6.9 g/dL, hematocrit of 22.8%, and white blood cell count of 1200/μL. Neutrophis 60%, bands 2%, monocytes 18%, lymphocytes 15%, eosinophis 5%. Platelet count was 140,000/μL. MCV was 116fl.

Question 1. What is your first job here?

Answer. The patient should be assessed for hemodynamic instability. Upon standing as well as sitting, no orthostatic changes were found in pulse or blood preassure.

Question 2. What should you consider as the major causes for this patient's anemia and leukopenia?

Answer. *Hypoproliferation* of bone marrow secondary to infections (B-19 parvovirus, MAI), malignant infiltration (from lymphoma or KS) and medications (Zidovudine, TMP/SMX). White blood cell and red blood cell precursors could be affected.

Destruction of red blood cells and white blood cells from autoimmune or drug-induced mechanisms.

Blood loss: Acute or chronic blood loss could cause anemia here.

Question 3. What should you do next?

Answer. The peripheral blood smear should be carefully examined. First, the red cells, looking for polychromasia. (Lack of polychromasia indicates a poor bone marrow erythropoietic response). Spherocytes would indicate immune destruction. Fragments would indicate micrroangiopathic hemolytic anemia. Macrocytosis can occur from many possible mechanisims, microcytosis or hypochromia might indicate iron deficiency (Table 3-3). White cell abnormalities as well as platelet abnormalities should also be rearched for.

Question 4. What was found on peripheral blood smear?

Answer. The peripheral blood smear revealed macrocytes and a paucity of polychromatophilic cells. No small or pale red cells were noted. There were no schistocytes. White cells were few in number, but otherwise appeared normal. No hypersegmented neutrophils were seen. Platelet count was mildly reduced.

Question 5. What other laboratory testing should be obtained?

Answer. SerumB_{12} and folate levels, serum LDH, indirect bilirubin, haptoglobin, and Coombs testing might be done. These were all normal. However, a reticulocyte count which was performed returned at 0.

Question 6. What should your thinking focus on now?

Answer. Because of the lack of polychromatophilia (polychromasia) and lack of reticulocytes as well as other normal studies, it seems that a marrow production problem is the most probable reason for this patients anemia and leukopenia as well.

Qustion 7. What should be done next?

Answer. Bone marrow examination should be performed to assess nutritional deficiences, infectious or infiltrative causes. This test was done and showed normal cellularity but few erythroid precursors were noted. No giant pronormoblasts were seen. White blood cell precursors and megakaryocytes were normal. Testing for B-19 parvovirus in the bone marrow and peripheral blood was negative. Specimens of the biopsy revealed no infiltration by malignancy.

Question 8. Should any other testing be done?

Answer. Yes, an erythopoietin (EPO) level came back at 27 IU indicating that supplemental EPO might be helpful. It was decided to discontinue Zidovudine and TMP/SMX and begin EPO treatment. Because Zidovudine and TMP/SMX can cause anemia and leukopenia by marrow suppression mechanisms which are only partially understood, patients on these medications may need close monitoring.

Follow-up:

The patient was given other anti-retroviral and PCP prophylaxis medications. Her hematocrit and WBC rose to normal levels and then stabilized. EPO injections were discontinued. She is doing well 10 months after her hospital discharge.

SELECTED READING

Aboulafia DM, Mitsuyasu RT. Hematologic abnormalities in AIDS. *Hematol Oncol Clin North Am* 1991;5:195–215.
A clinically oriented overview of the hematologic manifestations of HIV infection.

Canellos GP, Lister TA, Sklar JL. The lymphomas. Philadelphia: WB Saunders, 1998.
Several well-written sections are included on HIV-related lymphomas.

Carpenter CCJ, Fischl MA,Hammer SM, et al. Antiretoviral therapy for HIV infection in 1997 Updated Recommendations of the International AIDS-Society—USA panel. *JAMA* 277 : 1962–1969, 1997.
Current guidelines for the use of antiretrovirals in the treatment of HIV infection.

Centers for Disease Control. First 500,000 AIDS cases. U.S. 1995. *MMWR* 1995, 849–851.
Provides an up-to-date epidemiologic survey of HIV infection in the United States.

Coyle TE. Hematologic complications of human immunodeficiency virus infection and the acquired immunodeficiency syndrome. *Med Clin North Am* 81:449–470, 1997.
A concise, up-to-date review.

Fauci AS, Pantaleo G, Stanley S, Weissman D. Immunopathogenic mechanisms of HIV infection. *Ann Intern Med* 1996;124:654–663.
A well-written overview of the pathogenesis of HIV infection.

Forsyth PA, DeAngelis LM. Biology and management of AIDS-associated primary CNS lymphomas. *Hematol Oncol Clin North Am* 1996;10:1125–1134.
A concise review on the biology and treatment of HIV-related CNS lymphoma.

Glaspy JA, Chap L. The clinical application of recombinant erythropoietin in the HIV-infected patient. *Hematol Oncol Clin North Am* 1994;8:945–957.
A clinical overview of the indications for recombinant erythropoietin use in HIV infection.

Glatt AE, Anand A. Thrombocytopenia in patients infected with human immunodeficiency virus: treatment update. *Clin Infect Dis* 1995; 21:415–423.
A well-written review of the management of HIV-related thrombocytopenia.

Hoxie JA. Hematologic manifestations of AIDS In: Hoffman R, Benz EJ, Shattil SJ, Furie B, Cohen HJ, Silberstein LE, eds. *Hematology: Basic Principles and Practice.* New York: Churchill Livingstone; 1995:2171–2200.
A detailed overview of HIV-related hematologic pathophysiology.

Knowles DM. Etiology and pathogenesis of AIDS-related non-Hodgkin's lymphoma. *Hematol Oncol Clin North Am* 1996;10:1081–1109.
An overview of NHL in AIDS.

Koch MA, Volberding PA, Lagakos SW, et al. Toxic effects of zidovudine in asymptomatic human immunodeficiency virus-infected individuals with CD4 cell counts of $0.50 \times 10^9/L$ or less. *Arch Intern Med* 1992;152:1992.
A prospective trial of zidovudine that clearly demonstrated its hematotoxic effects.

Ramratnam B, Parameswaran J, Elliot B, et al. Short course dexamethasone for thrombocytopenia in AIDS. *Am J Med* 1996;100:117–118.
Outlines steroid-based treatment for HIV-related thrombocytopenia refractory to zidovudine.

Scadden DT. The clinical applications of colony-stimulating factors in acquired immunodeficiency syndrome. *Semin Hematol* 1992;29:33–37.
A clearly written summary of the indications for CSF use in AIDS.

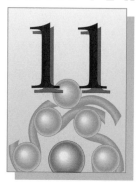

Clinical Laboratory Hematology

Peter McPhedran and Natalie Ortoli-Drew

Laboratory hematology is presented in a series of tables, with the tests grouped in categories:

Table 11-1. Hematology laboratory tests; routine, high volume;
Table 11-2. Tests for evaluation of anemia;
Table 11-3. Tests for detection of iron deficiency;
Table 11-4. Tests for detection of abnormal hemoglobins;
Table 11-5. Tests primarily for leukemia/lymphoma and myeloproliferative disorders;
Table 11-6. Coagulation tests (beyond PT, aPTT);
Table 11-7. Tests for evaluation of platelet function and thrombocytopenia;
Table 11-8. Tests for hypercoagulability.

The following tables describe each test by name and definition, normal values in adults (with commonly used units), main purposes, method, approximate test volume and cost (in an 800 bed teaching hospital in 1997), and problems with the test. The tests in these tables represent the majority used to evaluate any patient hematologically, as well as those useful in the evaluation of patients with specific, recognized hematologic problems.

Other hematology tests done by nonhematology labs have not been fully described here, but have been referred to.

The following are table-by-table specific comments:

Table 11-1 Hematology Laboratory Tests, Routine, High Volume. (Chapter 3.) A "*complete blood count*" (CBC) has a variety of meanings. We choose to define it as a set of tests of the sufficiency of red and white cells, along with red cell size and size distribution. Platelet count is not included in the CBC in our lab, in order to control charges, although the test is added to the report if the cell counter operator sees that the platelet count is abnormal. The automated differential count is treated differently. We don't *call* it part of the CBC, but we do report it without additional charge unless a manual differential count is ordered. We regard the automated differential count as equally useful for counting neutrophils/granulocytes, lymphocytes, and eosinophils as the manual test. The actual monocyte count is rarely important, though a mono count is offered by the machine.

Automated cell counters usually offer more red cell indices than are listed in the table (or in our lab reports). We consider the *mean corpuscular volume* (MCV) as of established usefulness in the differentiated diagnosis of anemia: high MCVs suggest reticulocytosis, alcoholic liver disease, folic acid or B_{12} deficiency, or treatment with certain drugs. Low MCVs suggest iron deficiency, thalassemia trait, anemia of chronic disease, and some others. Abnormal red blood cell distribution width (RDW) is a more sensitive but less specific test for the deficiency states.

Other red cell parameters offered by automated equipment and reported by most laboratories with their CBCs are *red blood count* (RBC) per microliter; *mean corpuscular hemoglobin* (MCH), which is hemoglobin divided by RBC; and *mean corpuscular hemoglobin concentration* (MCHC), which is the hemoglobin concentration of the packed red cells, the opposite of cell water (Appendix 1). Many laboratories report all these on their paper reports, on their computer networks, and by phone. The MCHC may have some value for checking quality control in the laboratory. None of these last (RBC, MCH, MCHC) are independently useful in evaluating anemia now. *Hemoglobin* and *hematocrit* have a fixed one to three ratio and are somewhat redundant, but some clinicians "think" in hemoglobin, some in hematocrit. Rarely the usual ratio is disrupted, as by gross hemolysis.

In addition to the automated white cell differential, there is the traditional differential done by the technologist who tallies white cell types seen on a stained blood smear, the "manual differential." As far as who needs a manual differential blood count, the automated differential count does as well or better at the gross cell type tallies, especially counts of neutrophils/granulocytes, lymphocytes, eosinophils, and at delineation of the absolute neutrophil count (ANC). (An automated differential count is better for the ANC, because the lab computer can easily calculate it from WBC × granulocyte %.) Manual differential counts are needed to be sure of abnormal cells (e.g., blasts, atypical lymphocytes, myelocytes, metamyelocytes, and Sezary cells), inclusions (e.g., those of malaria), and many other unusual cells, inclusions, and cell shapes. (Chapters 3 and 4.) Red cell morphology, including morphologies associated with hemolysis, are only well assessed using a manual differential. (Chapter 3.). Manual differential counts also offer the possibility of a tally of band neutrophils, called *stabs* in some places. Increased bands have been considered by many clinicians to be an aid in the diagnosis of bacterial infections, though current literature does not support the band count as either a sensitive or a specific test for such infection. Leukocytosis or granulocytosis serve as well, or better, as crude indices of infection, and require fewer resources. Granulocytosis or neutrophilia support a diagnosis of infection. Reduction in granulocytes or neutrophils is called *granulocytopenia* or *neutropenia* and shows the patient to be at risk for infection, especially if the ANC is lower than $500/\mu L$. Lymphocytosis in an adult is suspicious for chronic lymphocytic leukemia. Eosinophilia suggests a menu of possible conditions, including allergy, certain lung diseases (e.g., asthma), skin diseases, invasive parasitic infestations, and, rarely, certain malignancies, including hypereosinophilic syndrome. However, many variations in the white blood cell differential count are only occasionally interpretable, such as variations in monocyte count, or eosinopenia.

Platelet counts became routinely available with the CBC in many laboratories in the 1980s, with improvements in filtering of commercial cell-counter diluent. Although we are accustomed to evaluating marked elevations and reductions in platelet count (Chapter 5), there are now many more patients with borderline results, and it is often uncertain whether these patients should be subjected to further evaluation or simply watched (e.g., a pregnant woman with a platelet count of 125,000/μL).

The *prothrombin time* and *activated partial thromboplastin time* (PT and aPTT) have separate roles in anticoagulant monitoring. (Chapter 6.) They are sometimes appropriate for "screening" patients who, before an invasive procedure, cannot give a history, or who, by history, might be bleeders. They are also appropriate for evaluating patients with undiagnosed bleeding disorders. Since clotting factors are nearly all made in the liver, both PT and aPTT will be lengthened in severe liver disease. (The PT is the better to use for this purpose, as the range in healthy individuals is much tighter.) It is desirable to know the sensitivity of these screening tests for deficiency of individual clotting factors, though most laboratories do not have that information. For example, what degree of factor VIII deficiency will result in an aPTT above normal? (In our lab, less than 25% factor VIII is associated with an elevated aPTT.)

The reticulocyte count is a major branch point in the evaluation of anemia, separating anemias *without* adequate bone marrow response from those *with* a bone marrow response. (Chapter 3.) The same absolute number of reticulocytes per microliter will, of course, be a different percent of different red blood cell counts. In severe anemia, healthy kidneys boost erythropoietin output, pushing reticulocytes from the marrow into the blood. These two effects may give the illusion of a bone marrow response when there is none, so some laboratories issue a corrected reticulocyte count using the formulas outlined in Chapter 3. Other laboratories circumvent the complications by reporting an absolute reticulocyte count: (Chapter 3.)

The *erythrocyte sedimentation rate* (ESR) is simply the most available and cheapest "acute phase reactant" test, of which there are many others. It responds to increases in serum globulin or plasma fibrinogen. These proteins coat RBCs that are normally surrounded by negative charges called *zeta forces*. Thus insulated from their usual repulsion, RBCs easily associate with one another in forms of rouleaux (like stacks of coins). In this configuration they achieve a critical mass and overcome their buoyant density, which causes them to plummet to the bottom of the long ESR tube at a high velocity, thereby demonstrating an elevated ESR. It is a nonspecific test, but some consider it useful for detecting "illness" in patients who otherwise might appear to have none, and for following chronic inflammatory states, such as rheumatoid arthritis. It is most helpful in detecting and following temporal arthritis and may be an indicator of bony metastatic disease and widespread Hodgkin's lymphoma. It is elevated in the elderly and in anemic patients. It may yield falsely low values in patients with sickle cell anemia, trichinosis, congestive heart failure, disseminated intravascular coagulation (DIC), and low fibrinogen states—all conditions in which there is interference with protein coating of RBC, their association, and/or their stacking.

Table 11-2 Tests for Evaluation of Anemia (EXCEPT CBC, Retics, Bone Marrow). *Erythrocyte protoporphyrin* (EP) is not primarily an anemia test. It was popularized to fight lead poisoning in children. With the recent availability of simple microlead levels, the EP is now used less for that purpose. Iron deficiency, like lead poisoning, interferes with heme synthesis and causes the buildup of EP (usually termed either *free* or *zinc* protoporphyrin [i.e., FEP or ZPP]), although the test is not very sensitive to early iron deficiency. In a survey done in 1989, about one-fourth of patients with iron deficiency had ZPP levels above 100 μg/dL whole blood, a value higher than seen in any other type of anemia; so extreme values are buffered in the context of anemia.

Vitamin B$_{12}$ and *folic acid* tests are ordered for work-up of anemia, especially macrocytic anemia, but also for evaluation of malabsorption. B$_{12}$ levels are useful in evaluating patients with neuropathy and dementia. Among folate tests, the *red cell folate* is more reflective of tissue stores, *serum folate*, of recent diet; therefore a low red cell folate is the more useful test for diagnosis of folate-deficient erythropoiesis. Alcoholics with macrocytic anemia often have folate deficiency *and* liver disease, both causing large cells (Table 3-3). Alcohol use alone leads to an increase in the MCV as measured by automated cell counters.

Serum haptoglobin seems to be present to detoxify hemoglobin released in intravascular hemolysis. It is absent (zero) in intravascular hemolysis as well as high-grade extravascular hemolysis. Absent haptoglobin tends to be accompanied by elevated LDH (from lysed red cells) and elevated indirect bilirubin in these situations. Haptoglobin is an acute-phase reactant and *increases* sharply in patients with inflammatory states.

Erythropoietin (EPO) testing is a relatively recent and incompletely evaluated aid to differential diagnosis of anemia and erythrocytosis. An unexpectedly low EPO value in an anemic patient points to a failure of renal EPO response to anemia. In this situation, the EPO test may be more sensitive to decreased renal function than a serum creatinine and more convenient than the test called creatinine clearance. On the other hand, high EPO values in *anemia* indicate inability of marrow erythroid precursors to respond to body hypoxic drive. In *erythrocytosis*, low EPO values indicate a bone marrow disorder, polycythemia vera; high values indicate either hypoxia, an EPO secreting tumor, or marked anemia.

Glucose 6-phosphate dehydrogenase (G6PD) testing may help to explain hemolysis in patients of Mediterranean or African ancestry. The hemolysis may be *acute* (related to stress of an acute illness or to ingestion of medications, such as antimalarials or sulfas) or chronic-compensated. G6PD deficiency must also be screened for before the use of certain potentially hemolyzing drugs, such as Dapsone and BAL. It is appropriate also to consider other red cell enzymopenias in any hemolytic state that might be congenital. The next most common red cell enzyme deficiency is that of the enzyme *pyruvate kinase.*

Of the tests for paroxysmal nocturnal hemoglobinuria (PNH) the *sucrose hemolysis test* is manual, but extremely simple to perform, and as sensitive as the elaborate, time-consuming *Ham test* or the more costly flow cytometry test used to search for a lack of *CD55 decay accelerating factor* (DAF), on the patients cells. Most labs will rarely see a positive for any of these tests.

The osmotic fragility test, when it shows markedly increased sensitivity of the patient's red cells to osmotic lysis, is the gold standard for the diagnosis of hereditary spherocytosis and will be sensitive to several rarer congenital, cytoskeletal causes of hemolysis (stomatocytosis; some cases of elliptocytosis/ovalocytosis). Fragility is reduced in conditions causing red cells to be *thin* or have redundant membrane (e.g., iron deficiency) and in conditions with many target cells (e.g., hemoglobinopathies or severe liver disease).

Serum or plasma free hemoglobin tests for the detection of low levels of hemoglobin are traditionally and potentially useful for the evaluation of intravascular hemolysis. A major problem is that common blood drawing and specimen transport techniques commonly cause *in vitro* hemolysis. If it is desired to do this test, blood must be drawn by butterfly needle and syringe. The needle and tube-cork on the blood tube should be removed, the tube filled by slowly dribbling the blood down the side of the tube, recorking, and taping the cork. The blood should be carried by hand to the lab, where precautions must also be taken. Otherwise a positive test (elevated serum hemoglobin) is uninterpretable.

Hemosiderinuria, or iron granules seen in urine sediment, is a convincing demonstration of chronic intravascular hemolysis. This is especially so if the iron granules are seen within shed renal tubular cells.

Table 11-3. Tests for Detection of Iron Deficiency. (Chapter 3.) There are many tests for iron deficiency, none completely satisfactory. It is easy to diagnose iron deficiency in a patient with a hematocrit of 25%, an MCV of 70 fL, a hypochromic blood smear, and a ferritin of 10 ng/mL. However, the MCV is not sensitive to early iron deficiency, the smear is subject to artifact, and the ferritin is raised at least to ambiguous levels by fever or inflammation. Bone marrow testing is usually not done (because of the pain and expense), and even if it is done, it is not entirely specific. The marrow can be depleted, without yet causing iron deficiency anemia. If a diagnosis of iron deficiency is made and treated, it is important to clinically follow the hemoglobin or hematocrit serially. It is critical that the GI tract be evaluated with stool blood testing, endoscopy or barium studies in men (and women who appear to have lost iron not solely through menstruation). Iron deficiency in adults *almost always* indicate that blood has been lost from GI or genitourinary tracts. The serum iron test cannot be trusted in febrile patients. (It decreases consistently to apparently iron-deficient levels in patients with fever.) It also shows a diurnal variation and may change with inflammation.

Table 11-4. Tests for Detection of Abnormal Hemoglobins. (Chapter 3.) There are hundreds of hemoglobin structural variants. Many do not cause symptoms. Those that do or may cause problems for the patient can be classified among sickling disorders, hemoglobins causing erythrocytosis due to high oxygen affinity, hemoglobins causing cyanosis due to methemoglobinemia, unstable hemoglobins causing hemolysis, and hemoglobins C and E, which cause splenomegaly, mild hemolysis, and microcytosis. In addition, the thalassemias in which there is deficient production of one or another globin chain, cause early mortality in homozygotes and microcytic anemia in heterozygotes.

Many of the clinically significant hemoglobinopathies are suggested by abnormal hemoglobin and hematocrit (low, or rarely high), microcytosis, target cells on the blood smear, or all of these. The pivotal and essential test in identifying and evaluating most hemoglobinopathies is hemoglobin electrophoresis at alkaline pH (usually 8.4 or 8.6), which will usually show an abnormal hemoglobin band if there is a clinically significant hemoglobin abnormality.

Hemoglobinopathies causing erythrocytosis do not usually have abnormal electrophoretic mobility, and usually must be detected by hemoglobin-oxygen affinity studies ("p50," or pO$_2$ at which hemoglobin is 50% saturated with oxygen). For other types of hemoglobinopathies, separate algorithms for work-up depend on the clinical picture and the position of the abnormal band on the electrophoresis-supporting medium as compared to a set of known normal and variant hemoglobins, such as an artificial mixture of hemoglobins A, F, S, and C. For example, if an S band is seen, the laboratory would do either (or all) of several tests, such as hemoglobin electrophoresis at acid pH (6.2) to confirm that the S band represents sickle hemoglobin. At acid pH, S will still be separate, whereas common competitors (D, G-Philadelphia) will not. Alternatively, a functional study such as (1) a sodium metabisulfite "sickle prep"(looking for red cell shape change in a hypoxic solution, in the presence of a strong reducing agent) or (2) hemoglobin solubility in phosphate buffer. (Hemoglobin A and most others are soluble; S is not.)

Cyanosis-producing methemoglobins are detected or confirmed by spectroscopic evaluation of the specimen. Unstable hemoglobins are detected electrophoretically, and/or by supravital staining for Heinz bodies. β thalassemias are identified by measuring hemoglobins A$_2$ and F; α thalassemias, by dominantly inherited microcytosis in a patient without β thal (or iron deficiency) or by detection of rapidly migrating hemoglobin H. Hemoglobins C and E, both common, are easily distinguished by hemoglobin electrophoresis at alkaline and acid pH.

Table 11-5. Tests Primarily for Leukemia/Lymphoma and Myeloproliferative Disorders. (Chapter 9.) Initial identification of leukemia is made by looking at routine, Wright-stained slides of peripheral blood and bone marrow. Identification of the specific type of an acute leukemia can be made by flow cytometry using monoclonal antibodies to cell line–selective surface antigens. Flow cytometry is essential for positive identification of lymphoblastic leukemias. Identification of myeloblastic and monocytic leukemias, and erythroleukemias may be adequate, and is less costly, using cytochemical stains. These stains help in allocating acute leukemias among different FAB types, which are sometimes prognostically helpful.(See Chapter 9.) Use of both flow cytometry and cytochemistry can be redundant, but may be useful.

Another test often helpful in discrimination among types of acute leukemia is serum or urine lysozyme, which is elevated in AML variants, and especially so in monocytic acute leukemias, but not in lymphoblastic leukemia. Other tests useful in different leukemias are listed in the table. Chromosome studies are particularly useful in identifying promyelocytic leukemia, Burkitt's leukemia-lymphoma, chronic myelocytic leukemia, and certain favorable and unfavorable subtypes of myeloblastic leukemia.

A few chromosome patterns follow which may be helpful in diagnosing or prognosticating about leukemias

Leukemia Type	Karyotype	Implication
CML	"Philadelphia" or 9-22 translocation (t9; 22) (q34; q11)	Diagnostic of CML
Acute promyelocytic leukemia	15–17 translocation (t15; 17) (q22; q12)	Diagnostic of APL
Burkitt's leukemia lymphoma	8–14 translocation (t8; 14) (q24; q32)	Diagnostic of Burkitt's lymphoma
AML	16 inversion (p13; q22)	Good prognosis
	8-21 translocation (q22; q22)	
	Trisomy 8 deletion of 5 or 7	Bad prognosis

Table 11-6. Coagulation Tests. (Chapter 6.) Choice of coagulation testing is most likely to be dictated either by the clinical situation (bleeding, or a history of bleeding) or by results of screening clotting tests, the PT, and aPTT. Initial evaluation of a bleeder is often done using PT, aPTT, and platelet count and bleeding time. Results of this battery are then followed up as appropriate. If the PT and aPTT are prolonged, the first responses after confirmation by repeat testing, may be checking liver function tests, administering vitamin K, and adding other "DIC screen" tests: fibrinogen, FSPs, or D-dimer. If the aPTT alone is prolonged, initial maneuvers are often a repeat aPTT, and/or if the specimen is from an in-patient who might have an intravenous line, *in vitro* heparin correction (in our lab, using polybrene). If the prolonged aPTT is confirmed, and not due to heparin, the patient's plasma is mixed with normal plasma and the PTT is repeated. *Correction* by the 1:1 mix indicates deficiency of a clotting factor (VIII, IX, XI or XII). Failure to correct the aPTT by an equal volume of normal plasma indicates an inhibitor, usually either the lupus "anticoagulant," which sometimes causes hypercoagulability, or an antibody to a clotting factor, such as factor VIII. Algorithims for work-up of a lupus anticoagulant and of clotting factor inhibitors are well established. (Figs. 6-18 and 6-19.)

Table 11-7. Tests for Evaluation of Platelet Function and Thrombocytopenia. (Chapter 5.) Patients with platelet dysfunction commonly have mild bleeding disorders (MBD). Platelets participate in initial or "primary" hemostasis by sticking to the edges of cut vessels and to each other, with the aid of plasma von Willebrand factor (vWf) and fibrinogen. The fact that a MBD is due to platelet dysfunction is normally detected by a prolonged bleeding time test. When a long bleeding time is noted, the most likely causes (after thrombocytopenia is excluded) are medications, especially aspirin and nonsteroidal anti-inflammatory drugs, and renal insufficiency. If these possibilities are excluded, one needs to consider other less commonly important medications, including high doses of penicillin-like drugs and sodium nitroprusside (Nipride). Congenital platelet defects, such as platelet storage pool deficiencies causing especially a lack of ADP for platelet aggregation, or deficiency or dysfunction of the enzyme cyclo-oxygenase, which normally produces the platelet-aggregating substance thromboxane. Hereditary deficiency of specific platelet surface glycoproteins can result in the rare recessive disorders of platelet function, Glanzmann's thrombasthenia, and Bernard-Soulier syndrome. Platelet function is also affected by reduced levels of von Willebrand factor in von Willebrand disease, and less commonly, lack of fibrinogen.

Low platelet count, or thrombocytopenia, is very common. Initial etiologic considerations are medications, recent infections, and autoimmune or idiopathic thrombocytopenia (ITP). Hematologic neoplasms lurk in the background but rarely cause *isolated* thrombocytopenia, that is, thrombocytopenia without anemia or leukopenia.

Medications and infections as causes of the thrombocytopenia can be approached by history. Any medications started in the last 2 months, and continuing at presentation are suspect (but even long-term medications can be causative), as are acute infections with onset in the previous week or two. Tests useful in identification of the cause of thrombocytopenia, and important if the low platelets are not easily explained, include bone marrow aspiration, looking for abundant platelet precursor cells, or megakaryocytes, which confirm a platelet destructive process; possibly, platelet antibody tests; platelet reticulocyte count; and serial platelet counts during a 2-week trial of therapy such as corticosteroids or intravenous gamma globulin.

Bone marrow testing, though providing helpful information, is uncomfortable and costly. Most platelet antibody tests lack sensitivity and specificity, although testing for IgG and IgM antibody protein sticking to specific platelet glycoproteins is reported to have a 70–80% sensitivity and specificity for ITP. Normally, the "platelet reticulocyte" count (large immature-appearing platelets) is under 10%. If it is 40–50%, high platelet turnover is confirmed. These tests, and especially the more invasive ones, become particularly important if the low platelet count is a serious threat to life and health.

Thrombocytopenia developing in the hospital is a special topic. It is likely to be due to drugs such as marrow-suppressive chemotherapy, or an idiosyncratic effect of a drug. The drug most commonly implicated is the anticoagulant heparin. Several tests are available for heparin platelet antibody. We do heparin platelet aggregation, which is only 50% sensitive but quite specific. Also important as a cause of hospital-acquired thrombocytopenia is bacterial sepsis. Thrombocytopenia is an earlier marker of sepsis than the consumption of clotting factors or DIC, shown by an elevated prothrombin time or low fibrinogen.

Table 11-8. Tests for Hypercoagulability. (See Chapter 6.) Currently, a hematology work-up for thrombotic tendency is most useful in the evaluation of patients with venous thrombosis, especially in young patients without clinical risk factors (the latter include obesity, trauma, stasis of blood), especially patients with recurrent thrombosis and/or positive family history. Assessment then should focus on activated protein C resistance or factor V Leiden, and deficiency of natural anticoagulants (anti–thrombin III, protein C, protein S). These tests are affected by anticoagulants and liver disease, and perhaps by DIC and active clotting. Timing of testing is critically important. Homocysteinemia/uria is a new comer to the list, possibly an important one.

If the thrombotic state is *acquired* and/or includes *arterial* and central nervous system events, antiphospholipid antibodies and lupus anticoagulant are worth pursuing through aPTT, the Russell's viper venom clotting time, and anticardiolipin antibodies. Older patients with venous and/or arterial events may have "Trousseau's syndrome," or thrombosis as a sign of cancer, sometimes early in the course.

There are other causes of hypercoagulable states, sometimes reflected in aspects of normal fibrinolysis that can be tested. Deficiency of endogenous tissue plasminogen activator (tPA) or an excess of naturally occurring tPA inhibitor (tPAI) are two such causes. Deficiency of plasminogen itself may be a cause of hypercoagulability.

TABLE 11-1. *HEMATOLOGY LABORATORY TESTS, ROUTINE, HIGH VOLUME*

TEST	NORMAL VALUES (ADULTS)	MAIN PURPOSES	METHOD	TEST VOLUME AND COST*	PROBLEMS WITH TEST
Complete blood count: (CBC) and red cell indices		Testing for low and high blood cell counts: anemia, polycythemia; leukopenia, leukocytosis. MCV and RDW attempt to *classify* anemias.	Automated particle counting instruments aspirate, dilute, and analyze one blood specimen in about a minute; impedance, laser, and/or radiofrequency-based methods are used for cell counts. Backup manual methods include "hemoglobinometer" spectrophotometry of cyanmehemoglobin, hematocrit centrifugation, hemocytometer chamber cell counts, blood smear estimates of WBCs.	>100/day, ($10–20)	Correct specimen identification is critical, as with any lab test. For inpatients with IV lines: dilution of blood with IV fluids will reduce counts. Partial clotting of a specimen lowers blood counts, especially the platelet count. Cold agglutinins cause apparent macrocytosis, artifactual anemia.
Hemoglobin: men	13.5–17.5 g/dL				
women	12–16 g/dL				
pregnancy	>10 g/dL				
Hematocrit: men	41–53%				
women	36–46%				
pregnancy	>30%				
Mean corpuscular volume (MCV)	80–95 fL				
Red cell distribution width (RDW)	13 ± 1%				
White count (WBC)	4,000–10,000/μL				
Differential (automated)	See manual test later	Counting granulocytes, lymphocytes, monocytes and eosinophils—testing for abnormal distributions. Screens for and flags blasts, nucleated red cells, atypical lymphocytes.	CBC instrument; a simplified differential based on analysis of 10,000 cells.	>100/day, (Part of CBC)	Does not identify abnormal cells.

Test	Normal values	Purpose	Method	Frequency (Cost)	Comments
Absolute neutrophil count (ANC) [a calculation: WBC × % granulocytes/100]	1,800–7,000/μL	Identifying dangerous neutropenia: <500/μL ANC is generally emphasized.	Automated differential (impedance/laser/ radiofrequency).	>100/day (Part of CBC)	Must hand-calculate if derived from manual differential.
Differential (manual) Segmented neutrophils Band neutrophils Lymphocytes Monocytes Eosinophils Basophils Atypical lymphocytes Metamyelocytes Others	(90% ranges in adults) 38–71% 0–10 14–46 2–15 0–5 0–2 0–7 0–1 None	Looks for patterns of infection, bacterial or viral; allergy; or leukemia. Sometimes this is *the* definitive diagnostic test.	A drop of blood is smeared on a glass slide and stained with Wright's stain. White cells seen are tallied into categories while the smear is scanned under a microscope. Meanwhile, WBC and platelet count can be estimated, red cell morphology reviewed.	>100/day, ($10–20)	Time-consuming, therefore expensive. Band counts, often sought by clinicians as a marker for bacterial infection, are nonspecific, but continue to be requested.
Red cell morphology on Wright-stained blood smear.	Normal size, color, shape, association of red cells on smear; no inclusions	Looks for cause of anemia: inflammation, deficiency, hemolysis, etc.	Evaluation of blood smear for abnormalities of size, color, shapes, inclusions, cell association.	>100/day (Part of diff)	Interpretation of blood smears is subjective; there are many artifacts of smearing and staining.
Platelet count	150,000–400,000/μL	Often done as screening, which is not recommended. More usefully done to look for the cause of bruising or bleeding, which is common with very low counts, or, less commonly, thrombosis.	Automated particle counter; backup tests are chamber count or blood smear estimate (average number of platelets/microscope field at 1,000× multiplied by 13,000 = platelets/μL).	>100/day (<$10)	Formerly, nonplatelet particles in the diluent caused counting errors. Now, small clots in Vacutainer tube can cause spurious thrombocytopenia.

(continued)

TABLE 11-1. (continued)

TEST	NORMAL VALUES (ADULTS)	MAIN PURPOSES	METHOD	TEST VOLUME AND COST*	PROBLEMS WITH TEST
Prothrombin time (PT)	13 ± 1	Both PT and aPTT are used for anticoagulant control (PT for warfarin, aPTT for heparin); for preprocedure hemostasis screening; and for looking for the cause of bleeding, in a bleeder. PT is also used in evaluating patients with severe liver disease.	Patient's decalcified plasma, calcium chloride, and the appropriate thromboplastin or partial thromboplastin are mixed and the specimen is observed for turbidity change in an automated clot timer; there are backup manual methods.	>100/day, ($10–20)	Various PT activators are available, sensitivities vary. Comparisons of PTs done with different activators are aided by the international normalized ratio or INR. Using this method the ratio of the patients PT is compared to a control PT. The ratio is adjusted for the sensitivity of the thromboplastin used by the laboratory as determined by the International Sensitivity Index (ISI). The INR allows standardization of PT between different laboratories.

Test	Normal value	Use	Method	Test volume (cost)*	Comments
Actuated partial thromboplastin time (aPTT)	25–38 sec			>100/day, ($20–50)	Wide range of normal; activator variation shows the unmet need for aPTT-INR; heparin contamination of patient's blood specimen is problematic.
Reticulocyte count	0.6–2.7% of red blood cells. The reticulocyte percentage is sometimes corrected to a "reticulocyte index" (Chapter 3).	Determining category of anemia: hypo- vs. hyperproliferative. "Hyper" includes patients who have been bleeding as well as those with hemolysis.	Automated and manual methods are available; both use RNA detecting stain (new methylene blue)	10–100/day, ($10–20)	Manual test is tedious and poorly reproducible. Automated test must be batched.
Erythrocyte sedimentation rate (Westergren)	<20 mm/hr	Screening for illness (especially, inflammatory). Inflammatory states cause increase in fibrinogen and serum globulins that allow red cells to form rouleaux, which sediment rapidly.	Blood cells are allowed to sediment for one hour in a calibrated tube.	10–100/day, ($10–20)	Result is nonspecific. Sedimenting tendency diminishes in old blood (>4 hr).

* Test volume cost in an 800-bed teaching hospital, 1997.

TABLE 11-2. *TESTS FOR EVALUATION OF ANEMIA (OTHER THAN CBC, RETICULOCYTES, BONE MARROW)*

TEST	NORMAL VALUES	MAIN PURPOSES	METHOD	TEST VOLUME AND COST	PROBLEMS WITH TEST
Erythrocyte protoporphyrin (EP) A heme precursor. This is also known as "free erythrocyte protoporphyrin" (FEP). In intact red cells, protoporphyrin combines with zinc (ZPP).	10–28 μg/dL whole blood	The test screens for lead poisoning in infants, iron deficiency in infants, children, and adults.	Extracted EP is measured in a fluorometer; ZPP may be measured quickly in a "front face fluorometer" using whole blood.	10–100/day, ($10–20)	ZPP is moderately elevated in anemia of inflammatory disease, overlapping with iron deficiency. Bilirubinemia causes false positives.
Vitamin B_{12}	200–1200 pg/mL of serum or plasma	Search for B_{12} deficiency as the cause of anemia, especially macrocytic, and/or neurologic symptoms (neuropathy, dementia). B_{12} malabsorption is usually responsible.	Radioimmuno assay for example (RIA): B_{12} in patient's serum competes with isotopic B_{12} for sites on a binder such as gastric intrinsic factor.	1–10/day, ($20–50)	Test has a low diagnosis yield except in macrocytosis, where it has a higher yield if alternative causes of macrocytosis are excluded: AZT, liver disease, folate deficiency, reticulocytosis, etc.
Folic acid RBC (preferred) Serum	>160 ng/mL >3 ng/mL	Search for folate deficiency as the cause of anemia, usually macrocytic, especially in malnourished alcoholics and patients with malabsorption.	RIA: folate from patient's red cells competes with isotopic folate for binding sites on milk protein.	1–10/day, ($20–50)	Transfused red cells retain their folate, giving a misleading normal RBC folate posttransfusion. Serum folate reflects diet in the last 2 weeks.
Haptoglobin (a serum protein that binds free hemoglobin; the complex is then cleared by the R-E system)	20–200 μg/dL Hb-binding capacity (most other labs measure total haptoglobin protein)	Sensitive test for hemolysis, especially intravascular; haptoglobin is also an acute-phase reactant.	Patient's serum is mixed with excess hemoglobin; *unbound* hemoglobin is destroyed. The bound (protected) hemoglobin is measured chemically.	1–10/day ($20–50)	Would be useful stat, but present tests done in batches. Sensitivity and specificity for diverse types of hemolytic states is not fully established.

Test	Reference range	Indication	Method	Frequency (cost)	Comments
Erythropoietin (a hormone made by the kidneys that causes the bone marrow to increase erythropoiesis)	8–21 mU/mL	Evaluation of anemia in patients with marginal kidney function, and in polycythemia (EPO is low in these). Often high in anemias of bone marrow failure, and associated with mild macrocytosis.	RIA; enzyme linked immunoassay (ELISA).	1–10/day, ($50–100)	Usefulness in workup of general run of anemias not yet evaluated.
Glucose-6-phosphate dehydrogenase (G6PD)	6–11 IU/gm Hb	Evaluation of episodic or continuous hemolytic anemia, especially in African American or Mediterranean subjects.	Assay system is a mixture of chemicals that is dependent on hemolysate for G6PD enzyme; it generates NADPH, which is detected spectrophotometrically by absorbance change at 340 nM. Screening tests also available.	<1 day, ($120–150)	Reticulocytosis will cause false-normal values in African-type deficiency. G6PD deficiency is easily missed in heterozygotes.
Tests for paroxysmal nocturnal hemoglobinemia (PNH) Ham test	Normal red cells do not hemolyze in test mixtures. PNH red blood cells do hemolyze.	Detection/confirmation of a rare cause of anemia, pancytopenia, phlebitis.	Ham test: patient's red cells are exposed to complement (normal serum) in an acidified solution of low ionic strength and observed for hemolysis.	<1/week, ($50–100)	Ham test is cumbersome; relative sensitivities of the two tests not known. PNH is rare. Average lab goes years without seeing an abnormal. Flow cytometry tests to detect DAF may be better.
Sucrose hemolysis test			Sucrose hemolysis test: patient's blood is put in a solution of sugar water and observed for hemolysis.	<1/week, (<$10)	
Osmotic fragility (OF) (sensitivity of red cells to hemolysis in a series of progressively more hypotonic solutions)	Fresh red cells hemolyze between 0.55 and 0.35% saline; red cells incubated 24 hr at 37°C hemolyze between 0.7 and 0.3% saline	Detection of several causes of hemolytic anemia: spherocytosis, hereditary or acquired, hemolytic elliptocytosis and stomatocytosis.	Patient's red cells are put in saline solutions of decreasing concentration and observed for hemolysis.	<1/week, ($50–100)	Screening by blood smear evaluation is insensitive to spherocytosis. This test (OF) is manual and cumbersome, but definitive when positive.

(continued)

TABLE 11-2. *(continued)*

TEST	NORMAL VALUES	MAIN PURPOSES	METHOD	TEST VOLUME AND COST	PROBLEMS WITH TEST
Plasma or serum-free hemoglobin	<4 mg/dl	Detection of intravascular hemolysis.	Patient's plasma or serum is mixed with a chemical that generates color in the presence of the peroxidase activity of hemoglobin (for example, o-dianisidine).	<1/week, ($10–20)	Standard blood drawing techniques and specimen transport by pneumatic tube system often cause in vitro hemolysis detectable by this test. The test is useless unless special precautions are taken in drawing and transport.
Hemosiderin in urine (iron particles in urine, especially within renal epithelial cells in urine)	None seen in centrifuged first AM, or any other, urine	Detection of recent, usually persistent, intravascular hemolysis.	Urine sediment is stained by Prussian Blue technique and examined microscopically for iron particles.	<1/week, ($10–20)	Specimen must be obtained in iron free, washed vessel. Test is only positive in chronic intravascular hemolysis.
Pyruvate kinase screen (test for red cell enzyme)	Normal activity—disappearance of fluorescence (Beutler screening test)	Detection of congenital deficiency of PK enzyme that causes hemolytic anemia.	Patient's hemolysate is mixed with chemicals that will destroy NADPH fluorescence if PK is present.	<1/week, ($50–100)	Screening test, done occasionally, is not particularly sensitive; must do full assay if suspicious.
Red cell enzyme panel (for critical red cell enzymes)	Normal activity of about 15 RBC enzymes	Detection of cause of congenital hemolytic anemia.	Many and elegant; these tests are referred to specialized laboratories.	<1/week, ($100)	Most of these deficiencies are rare, making it impractical to maintain testing locally.

Also important to anemia evaluation, but done in other laboratories, are creatinine, LDH, bilirubin, and thyroid indices; serum iron, iron-binding capacity, and ferritin (Table 11-3); creatinine. Coomb's test, and cold agglutinin titer; methylmalonic acid in urine; parvovirus antibodies; and, occasionally, red cell survival by ^{51}Cr labelling. (See Chapter 3.)

TABLE 11-3. *TESTS FOR DETECTION OF IRON DEFICIENCY*

TEST	NORMAL VALUES	MAIN PURPOSES	METHOD	LOCAL VOLUME AND COST	PROBLEMS WITH TEST
MCV (see Table 11-1 and Appendix 1)	80–95 fL	One form of initial categorization of type of anemia, i.e., "macrocytic, normocytic, microcytic."	Impedance or laser light scattering ("narrow angle") determination in automated instruments; formerly, calculated from hematocrit and red count.	>100/day (part of CBC)	Sensitivity of MCV <78 for iron deficiency is about 50%; specificity is about 60%, in our population (also detects thalassemia, anemia of chronic disease).
RDW, or red cell distribution width	13% ± 1	Detection of anisocytosis, or variation of red cell size.	Same as MCV: impedance or scatter of laser light	See MCV	Elevated RDW does not appear to be sensitive or specific for iron deficiency (controversial).
Red cell morphology (Table 11-1; see also Chapter 3)	Normochromic normocytic red cells; central pallor should be <1/3 of cell diameter, for example.	The cause of many anemias is reflected by deviations from normal biconcave discocytes; enlarged central pallor and long elliptocytes (pencil forms) accompanied by thrombocytosis are characteristic of iron deficiency, for example.	A drop of blood is smeared on a glass slide, dried, and stained with Wright's stain. Red cell morphology is evaluated microscopically.	>100/day (part of diff)	Hypochromia detection is subjective; hypochromia can be simulated by artifact, to mention one example.
Fecal occult blood, Hemoccult® etc	Negative, no blood detected (stool brown)	Detection of GI blood loss, a common cause of iron deficiency. (Iron deficiency in men is usually due to GI losses and requires endoscopy and/or imaging, regardless of Hemoccult result.)	Stool specimen is spread on guaiac–impregnated paper such as Hemoccult, peroxide added, blue color develops if blood is present (peroxidase activity of blood).	Part of general physical exam: >100/day done at bedside. (Not charged by laboratory)	Test is very sensitive; reaction can be triggered by vegetable peroxidases. GI bleeding often intermittent. Peroxide goes flat.
Erythrocyte protoporphyrin (EP) (see Table 11-2)	10–28 µg/dL whole blood	Screens for lead poisoning and iron deficiency.	EP extraction and fluorometry; zinc protoporphyrin by front-face fluorometer.	10–100/day, ($10–20)	Mildly elevated in anemia of chronic disease. Marked elevation in a minority of iron-deficient subjects. Large overlap.

(continued)

347

TABLE 11-3. *(continued)*

TEST	NORMAL VALUES	MAIN PURPOSES	METHOD	LOCAL VOLUME AND COST	PROBLEMS WITH TEST
Serum iron Iron binding capacity (IBC) % IBC saturation (% Sat)	Iron 50–180 μg/dL IBC 250–450 μg/dL % Sat: 20–40%	Detection of iron deficiency (low iron, high IBC, low % Sat) or iron overload (high iron, high % Sat).	Automated chemistry instruments; detected by color change after combining with the chromogen Ferrozine.	1–10/day, ($10–20), 1–10/day, ($10–20)	Serum iron and % Sat. declines steeply in patients with fever or inflammation; serum iron varies diurnally; IBC rises in pregnancy.
Evaluation of GI tract for bleeding sites: upper endoscopy (EGD) and colonoscopy	No bleeding sites—no ulcers or erosions, no polyps, cancers, or arteriovenous malformations.	Finding the source of blood loss that caused iron deficiency.	Fiberoptic endoscope and/or colonoscope passed from above or below by gastroenterologist or surgeon.	1–10/day, ($1000+)	Invasive, uncomfortable, expensive; not to be undertaken before anemia is shown to be iron deficient.
Serum ferritin	12–300 ng/mL (some sex variation, probably due to prevalent iron deficiency in women)	Detection of iron deficiency and iron overload. The test is less labile than serum iron (see "Problems").	Radioimmunoassay; alternatively the IMX instrument sandwich technique with an ELISA endpoint.	1–10/day, ($50–100)	Elevated by inflammatory states (but only slightly, usually still <50 ng/mL, if patient is actually iron deficient); dramatic rises in liver necrosis.
Therapeutic trial of iron treatment: (prescribing iron and checking Hct and Retic count 1–2 weeks to 1 month after starting iron.)	There should be no rise in reticulocytes or hematocrit unless the patient was iron deficient.	Confirmation of diagnosis of iron deficiency anemia, while correcting it.	FeSO$_4$ 325 mg t.i.d.; a pill 1 hour before each meal. Ferrous gluconate, iron dextran i.v. are also options.	1–10/day, ($20–50*)	Rise in hematocrit during iron treatment may occur due to other factors such as correction of febrile state, or wound healing. Confounding factors may prevent reticulocytosis even if iron deficiency is present.
Bone marrow aspirate, and/or biopsy, stained for iron	Iron is normally present in moderate amounts in marrow histiocytes, many of which are broken when marrow is smeared, leaving a scattering of variable-sized granules.	Confirmation of iron stores (commonly taken as the definitive test). Patients do not develop iron deficiency anemia until after bone marrow iron stores are used up; presence of *any* iron in the marrow proves that anemia is not due to iron deficiency.	"Prussian Blue." A standard histologic stain.	<1/day (done with bone marrow aspirate, and/or biopsy, without a separate charge)	Marrow tests are painful and expensive. False *negatives* and false *positive* tests do occur. Sensitivity and specificity are not perfect.

* The cost of the pills and follow-up Hct and reticulocyte counts.

TABLE 11-4. *TESTS FOR DETECTION OF ABNORMAL HEMOGLOBINS*

TEST	NORMAL VALUES	MAIN PURPOSES	METHOD	TEST VOLUME AND COST	PROBLEMS WITH TEST
Hemoglobin electrophoresis, alkaline (pH 8.6); supporting media include cellulose acetate, agarose, or acrylamide, locally	Hemoglobins A, F, and A₂, in that order, are usually seen as separate bands.	Detection of hemoglobinopathies able to cause anemia, hemolysis, sickling complications, cyanosis, polycythemia.	Red cells are washed with saline, then lysed with water ± toluene; hemoglobin is separated from RBC membrane by centrifugation then applied to the buffer-saturated supporting medium and subjected to an electric current for 20 min or more. Hbs move toward the positive pole at alkaline pH. Bands are quantitated by densitometer.	1–10/day, (<$10)	If abnormal Hb bands are present, further testing is necessary (including functional). The challenge is to detect a few important hemoglobinopathies among many that are clinically insignificant.
Hemoglobin electrophoresis, acid (pH 6.2)—agarose	Hemoglobins F, A, and A₂ are seen	Further definition of abnormal hemoglobins seen at pH 8.6. Discriminates Hb S from D and G; C from E, and O Arab. Discriminates well between AS and SS in newborns.	Hemolysate prepared as above is applied to an agarose gel and subjected to an electric current. Hbs move toward negative pole.	<1/day, ($20–50)	Batched test (delayed) in our hospital; definitive "S" and "C" results await two test cycles.
Hb A₂ quantitation by minicolumn	<3.8% of total Hb	By identifying patients with elevated Hb A₂, one detects β-thalassemia trait.	Prepared column is allowed to settle in upright position. Hb applied to top; buffers poured through; Hb fractions collected; Hb levels read using Drabkin's solution, % Hb A₂ calculated.	<1/day, ($20–50)	Moderately time-consuming, manual test. Insufficient Hb workup for non-iron-deficient microcytosis. (Iron deficiency causes falsely low Hb A₂) Hb C elutes with Hb A₂.
Hb S quantitation by minicolumn	"Normally," none is present; in patients transfused for a sickle cell disease complication, goal is usually to transfuse until <50% S present.	Following Hb S levels in sickle cell patients who are on chronic transfusion programs.	Like A₂ columns.	<1/day, ($50–100)	% S is less reproducible, in our hands, than by electrophoresis.
Sickle cell preparation	No sickling	Detection of sicklable red cells (Hb S; rarely Hb C-Harlem).	Red cells are mixed with a strong reducing agent, sodium metabisulfite, and watched, off and on, for 1 hour sealed under a cover slip for characteristic shape change.	2/weeks, (not charged)	False positives and negatives are common unless controls are run and technologist has experience. Echinocytes in old blood specimens may confuse. Need a fresh sickle-positive control.

(continued)

TEST	NORMAL VALUES	MAIN PURPOSES	METHOD	TEST VOLUME AND COST	PROBLEMS WITH TEST
Fetal hemoglobin	<2% after the age of 6 months	Detection of thalassemias major and minor, including beta-delta thal and hereditary persistence of fetal Hb. Monitoring of patients with sickle cell anemia treated with hydroxyurea (Hb F may increase to 25%).	Dilute, KCN treated hemolysate is mixed with 1/15 vol of 1.2 N sodium hydroxide, which denatures nonfetal hemoglobins, precipitated with ammonium sulfate, then poured through a filter. The amount of hemoglobin filtered is compared with hemoglobin in the starting material.	<1/day, ($10–20)	NaOH concentration and timing must be right.
Fetal red cell stain: Kleihauer–Betke	In adults, there are no fetal RBCs (strongly staining) on smear except in thalassemia trait	Detection of fetal red cells in maternal blood; identification of red cells in amniotic fluid; study of distribution of fetal Hb among red cells. Used for dosing Rhogam after Rh incompatible delivery and for diagnosis of hereditary persistence of fetal hemoglobin (HPFH).	Blood smear is prepared; adult Hb is eluted selectively using citrate buffer. Residual Hb is stained. In Rh incompatibility, fetal Hb containing RBCs are counted. In HPFH diagnosis distribution of fetal Hb among RBCs is evaluated.	<1/day, ($10–20)	Subjective discrimination of amounts of fetal Hb; smears and buffers must be fresh. Good controls needed. Counting of fetal RBCs is tedious. Retics are falsely positive.
Heinz body, supravital RBC stain	No Heinz bodies	Detection of unstable Hbs (e.g., Hb Köln) or mechanism of oxidant-mediated hemolysis by discovery of denatured Hb bodies in RBCs.	Red cells are mixed with crystal violet stain in a test tube, incubated, then inspected for Heinz bodies. Positive controls are made by treating normal RBCs with acetyl phenyl hydrazine.	<1/week, (<$10)	Experience is useful in interpretation, as is a positive control. Retics are falsely positive.
Hb H inclusions, supravital stain	No inclusions	Confirmation of Hb H (or Hb Barts) inclusions.	Red cells are mixed with brilliant cresyl blue stain, incubated, smeared, inspected for characteristic inclusions.	<1/week, ($10–20)	Positives are rare in our lab, creating insecurity in interpretation.
Tests for unstable hemoglobin: isopropanol or heat precipitation of Hb	No precipitate; test supernate has same Hb as untreated hemolysate	Detection of any of 50 or so Hbs able to cause episodic anemia by episodic hemolysis (see also Heinz body test above).	Hemolysate is mixed with isopropanol, or heated at 50°C for 3 hr, and evaluated for Hb precipitation. Treated hemolysate is then centrifuged and Hb is supernate compared with baseline.	<1/week, ($20–50)	Positives are rare; red cell stroma may give turbid appearance of unstable Hb.
Hemoglobin-oxygen affinity "p50"	Hemoglobin is 50% saturated with O_2 at pO_2 of 26 mm Hg ± 1	Detection of abnormal hemoglobins of high or low oxygen affinity able to cause polycythemia or apparent anemia, respectively.	Hemolysate, either whole or separated chromatographically according to hemoglobin fraction, is exposed to various levels of pO_2; Hb O_2 saturation is determined at each pO_2.	<1/week, (not charged)	Too infrequently requested to be easily done.

Other tests: isoelectric focusing of hemoglobins, Sickledex® detection of sickle hemoglobin, definitive identification of abnormal hemoglobins by amino acid sequencing, prenatal diagnosis by DNA analysis.

TEST	NORMAL VALUES	MAIN PURPOSES	METHOD	TEST VOLUME AND COST	PROBLEMS WITH TEST
Flow cytometry	Normal and abnormal blood cells have characteristic arrays of surface antigens by which they can be identified, tallied, and separated if necessary	Detection and identification of leukemia and lymphoma, including subtyping of these conditions. Detection of residual disease after treatment. Assessment of marrow recovery after transplantation. Tallying of CD 4 and CD 8 cells in HIV disease and of CD 34 cells in stem cell collections for marrow transplantation. Diagnosis of congenital immunodeficiencies.	Mononuclear cells are collected from blood or bone marrow by Ficoll–Hypaque separation or electronically, after lysing red cells. They are labeled or multiply-labeled with fluorescent-tagged monoclonal antibodies (MABs) and passed through a laser beam. Light is scattered to fluorescence detectors and cells with different surface antigens are tallied.	10–100/day, ($100+)	Expensive reagents; hard to limit the number of MABs used per case. Interpretation requires experience, may be subjective.
T- and B-cell gene rearrangement: T-cell receptor or immunoglobulin gene	Germline pattern, only. Absence of abnormal bands representing new clones.	Detection of lymphoma and other lymphoid neoplasms in blood and bone marrow.	DNA is extracted from blood or marrow cells, cut with a standard set of about three restriction endonuclease enzymes, separated on a gel, and evaluated for extra bands, in comparison with a control.	<1/week, ($100+)	This is a new technology, often done with expensive reagent kits. Evidence of clonal gene rearrangements is not absolute proof of neoplasm.
Lysozyme (serum or urine)	S: 7–14 μg/mL U: 0–2.5	Increase, in a patient with leukemia, indicates nonlymphocytic type; marked increase, monocytic leukemia. Elevated values also found in *M. tuberculosis*, sarcoid, and Crohn's disease.	A suspension of lyophilized bacteria ("micrococcus lysodekticus") is mixed with patient's serum or urine and observed for clearing, in comparison with egg white lysozyme standards.	<1/week, ($50–100)	Reliable test, limited application. Not always elevated in AMLs.

(continued)

TABLE 11-5. *(continued)*

TEST	NORMAL VALUES	MAIN PURPOSES	METHOD	TEST VOLUME AND COST	PROBLEMS WITH TEST
Bone marrow aspiration (often combined with marrow biopsy, flow cytometry, special cytochemical stains, chromosome analysis, cultures)	Semiquantitative evaluation of cellularity, megakaryocytes (3–5/central field), myeloid: erythroid ratio (3–4:1 in adults), lymphocyte % (<15), plasma cell % (<3). Full maturation of myeloid and erythroid cells. Iron present, no ring sideroblasts.	Looking for causes of abnormal blood counts, benign and malignant. Occasionally, staging malignancies despite normal counts; obtaining specimens for culture.	Marrow is aspirated into syringe containing 1% EDTA anticoagulant, smeared, stained with Wright–Giemsa and Prussian Blue stains (separately) and reviewed by hematologist or pathologist.	1–10/day, ($100+)	Patient discomfort may impair ability to get good specimen, skill of operators vary. Techniques of smearing and staining are critical. Cost can easily amount to $2,000 if full test menu is done.
Cytochemical stains For acute leukemia: Peroxidase, Sudan B, PAS Monocyte esterase (alpha naphthyl butyrate esterase, for example)	Stain neutrophils and neutrophil precursors, back to promyelocytes. PAS also stains megakaryocytes and platelets. Monocyte esterase stains show monos and marrow histiocytes.	If blasts are present and stained, leukemic cell type can be identified.	Marrow and PB smears are stained by various methods (peripheral blood often useful if cells of interest are present)	<1/day, ($20–50)	Lymphoblastic leukemias often stain negative (50% of cases). Sensitivity of staining improves with number of blasts. Interpretation subjective.
For hairy cell leukemia: acid phosphatase with tartrate	Nucleated cells are all acid phosphatase positive, which usually disappears in presence of tartrate.	Diagnosis of hairy cell leukemia.	Isoenzyme of acid phosphatase in hairy cells "resists" tartrate inhibition.	<1/week, ($20–50)	Monocytes may stain TRAP positive.
For mastocytosis: toluidine blue	Occasional mast cells seen.	Diagnosis of mastocytosis.	Mast cells are uniquely stained (purple) in marrow.	<1/week, ($20–50)	Mast cells often prominent in other conditions such as aplastic anemia.
For CML and polycythemia: leukocyte alkaline phosphatase (LAP)	Stains neutrophils and bands in peripheral blood Kaplow score of 13–130 arbitrary units cumulated in 100 neutrophils.	Supports a diagnosis of CML (low LAP) and polycythemia vera (high LAP).	Peripheral blood smears stained, strength of cytoplasmic staining evaluated under the microscope (semiquantitatively 1–4+)	<1/day, ($20–50)	Limited scope: useful in CML and polycythemia vera
Unbound vitamin B$_{12}$ binding capacity ("transcobalamins")	600–1600 pg/mL serum (75–90% transcobalamin II; "R," or rapid, binders 9–25%)	Values elevated in myeloproliferative disorders, especially CML and polycythemia vera.	Serum is mixed with excess isotopic B$_{12}$; bound B$_{12}$ separated and measured; can be fractionated into TC I elevated in (CML) TC II (physiologically important), and R binders (said to be elevated in polycythemia vera)	<1/week, ($50–100)	Infrequent test, hard to maintain reagents and skills. Test largely superseded by other tests for the conditions of interest.

Other tests, referred: bone marrow biopsy, chromosome karyotyping

TABLE 11-6. *COAGULATION TESTS (BEYOND PT, PTT)*

TEST	NORMAL VALUES	MAIN PURPOSES	METHOD	TEST VOLUME AND COST	PROBLEMS WITH TEST
Fibrinogen (the substrate for the clotting cascade)	150–350 mg/dL higher in normal pregnancy and in inflammatory states	Screening for disseminated intravascular coagulation (DIC); checking validity of specimen if PT/aPTT prolonged in patient with an indwelling line. Also for controlling Ancrod (snake venom) anticoagulation.	*Derived* from PT clot density, seen by clot timer; or, tested by von Clauss method, a thrombin time–based test.	10–100/day, ($20–50)	Normal values do not exclude DIC, though fibrinogen *drop* may be helpful.
Thrombin time (clotting the substrate with the immediately relevant enzyme)	Adjustable, our version gives 20 sec ± 5	Detection of heparin effect, or abnormal fibrinogen, or fibrin split products; "lytic state" in fibrinolytic treatment. Can be used for heparin anticoagulation control.	Clotting time of patient's plasma, straight or diluted, after addition of dilute bovine thrombin.	<1/day, ($20–50)	Heparin presence; FDPs are identifiable in other ways. Dysfibrinogenemia is rare and usually insignificant.
Reptilase time (thrombin time substitute)	Adjusted like thrombin time: 20 sec ± 5	Detection of dysfibrinogenemia; especially useful in heparinized patients; test is not interfered with by heparin.	Clotting time of patient's plasma using a snake venom (acts directly on fibrinogen).	<1/week ($50–100)	Rarely necessary; reagent expensive, packaged for batches, rarely done that way.
Fibrin degradation or split products (FDP or FSP), fragments D and E (Thrombo–Wellco® test)	<10 µg/mL	Screening for DIC, fibrinolysis	Serum obtained from blood drawn and clotted in special tube is mixed with latex particles coated with antibody to fibrin or fibrinogen. Particles are then observed for clumping.	1–10/day, ($50–100)	Also elevated in liver disease, active thrombosis; will give false positive if blood does not clot; need to use special tube.
D-dimer (a fragment of fibrin generated when plasmin lyses fibrin)	<0.5 µg/mL	Screening for DIC; also may be useful in detection of venous thrombosis.	Latex beads coated with anti D-dimer are clumped on a glass plate if D-dimer is present in patient plasma.	<1/day, ($20–50)	Relative merits of this test and FDPs are not clear. Sensitivity and specificity for DIC and thrombosis not clear.

(continued)

TABLE 11-6. (continued)

TEST	NORMAL VALUES	MAIN PURPOSES	METHOD	TEST VOLUME AND COST	PROBLEMS WITH TEST
Coagulation factor assays (II, V, VI, VIII, IX, X, XI, XII)	50–150% (most) 50–200% (VIII)	Testing for congenital and acquired coagulation disorders.	Clotting, detected by time to turbidity change, of factor-deficient plasma; "substrate" is corrected, or not corrected, by patient's plasma as the source of the factor being tested (automated or manual test). If a substrate factor VIII–deficient plasma (for example) does not clot faster after addition of the patient's plasma, the patient is also factor VIII deficient.	1–10/day, ($50–100)	Commercial test systems (machines, substrates, activators) are necessary to pass official testing. They are expensive to maintain. Interpretation of assay results requires experience. Stability/accuracy of factors in plasma mailed to reference labs is sometimes questioned.
Coagulation factor XIII screening test	Clot persists overnight	Detection of factor XIII deficiency or XIII inhibitor.	Stability of patient's plasma clot in 5 M urea.	<1/week, ($50–100)	Rarely abnormal.
Von Willebrand factor activity or Ristocetin cofactor activity	50–200% of average normal pool (Fig. 6-20)	Detection of von Willebrand's "disease," usually accepted as present if <50% vWf activity.	Aggregation of washed platelets by Ristocetin in the presence of dilute normal vs patient plasma.	<1/day, ($50–100)	Exact definition of "vW disease" is unclear; 40–50% levels of vWf are common and hard to interpret. Levels vary over time; may vary with patient blood type.
vW antigen	Same	Same.	Laurell rocket: location of precipitate made by vW antigen from patient's plasma migrating into agarose gel containing anti-vWf antibody. Precipitate forms at zone of equivalence.	<1/day, ($100+)	Same as above. Antigen test now may be redundant. Both antigen and activity of vWf are acute-phase reactants. Antigen–range appears to vary with blood type.
von Willebrand factor multimers	Full "ladder" pattern on SDS molecular sizing gel (Fig. 6-20)	Discrimination of different types of vW disease; especially, detection of vW type IIb, for which a common treatment, DDAVP, may be contraindicated.	SDS gel electrophoresis followed by anti-vW Western blot linked to isotope or ELISA for detection. (Tables 6-5 and 6-6)	<1/week, ($100+)	Referred test (delays in reporting); rarely necessary.

Test	Normal values	Use	Method	Frequency (cost)	Comments
Mixing study, aPTT or PT	aPTT or PT must be abnormal to do test.	Mixing studies are done to determine whether aPTT or PT are prolonged due to deficiency of clotting factors or a clotting inhibitor.	1 + 1 mixture of patient plasma with normal plasma is clotted by aPTT (or PT) activator. If normal plasma corrects patient's prolonged aPTT (or PT), a deficiency is present.	<1/day, ($20–50)	aPTT prolonged by an inhibitor may also be partly corrected by normal plasma.
Coagulation factor inhibitor titer (usually, an antibody to factor VIII)	No inhibitor present; if an inhibitor is present, it is measured in Bethesda units.	Establishment of level of inhibitor helps to determine appropriate treatment. Low-level inhibitors can be overwhelmed by clotting factor concentrates. High-level inhibitors must be "bypassed" if patient is bleeding.	Patient's plasma is serially diluted in normal plasma until 50% of the factor of interest persists.	<1/week, ($100+)	Time-consuming to perform, confusing if done in *treated* patient.
Heparin assay (anti-factor Xa assay)	None present; target values for anticoagulation are 0.2–0.4 U/mL of plasma. With regular, unfractionated heparin, higher with low molecular weight heparin.	Control of heparin anticoagulation for patients requiring unexpectedly large doses of heparin to lengthen aPTT, for patients with lupus anticoagulant, and for patients receiving low molecular weight heparin.	Factor Xa mixed with a chromogenic substrate yields a color: heparin in patient's plasma impedes color generation.	<1/week, ($20–50)	Harder to do, more expensive, less established than aPTT. Standard curve must be prepared with type of heparin that patient is receiving.
Euglobulin lysis time: (stability of clot in a fraction of patient's plasma.)	Clot persists for 3 hours.	Detection of fibrinolytic activity in patient's plasma: during fibrinolytic treatment (SK, UK, TPA); DIC, or "primary fibrinolysis" will shorten the euglobulin lysis time.	Patient's euglobulins are precipitated and washed free of endogenous fibrinolytic inhibitors; they are then observed for lysis.	<1/week, ($20–50)	A stat result would be desirable in this situation. This test cannot be done stat. Thromboelastograph, which also detects fibrinolysis, may be faster.
Anti-plasmin ("alpha-2"); the endogenous fibrinolysis inhibitor	50–150% of average normal	Detection of deficiency, which causes a bleeding tendency; part of the search for unusual causes of bleeding in bleeders with normal screening tests.	Plasmin lyses an artificial chromogenic substrate, yielding a color. Plasma from normals, and the patient, are compared for their ability to inhibit this reaction.	<1/week, ($50–100)	Uncommonly done, therefore, slow turnaround.

TABLE 11-7. *TESTS FOR EVALUATION OF PLATELET FUNCTION AND THROMBOCYTOPENIA (OTHER THAN PLATELET MORPHOLOGY, BONE MARROW, CREATININE, VON WILLEBRAND FACTOR, ETC)*

TEST	NORMAL VALUES	MAIN PURPOSES	METHOD	TEST VOLUME AND COST	PROBLEMS WITH TEST
Bleeding time, Ivy, Simplate® (an alternative commercial device is called Surgicutt)	<9 min (some authors give shorter times)	Screening test for the detection of platelet dysfunction.	Scratch(es) or cuts 5 mm long × 1 mm deep are made on the volar aspect of the forearm under BP cuff compression at 40 mm Hg. Cuts are observed until bleeding stops.	1–10/day, ($20–50)	Affected by platelet count, air and skin temperature, edema technique. Not shown to be predictive of bleeding at surgery.
Heparin-platelet aggregation	<25% clearing of donor platelet rich plasma (PRP) after addition of patient's plasma and heparin	Detection of heparin platelet antibody developing in about 5% of patients on therapeutic heparin, which can cause thrombocytopenia, with or without thrombosis ("HIT" or "HITT").	Mixture of healthy donor's PRP, patient's platelet-poor plasma, and heparin: mixture is observed for aggregation of donor platelets.	<1/day, ($100+)	Insensitive: detects ~50% of affected patients. Serotonin, or ATP, release tests probably are more sensitive and increasingly available and accurate.
Platelet aggregation (with collagen, ADP, epinephrine, Ristocetin, arachidonic acid)	>50% clearing of patient's PRP after addition of each agent	Detection and partial characterization of platelet dysfunction.	Patient's blood is gently centrifuged to prepare platelet-rich plasma (PRP); aggregating agents are added to aliquots of PRP, and PRP is monitored for aggregation (increased light transmission).	<1/day, ($100+)	Technically demanding and time-consuming. Results are nonspecific. Sensitivity and specificity for significant platelet dysfunction are not known.
Thromboxane B$_2$ (serum) (stable end product of arachidonic acid metabolism)	300–700 ng/mL of serum	Evaluation of function of arachidonic acid metabolic pathway, which is subject to enzyme deficiencies (cyclo-oxygenase, thromboxane synthase) or dysfunction due to medication	Radio-immuno assay (RIA) of thromboxane B$_2$ in serum of patient's clotted blood.	<1/day, (not charged)	Not widely available. RIA kit is expensive and getting more so.

Test	Normal value	Purpose	Method	Turnaround (cost)	Comments
Serotonin (blood serotonin; mostly in platelet-"dense" bodies)	80–180 ng/mL of blood	Detection of platelet storage pool disease(s) (delta SPD, or dense body deficiency).	High pressure liquid chromatography (HPLC)	<1/day, (not charged)	Not widely or rapidly available; affected by serotonin reuptake inhibitor drugs, which probably do not affect hemostasis (Prozac, Zoloft).
Platelet antibody tests					
Qualitative serum antiplatelet IgG, IgM (indirect)	No (visible) fluorescence		Fluorescence microscopy: washed donor platelets are exposed to patient's serum, then fluorescent anti IgG, IgM	<1/week, ($20–50)	
Antibody to platelet membrane glycoproteins: MAIPA test; indirect, or direct	No antibody	Detection of antibody able to cause immune thrombocytopenia (ITP).	Western blot: normal platelet membrane GPs are separated on a gel, exposed to patient's serum or plasma, then to anti IgG or IgM attached to an indicator.	<1/day, ($100+)	Sensitivity and specificity of these tests is still unknown; tests are not well standardized between institutions. Slow turnaround. Not known to be useful in HIV–ITP.
Antiplatelet antibody, indirect or direct	No antibody		Flow cytometry, using donor platelets with patient's serum or patient's platelets, and fluorescent anti IgG.	<1/week, ($100+)	
Platelet reticulocytes (analogous to RBC reticulocytes)	<5%	Differentiation of hyperproliferative from hypoproliferative thrombocytopenia	Flow cytometry: patient's PRP is first mixed with a fluorescent dye (thiazole orange) with affinity for RNA	<1/week, ($100+)	Not generally or rapidly available; test deserves wider evaluation and use.
Platelet morphology (part of the manual differential)	Normal morphology: platelets appear as a cluster of purple and red granules. The cluster is <2 μm in diameter	Detection of gray platelet, Bernard Soulier, and May Hegglin syndromes. Gray platelets are pale and bluish-gray, lack α granules on EM. The others are *giant* and *reduced in number.*	Evaluation of platelets on Wright stained blood smear	See manual differential	Light microscopy is insensitive. Dysfunctional platelets nearly always appear normal.

Other tests, including referred tests: ^{14}C platelet serotonin release for heparin induced thrombocytopenia ("HIT"), prothrombin consumption, tourniquet test, platelet factor 4, beta thromboglobulin platelet surface antigen PLA-1, and antibody to PLA-1.

TABLE 11-8. *TESTS FOR HYPERCOAGULABILITY (OTHER THAN PTT, TT, MIXING STUDY)*

TEST	NORMAL VALUES	MAIN PURPOSES	METHOD	TEST VOLUME AND COST	PROBLEMS WITH TEST
Lupus anticoagulant (LAC): phospholipid correction of a prolonged aPTT.	A normal aPTT and Russell's viper venom clotting time rule it out, though they don't rule out anticardiolipin antibodies.	Confirmation of lupus anticoagulant, an antiphospholipid antibody and commonly associated with thrombosis	Starting with patient's plasma giving a long aPTT add increasing amounts of phospholipid to plasma, look for a shortening of prolonged aPTT	1–10/day, ($50–100)	One of many causes of prolonged aPTT; aPTT prolongation doesn't detect all LACs.
Antithrombin III (natural anticoagulant that inhibits thrombin, factor Xa, others; it is activated by exogenous heparin and by endogenous "heparans").	70–130%	Detection of AT III deficiency or dysfunction	Patient's plasma is used for anti factor Xa effect after mixing plasma with Xa, heparin, chromogenic substrate	<1/day, ($100)	
Protein C (natural anticoagulant that, when activated, degrades activated clotting factors V and VIII)	70–130%	Detection of protein C deficiency or dysfunction	Patient's protein C is activated and in turn converts a chromogenic substrate.	<1/day, ($100)	
Protein S (PS), total, and free (a natural anticoagulant, a protein C cofactor; some is bound to complement, some is "free")	70–130%	Detection of deficiency of free protein S	Laurell rocket antigen precipitation before and after an initial PEG precipitation of *bound* PS. Gel has antibody to PS.	<1/day, ($100+)	Affected (lowered) by liver disease, anticoagulants, DIC, ongoing thrombosis.

Test	Reference value	Use	Method	Frequency (Cost)	Comments
Protein C resistance, or "activated protein C resistance" (usually turns out to be "factor V Leiden"; the latter is identified by PCR of patient's DNA.)	Ratio >2.3; 2.0–2.3 borderline	Detection of the most common inherited cause of venous thromboembolic disease.	The patient's aPTT is run before and after addition of activated protein C. The aPTT after APC addition should be twice as long, or longer. If it fails to lengthen, APC resistance is present.	<1/day, ($100+)	Requires addition of factor V deficient plasma to work in the presence of anticoagulants. Importance of the condition not universally appreciated yet.
Anti-cardiolipin antibody (ACA)	Lower than control	Detection of anti phospholipid syndrome; patients with the lupus anticoagulant usually have ACAs	RIA or ELISA	1–10/day, ($100+)	Levels are a continuum; post infectious ACAs appear to be benign.
Plasminogen (plasmin precursor)	80–120%	Detection of deficiency or dysfunction	Plasminogen from plasma is activated by streptokinase; the plasmin generated acts on a chromogen	<1/day, ($50)	Recent streptococcal infection can cause anti SK antibodies which will look like absent plasminogen with this method.
Plasminogen activator (PA or TPA) (endogenous)	TPA should be detectable (average may be 0.3 IU/mL); level doubles after venous compression 90 mm Hg × 10 min.	Detection of lack of response of plasma TPA level to venous compression, which implies deficiency of normal fibrinolysis	Patient's plasma is used as a source of TPA to convert plasminogen to plasmin, which in turn converts a chromogen.	<1/week, ($100+)	Not a routine blood draw. Relevance not universally accepted.
Plasminogen activator inhibitor (PAI)	<10 "arbitrary units"/mL	Detection of excess PAI, which would imply deficiency of normal fibrinolysis	Urokinase is mixed with patient's plasma, then allowed to act on plasminogen. Plasmin released is mixed with a chromogen. Less plasmin will be released if patient's PAI is elevated.	<1/week, ($100+)	Acute phase reactant: inflammation causes high values.

Also note that hematocrit and platelets are not elevated; consider Trousseau's syndrome (cancer-associated venous and arterial thrombosis) in patients over 50 years.

Appendix 1. Red Blood Cell Indices

Index		Formula	Normal Value
*Mean corpuscular volume (MCV)	=	$\dfrac{\text{hematocrit (L/L)} \times 1000}{\text{*red cell count } (\times 10^{12}/L)}$	80–95 fL
Mean corpuscular hemoglobin (MCH)	=	$\dfrac{\text{*hemoglobin (g/L)}}{\text{*red cell count } (\times 10^{12}/L)}$	25.4–34.6 pg/cell
Mean corpuscular hemoglobin concentration (MCH)	=	$\dfrac{\text{*hemoglobin (g/dL)}}{\text{hematocrit (L/L)}}$	31–36 g/dL packed cells

* = Measured directly by Coulter counter.

Appendix 2. Blood Cell Generation Times

	Approximate Time in Compartment		
Cell Line	*Bone Marrow*	*Blood*	*Tissue*
Red blood cell	7.5 days	120 days	
White blood cell (granulocyte)	14 days	<1 day	1–2 days
Platelet	5 days	10 days	
Monocyte	55 hr	12 hr	

Appendix 3. The Porphyrias

The neurologic system and skin are the primary targets of the porphyrias, a group of metabolic disorders in which heme biosynthesis pathway enzyme defects cause the excess accumulation and excretion of porphyrias and their precursors. Clinical manifestations may be quite overt or subtle and often puzzle even experienced clinicians. The hematologic system is involved in many types of porphyria.

The following table shows the heme synthetic pathway and the sites of enzyme defects in the different porphyrias.

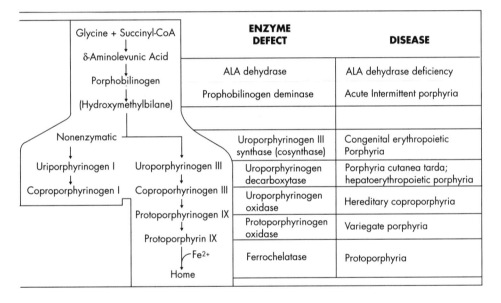

	ENZYME DEFECT	DISEASE
Glycine + Succinyl-CoA ↓ δ-Aminolevunic Acid ↓ Porphobilinogen ↓ (Hydroxymethylbilane)	ALA dehydrase	ALA dehydrase deficiency
	Prophobilinogen deminase	Acute Intermittent porphyria
Nonenzymatic ↓ Uriporphyrinogen I ↓ Coproporphyrinogen I	Uroporphyrinogen III synthase (cosynthase)	Congenital erythropoietic Porphyria
Uroporphyrinogen III ↓ Coproporhyrinogen III ↓ Protoporphyrinogen IX ↓ Protoporphyrin IX	Uroporphyrinogen decarboxytase	Porphyria cutanea tarda; hepatoerythropoietic porphyria
	Uroporphyrinogen oxidase	Hereditary coproporphyria
	Protoporphyrinogen oxidase	Variegate porphyria
Fe²⁺ Home	Ferrochelatase	Protoporphyria

SELECTED READING

Bloomer JR, Bonkovsky HL: The porphyrias. *Disease-a-Month,* 1984; 3-56.

Desnick RJ, Anderson KE: Heme biosynthesis and its disorders: The porphyrias and endoblastic anemias. In Hoffman R, Benz EJ Jr, Shattil SJ, et al, eds. *Hematology. Basic Principles and Practice,* 2nd ed. Churchill-Livingstone; 1995:350–367.

Appendix 4. Morphologic Characteristics of the Leukocytes (Wright's Stain)

TYPE OF CELL		Size μm	NUCLEUS			
			Position	Shape	Color	Chromatin
1. **Granulocytes:** Myeloblast*		10–18	Eccentric or central	Round or oval	Light reddish-purple	Very fine meshwork
Promyelocyte*		12–20	Eccentric or central	Round or oval	Light reddish-purple	Very fine meshwork
Myelocyte*		12–18	Eccentric	Oval or slightly indented	Reddish-purple	Fine but becomes gradually coarser
Metamyelocyte*		10–18	Central or eccentric	Thick horse-shoe or indented	Light purplish-blue	Basi- and oxy-chromatin clearly distinguished
"Juvenile" or band form		10–16	Central or eccentric	Band shape of uniform thickness	Light purplish-blue	Basi- and oxy-chromatin clearly distinguished
Polymorphonuclear neutrophil		10–15	Central or eccentric	2–5 or more distinct lobes	Deep purplish-blue	Rather coarse
Polymorphonuclear eosinophil		10–15	Central or eccentric	2–3 lobes	Purplish-blue	Coarse
Polymorphonuclear basophil		10–15	Central	2–3 lobes	Purplish-blue	Coarse, overlaid with granules

(continued)

		CYTOPLASM			
Nuclear Membrane	**Nucleoli**	**Relative Amount**	**Color**	**Perinuclear Clear Zone**	**Granules**
Very fine	2–5	Scanty	Blue	None	None
Fine	2–5	Moderate	Blue	None	Primary (azurophilic, eosinophilic, or basophilic)
Indistinct	Rare	Moderate	Bluish-pink	None	Primary plus, in neutrophils secondary or specific granules
Present	None	Plentiful	Pink	None	Neutrophilic, eosinophilic, or basophilic
Present	None	Plentiful	Pink	None	Neutrophilic, eosinophilic, or basophilic
Present	None	Plentiful	Faint pink	None	Fine, pink, or violet pink
Present	None	Plentiful	Pink	None	Large, coarse, uniform in size crimson-red, numerous
Present	None	Plentiful	Faint-pink	None	Large, coarse, uniform, bluish-black

APPENDIX 4: Morphologic Characteristics of the Leukocytes (Wright's Stain)

TYPE OF CELL		Size μm	NUCLEUS			
			Position	Shape	Color	Chromatin
	2. **Lymphocytes** Lymphoblasts*	10–18	Eccentric or central	Round or oval	Light reddish-purple	Moderately coarse particles, "stippled"
	"Mature" lymphocyte	7–18	Eccentric	Round or slightly indented	Deep purplish-blue	Large masses of moderate or large size, or pyknotic
	3. Promonocyte*	12–20	Eccentric or central	Round or oval moderately indented	Pale bluish-violet	Fine reticulated, skeinlike, or lacy
	Monocyte	12–20	Eccentric or central	Round, oval, notched, or horseshoe	Pale bluish-violet	Fine reticulated, skeinlike, or lacy
	Macrophage*	15–80	Central	Elongated, indented, or oval	Pale bluish-violet	Spongy

* In healthy individuals, cells confined to bone marrow (not usually seen in peripheral blood smear).
From Lea, Febriges. Wintrobe's 8th ed.: Clinical hematology, 1981.

		CYTOPLASM			
Nuclear Membrane	**Nucleoli**	**Relative Amount**	**Color**	**Perinuclear Clear Zone**	**Granules**
Fairly dense	1–2	Scanty	Clear blue	Present	None
Dense	None	Scanty or plentiful	Sky blue, deep blue, or even very pale pink	Present if cytoplasm is dark	None or few, azurophilic
Present	1–2	Moderate	Grayish or cloudy blue	None	Few, fine, lilac or reddish
Present	None	Abundant	Grayish or cloudy blue	None	Abundant, fine, lilac or reddish blue
Distinct	None	Usually abundant	Opaque sky blue	None	Numerous, moderately coarse azure granules and vacuoles

SUBJECT INDEX

Page numbers followed by a *t* refer to tables; those followed by an *f* refer to figures.